MOSBY'S
COMPREHENSIVE REVIEW
OF RADIOGRAPHY

Mosby's
Comprehensive Review
of Radiography

William J. Callaway, BA, RT(R)
Director, Associate Degree Radiography
Lincoln Land Community College
Springfield, Illinois

with 112 illustrations

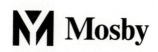

Mosby

St. Louis Baltimore Boston Carlsbad Chicago Naples New York Philadelphia Portland
London Madrid Mexico City Singapore Sydney Tokyo Toronto Wiesbaden

MK

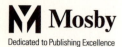
Mosby
Dedicated to Publishing Excellence

A Times Mirror Company

Editor: Jeanne Rowland
Developmental Editor: Lisa Potts
Project Manager: Gayle Morris
Editing: Winnie Sullivan
Design and Layout: Ken Wendling
Manufacturing Supervisor: Karen Lewis

Printed in the United States of America
Composition by Wordbench

Mosby–Year Book, Inc.
11830 Westline Industrial Drive
St. Louis, Missouri 63146

About the Author

William J. Callaway, BA, RT(R), is Director of the Associate Degree Radiography Program at Lincoln Land Community College in Springfield, Illinois. He has been involved in radiography education for nearly 20 years, directing both hospital-sponsored and associate degree programs. He is coauthor of *Introduction to Radiologic Technology*, also published by Mosby–Year Book, and has had articles published in state and national radiologic technology journals.

He has addressed groups of students, educators, and practicing technologists at international, national, state, and local radiologic technology meetings. His presentations include "Face to Face with Moments of Truth," "The Working Wounded: Survival in the Dysfunctional Workplace," "You'll Always Be an Only If You're Only an Only Now," "Practical Physics for the Radiographer (and You Thought Physics Had to Be Boring!)," "Understanding Conflict: Weapons or Tools," and "The You-Shaped Piece of the Puzzle."

Mr. Callaway also has an extensive background in staff development and has served as a management and quality services consultant to health care institutions all over the United States. He has coauthored a quality customer service guide for radiology and has presented more than 500 workshops on management, customer service, and communications in health care.

Reviewers

Sandra Alsop, RT(R)
Director
Radiographer Program
Clearfield Hospital
School of Radiologic Technology
Clearfield; Pennsylvania

Ronald Becker, LAS, BA, MS
Program Director
Shadyside Hospital/ Penn State University
Radiologic Technology Program
Pittsburgh, Pennsylvania

Alan Bode, MA, RT(R)
Program Director
Assistant Professor
Radiographer Program
College of St. Catherine
Minneapolis, Minnesota

Dorothy Bowers, MS, RT(R)
Director
Radiologic Technology Program
Belleville Area College
Belleville, Illinois

Irene Camp, BS, RT(R)
Program Director, Radiographer Program
Baylor University
Dallas, Texas

Michael Fugate, M.Ed., RT(R)
Lead Didactic Faculty
Radiography Program
Santa Fe Community College
Gainesville, Florida

Ginger S. Griffen
Program Director
Baptist Medical Center
School of Radiologic Technology
Jacksonville, Florida

Kenneth Helfrick, BA, RT(R)
Program Director
West Park Hospital
School of Radiologic Technology
Cody, Wyoming

Sheri L. Hosterman, RT(R) (CV)
Clinical Instructor
Holy Spirit Hospital
School of Radiologic Technology
Camp Hill, Pennsylvania

Douglas Hughes, BSRT, (R) (T)
St. Luke's Regional Medical Center
Mountain State Tumor Institute
Radiation Therapy Technology Program
Boise, Idaho

Douglas Larkin, RT(R)
Program Director
Sutter Community Hospitals
School of Radiologic Technology
Sacramento, California

Starla Mason, BS, RT(R)
Program Director
Laramie County Community College
Radiographer Program
Cheyenne, Wyoming

Michelle Miller, M.Ed., RT(R) (M)
Program Coordinator
Radiographer Program
Champlain College
Burlington, Vermont

Betty Palmer, RT(R)
Director, School of Radiologic Sciences
Portland Community College
Portland, Oregon

Debra Reese, MPH, RT(R)
Department Chairperson
Radiographer Program
Asheville-Buncombe Technical
Community College
Asheville, North Carolina

Gina Rigoni
Program Director
Radiography Program
College of DuPage
Glen Ellyn, Illinois

Donna Shehane
Program Director
School of Radiologic Technology
East Tennessee State University
Johnson City, Tennessee

Cheryl A. Thompson, BS, RT(R)
Program Director
Trinity Medical Center
Trinity School of Radiography
Moline, Illinois

Zoland "Skip" Zile, BS, MS, RT(R)
Professor
Northhampton Community College
Department of Radiologic Technology
Bethlehem, Pennsylvania

Evenings, weekends, holiday vacations, and college breaks provided the time for this monumental project. It is with deep appreciation that I dedicate this book to my wife, Karen, and to our children, Amy, Cara, David, Adam, and Kim.

Preface

Guiding my students through the process of reviewing for the radiography certification exam and preparing for careers in radiography has proved to be a source of great satisfaction. Over the years, the benefit of gathering information and making it available to all radiography students and educators became clear. The result of that effort is this review text, which is designed to be used either as a self-directed study guide and career planner or with the assistance of an instructor. This resource should not be viewed as a substitute for a textbook or for coursework that comprehensively covers a subject area. It should, however, provide a complete review and serve to complement instructors' advice to students who are approaching this career milestone.

The material in this guide is organized into three distinct areas: the review guide, a career preparation section, and a unit on career advancement. Part I, the review guide, represents the primary content that may be covered on the certification exam. It is presented in a thorough, but concise outline format to capture the key instructional points and to facilitate an efficient review. The study guide is written in response to the test specifications set forth by the American Registry of Radiologic Technologists (ARRT) and is structured to correspond to the ARRT's major test categories. The review chapters are amply illustrated and include questions that students may use to assess their knowledge of radiography topics. Chapter 7, a practice certification exam, provides another measure of content mastery that simulates the actual test-taking experience. Additional features of this section of the guide will help students plan the review process and familiarize themselves with the test application procedure and possible testing conditions.

The review questions have been written to stimulate creative thinking and to thoroughly evaluate understanding of the material. The test questions included in the study guide are, in my opinion, more difficult than those appearing on the certification exam. Each question and all of its answer choices require careful reading. However, this guide is intended to be more than a question and answer book. Students will need to think, study, answer the test questions, and study the outline again to accomplish a comprehensive review of the material. Answers to all of the review questions are provided in the appendix. Answers that are not understood should cause the student to return to that portion of the content for additional review. It is this type of interaction with the material—not just answering hundreds of review questions—that will result in depth of learning and long-term retention of information.

Parts II and III of the guide—the sections on preparation for employment and continuing education opportunities—are as important to career planning as Part I is to the review process. Many of the questions students ask me most often, about creating a résumé, interviewing for employment, fulfilling requirements for certification renewal, and advancing in the field of radiologic technology, are addressed in these sections. I have provided numerous sample documents (e.g., letters of inquiry, cover letters, sample résumés) to aid the transition from student to professional radiologic technologist.

A final note on the use of this guide: it is important to understand that variation in the details of test content will occur across certification exams; therefore, inclusion of specific content in this guide does not guarantee that it will be tested, nor is exclusion of content meant to suggest its absence from the exam. The ARRT does not review, evaluate, or endorse publications. Consequently, permission to reproduce copyrighted materials within this publication should not be construed as an endorsement of the publication by the ARRT.

Acknowledgments

This book is the culmination of a great team project involving the author and the professionals at Mosby–Year Book, Inc. Deep appreciation goes to Don Ladig and Jeanne Rowland who believed in this project from its inception and guided it into production. Special thanks go to Lisa Potts and Winnie Sullivan who led the book through its editorial stage and gave it form and polish. Nicole Alexander provided invaluable assistance by keeping the manuscript and illustrations at the right places at the right times. Given the talents of this group of people, any errors or omissions from this book are solely mine.

The support and encouragement of my colleagues at Lincoln Land Community College are greatly appreciated. I also wish to thank my fellow radiography educators who provided critique and guidance. Especially helpful were the students in my class of 1995 who used the study guide and "tested the tests" for me by pouring over the questions and answers included in this book as part of their review process.

Table of Contents

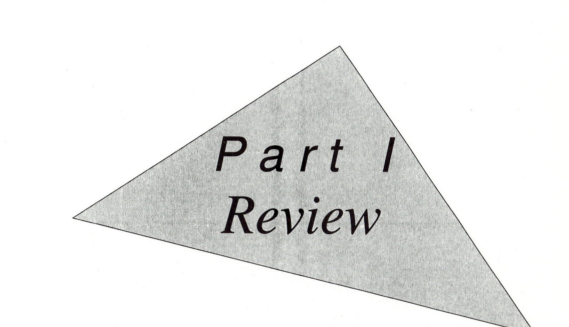

Part I
Review

Chapter 1

Preparation for Review

▲ Welcome to Your Review and Career Planner

> *The future belongs to those who believe in the beauty of their dreams.*

Congratulations on acquiring the most complete study guide available to prepare for the medical radiography examination. By reviewing major subject areas contained in Part I of this guide, answering and studying the test questions, and understanding the skills involved, you will be well on the way to achieving the goal of passing the radiography certification exam.

However, passing the examination is only one of several steps in building your new career. As you look toward graduation, you are probably contemplating your transition into the work environment or considering further education. In addition to thoroughly preparing you for the exam, this book helps you develop your career goals. In Part II, "Preparation for Employment," you will have an opportunity to describe the events and conditions that have been rewarding and motivating during your education. This activity will enable you to set goals for establishing your practice of medical radiography and to plan for either immediate employment or continued education.

The most important tools for use during the transition into the work force are the résumé and the interview, each of which is covered in separate chapters to thoroughly prepare you for marketing yourself in today's ever changing health care environment. So that you may be fully aware of your role as an entry-level radiographer, a complete chapter has been dedicated to helping you anticipate employer expectations for your first postgraduate job. The competitive, and at times chaotic, nature of health care delivery requires that you understand these expectations well before you write your first résumé or sit for your first interview. The goal of presenting this information is to ease the transition from student to entry-level radiographer.

Because the American Registry of Radiologic Technologists (ARRT) now requires proof of continuing education

for recertification, an entire chapter describes the process of acquiring continuing education credits in a manner that complies with ARRT regulations. Part III of the study guide also provides information about the content specifications and the requirements to sit for the ARRT's advanced-level examinations in mammography, computed tomography, magnetic resonance imaging, and cardiovascular-interventional radiography.

Increasing numbers of radiographers are choosing to further their education in diagnostic medical sonography, nuclear medicine technology, or radiation therapy technology. One of the most common questions asked by second-year radiography students is where such educational programs are located. Chapter 15 lists not only all of the accredited educational programs in these specialties in the United States, but also provides a sample letter to be used when requesting the information about these programs.

For those who wish to pursue higher academic degrees, the final chapter of this book describes the opportunities available for obtaining bachelor's or master's degrees in the field of radiologic technology. It also describes other degree options for those considering careers in management or education.

▲ Prioritizing Subjects and Scheduling Study Time

Determining the Length of Review

As you begin the exciting task of planning your review for the ARRT exam, you may wish to take a few moments to examine the study habits you will want to use. It is never too early to begin studying for the examination, but there can certainly be a time when it is too late. Most radiography educators would prefer that their students begin a well-thought-out review approximately six months before taking the exam. Not all students will require that much time to prepare adequately; those with better ability to retain the material they have already learned may complete their review more quickly.

Another factor that can greatly influence how far in advance to begin studying is the amount of time available. In all likelihood, you are beginning to review while still taking other courses in your educational program. Those courses must be given a high priority when budgeting your time. It does little good to review for the certification exam only to find that you are hopelessly behind in another required course. In addition, many students have employment obligations which take a considerable amount of time. Still others have marriage and family commitments that must not be allowed to falter while you prepare for the exam.

Use the six-month lead time as a guide. If you need to begin reviewing earlier, then do so. However, begin reviewing at least six months before the exam. If you finish your preparation sooner, you will have the option of ceasing your review or going back over the material lightly one more time. If you wait too long to begin reviewing—only four or five months ahead of time—you may find yourself with insufficient time to go over the material thoroughly. It is far better to finish early than to run out of time.

Before you begin budgeting your review time, consider the suggestions and encouragement provided by your instructors, who probably have several years' experience working with students about to prepare for the exam. Their wisdom and suggestions should be taken seriously. If you follow the routine they suggest, as well as the guidelines contained in this review book, you should be more than adequately prepared to pass the exam. Remember, however, that managing the quality and quantity of your review

time is, ultimately, up to you. Having successfully reached this point in your educational program, use your energy, time, and skills wisely during these final months of preparation. Just as with running a race, finish strong.

Scheduling Your Study Time

Next, let's go through the process of planning your study time and evaluating your commitment so that you may set goals for reviewing all of the material. Browse through Chapters 2, 3, 4, 5, and 6, and briefly refresh your memory about the material they contain. Are there large amounts of information that you can't seem to recall? Is there information there that you have never seen before? Does most of it look familiar and subject to fairly easy recall?

Try answering a few of the test questions after each section and sample some of the questions from the comprehensive exam in Chapter 7. Were you able to answer the questions easily? Do you feel confident about your answers or were they educated guesses? How many did you get correct compared with the number you missed? Also, are there specific subject areas in which you feel particularly strong or weak? Will you need to spend more time studying one area than another? All of these questions need to be answered as you attempt to budget your review time.

Sunday	Monday	Tuesday	Wednesday	Thursday	Friday	Saturday
				1 10:00 *Advanced Positioning* 1:00 *Pathology Class*	**2** 7:30 *Clinical Education* 7:00 *Review: Radiation Biol*	**3** *No Study Day*
4 7:00 *Review: Radiation Biol*	**5** 7:30 *Clinical Education*	**6** 10:00 *Advanced Positioning* 1:00 *Pathology Class*	**7** 7:30 *Clinical Education*	**8** 10:00 *Advanced Positioning* 1:00 *Pathology Class*	**9** 7:30 *Clinical Education* 7:00 *Review: Physics*	**10** *No Study Day*
11 7:00 *Review: Physics*	**12** 7:30 *Clinical Education*	**13** 10:00 *Advanced Positioning* 1:00 *Pathology Class*	**14** 7:30 *Clinical Education*	**15** 10:00 *Advanced Positioning* 1:00 *Pathology Class*	**16** 7:30 *Clinical Education* 7:00 *Review: Quality Control*	**17** *No Study Day*
18 7:00 *Review: Quality Control*	**19** 7:30 *Clinical Education*	**20** 10:00 *Advanced Positioning* 1:00 *Pathology Class*	**21** 7:30 *Clinical Education*	**22** 10:00 *Advanced Positioning* 1:00 *Pathology Class*	**23** 7:30 *Clinical Education* 7:00 *Review: Image Intensifier*	**24** *No Study Day*
25 7:00 *Review: Image Intensifier*	**26** 7:30 *Clinical Education*	**27** 10:00 *Advanced Positioning* 1:00 *Pathology Class*	**28** 7:30 *Clinical Education*	**29** 10:00 *Advanced Positioning* 1:00 *Pathology Class*	**30** 7:30 *Clinical Education* 7:00 *Review: Skull Anatomy*	

Figure 1-1 Calendar for scheduling study time.

Pause now to consider each of them carefully.

If you are already using some form of daily, weekly, or monthly calendar to plan your study time, you simply need to decide where within your study schedule you will include your review. If you have not been using a calendar to budget your time, this is a great place to start. It is not necessary to purchase an expensive time planner. Most students use a calendar with squares large enough to write in times and planned activities. Figure 1-1 is an example of a simple calendar which is being used to budget time for current classes as well as review.

The importance of writing this time on a calendar cannot be overstated. You are much more likely to adhere to a study schedule if you have thought it through, written it down, and posted it where you see it daily. It is highly recommended that once you plan your review time you make a copy of your calendar and provide it to your instructor. Educators can be powerful motivators by occasionally reminding the student of the written commitment to review. Filling in a calendar in this way is also a form of establishing a written contract with yourself. In so doing, you recognize that, ultimately, you are responsible only to yourself for covering this material.

When setting up a review calendar, it is most important to be regular and consistent. Be certain that you are setting aside specific time to review on a regular basis. Don't save review for those times when you have nothing else to do. State your commitment in terms such as the following: "I will review physics every Thursday evening for the next eight weeks for approximately two hours each time." This contract with yourself describes the activity, the time commitment, and the subject involved. Avoid such entries as: "I will study physics four times this month." There is little commitment to that statement and the ambiguous goal it sets forth likely will not be accomplished.

As an adult learner, you have probably developed an awareness of your strengths and weaknesses relative to time management and commitment to studies. Whatever your self-appraisal, the fact that you are using this book suggests that you are a successful student with good ability to manage your time effectively. Spend some time now applying your scheduling and time management skills to the planning of your review.

Keep in mind that if you are allotting at least six months to prepare for the exam, you should have plenty of time to cover all of the material and to take and review the tests in this book. Again, if you will do all that is expected of you in terms of your regular studies and review, you should have little difficulty on the exam. It is hoped that, by the time you take the test, you will regard it as just another quiz.

Planning the Review Process

> "*If one advances confidently in the direction of their dreams and endeavors to lead a life which they have imagined, they will meet with a success unexpected in common hours.*"
> Henry David Thoreau

It is now time to turn your attention to the actual review process. Look through the chapters containing the review material, if you have not already done so. In the space provided below, make a list of those subject areas in which you feel particularly strong or weak. By listing the subject areas in this manner, you will be able to prioritize the material that you need to cover. A common pitfall among second-year radiography students, as they prepare for the exam, is to review the easiest material first. This is the opposite of what you should do.

Strong Subjects

_____

_____

_____

_____

_____

_____

Weak Subjects

_____

_____

_____

_____

_____

_____

Look again at the entries you made above. Transfer these subjects to the spaces on the following page, ranking the weakest subjects first. Then progress, in order, to the subjects in which you are strongest.

Priority of Studies, Weakest to Strongest

I need to study the following subjects in this order:

1. _____

2. _____

3. _____

4. _____

5. _____

6. _____

7. _____

8. _____

9. _____

10. _____

11. _____

12. _____

This second prioritizing exercise helps to identify what you must study first. The rationale for studying more difficult content first is two-fold: the more difficult material is going to require more time, which you will have in greater supply at the beginning of the six-month period than at the end. Secondly, if you have had serious difficulty with some of the subject areas and you study those first, you will have additional time to seek explanation from your instructors and to read the material again.

Save the subjects with which you are the most comfortable for last. They will require the least amount of study and, should your time become limited, it will not be as critical if you have to move more quickly through the review chapter.

The time spent now on planning a study calendar and prioritizing your study needs will pay great dividends as you begin the review process. Such planning should allow you to proceed more efficiently and to dedicate more time to studying. If you are not filling in a calendar or prioritizing your study needs as you read this chapter, take the time right now to select a day and time when you will reread Chapter 1 and follow the directions for time management and prioritizing.

_____ I have completed my planner calendar and prioritized my subjects areas for study.

_____ I will complete my planner calendar and prioritize my subject areas for study on _____(day), _____(date) at _____a.m./p.m.

Now that you have established your priorities or made an appointment with yourself to plan your calendar, you have set your first goal for reviewing and passing the certification exam. What is even more exciting is that you have taken the initial step toward your first radiography job or continued education. Be sure to congratulate yourself on accomplishing this task and then finish reading this chapter.

Before turning to study habits, let's address concerns which many second-year students develop in response to feedback from others who recently have taken the exam. You may have been told to give little attention to certain subject areas because they did not appear on the test. You may hear that the exam was particularly easy and may be advised not to worry about it. While some may scoff at your calendar planning and the amount of time you choose to spend reviewing, others may feel that you are not spending enough time. For the student in this position, all of the suggestions, hints, and guidelines may become confusing. Again, you should refer to the suggestions made by your instructors and contained in this study guide.

Be aware that a test taker's recall of material from an examination can become greatly blurred with the passage of time. Though those who are providing you with feedback about the exam are surely well-intentioned, their memory of the test items is of questionable reliability. In addition, because of the size of the item bank for the exam, the questions vary each time the test is administered. Even if the individuals to whom you are speaking are accurate in their recall of the test content, you will not be taking the same test. Each radiography exam is different from the one that precedes it.

Discussing the exam with your classmates immediately after you complete it may prove interesting. You will be surprised to find, even two to three hours after completing the examination, how rapidly recall of specific test content has declined. In fact, many test takers become anxious immediately after the exam as they hear others referring to questions that they can't recall. A bystander overhearing such a conversation would conclude wrongly that these students had each taken a different exam. You may also be surprised, when speaking with individuals who have taken the exam in recent months, to hear that "There was almost no positioning on the test" or "My goodness, it was all physics!" Actually, the radiography exam follows content specifications which are included in this chapter. In most cases, when individuals think there were more questions in one category and almost none in another, it is a reflection of their command of the content or of their preparation for the exam.

Greet such advice with friendly skepticism. By choosing to ignore advice from even the most well-intentioned recent test takers and following the study routine that you are planning under the guidance of your instructors and this book, you will guarantee that you are the one controlling the test outcome and can be assured that you are undertaking the best preparation for the exam.

▲ Study Habits

Study habits mirror the individuality of each student. Some students prefer to study alone, reading small sections of a chapter at a time, pausing to reflect on the content, taking additional notes if necessary, or reciting the material aloud. Others choose to read over a section or an entire chapter many times, reviewing the material to facilitate their recall. Others find it helpful to study in groups, alternately quizzing one another and answering practice questions.

By now you probably have formed your own set of effective study habits. In using this book to prepare for the exam, you should consider every suggestion that may improve your method of study. Do not, however, greatly alter study habits that have proven successful. Also, keep in mind that as you review for the exam, you should not be learning new material. By definition, a review should be a revisiting of material that you have already learned and learned well.

A few reminders about study habits or study conditions are now in order. Remember to choose your most difficult subjects to study first. You have already listed these in the previous section. When you study, be sure you have time set aside during which you can be quiet with no interruptions. For some, soft music in the background can aid study, while others prefer silence. Other types of music, as well as television, simply interfere with concentration. Although you should be comfortable while studying, you should not be too comfortable. It is particularly important to remain upright.

Take regular but infrequent breaks. Be sure that you have adequate lighting and that the room temperature is controllable and comfortable. Arrange the study conditions so that you can focus all of your attention on what you are doing. Regardless of the study method used, quiet concentration is of utmost importance. You may wish to reinforce your learning by reciting the material aloud—a practice that requires a fairly isolated and distraction-free study setting. Also, study at the time of day when your mind is most alert. Some prefer to study early in the morning, whereas others study better later in the afternoon or in the early evening. Cramming late at night or into the early hours of the morning is ineffective for most individuals. Besides, if

review is a priority you will want to assign it a place of importance in your schedule.

▲ Test Specifications

This section contains the test specifications for the radiography examination administered by the American Registry of Radiologic Technologists (Table 1-1). While it does not divulge specific questions, it does give the reader an outline from which the test is constructed. In addition, the approximate number of questions in each category is listed to allow you to see the relative importance placed on the different subject areas.

You may wonder why these particular categories were selected for the exam and why they are weighted as such. The ARRT periodically undertakes an extensive study called a task inventory. The task inventory for radiographers lists all of the specific skills required of an entry-level radiographer. It is reproduced in Chapter 13, "Employer Expectations."

The skills in the task inventory should coincide with the terminal competencies of all approved educational programs. It is from this task inventory that the categories for the exam are constructed and the relative importance of each is weighted. The review of the major categories on the exam is covered in the next five chapters.

Analysis of Category Components

An approximate number of questions for each of the major subject areas is shown in the detailed listing below. The percentages of subcategory content within the major

Table 1-1 Content Specifications for the Radiography Examination

Content Category	Percent of Test	Number of Questions
Radiation Protection	15%	30
Equipment Operation and Maintenance	15%	30
Image Production and Evaluation	25%	50
Radiographic Procedures	30%	60
Patient Care	15%	30
	100%	200

Copyright ©1994, The American Registry of Radiologic Technologists.

areas are general guidelines and may vary to a certain extent with each test administration.

Radiation Protection—30 questions

A. Patient protection—12 questions
1. Biological effects of radiation
   a. Dose-effect relationships
   b. Long-term effects
      (1) Cancer (including leukemia)
      (2) Cataracts
      (3) Life span shortening
   c. Somatic effects
      (1) Embryonic and fetal effects
      (2) Bone marrow
      (3) Thyroid
      (4) Skin
   d. Genetic effects
      (1) Genetically significant dose (GSD)
      (2) Genetic effects
   e. Relative tissue radiosensitivities
2. Minimizing patient exposure
   a. Exposure factors
      (1) kVp
      (2) mAs
      (3) Single-phase, three-phase, and high-frequency generators
   b. Shielding
      (1) Rationale for use
      (2) Types of protective devices
      (3) Placement of protective devices
   c. Beam restriction
      (1) Purpose of primary beam restriction
      (2) Effect on secondary (scatter) radiation
      (3) Types (collimators, cones, aperture diaphragms)
   d. Filtration
      (1) Effect on skin and organ exposure
      (2) Effect on average beam energy
      (3) NCRP recommendations
   e. Patient positioning (i.e., PA versus AP)
   f. Film, screens, and film-screen combinations
   g. Grids; air gap techniques
   h. Automatic exposure control
B. Personnel protection—9 questions
1. Sources of radiation exposure
   a. Exposure to primary x-ray beam
   b. Secondary radiation
   c. Leakage radiation
2. Basic methods of protection
   a. Time
   b. Distance
   c. Shielding
3. NCRP recommendations for protective devices
4. Special considerations
   a. Portable (mobile) units

b. Fluoroscopy
   (1) Protective drapes
   (2) Protective Bucky slot cover
   (3) Cumulative timer
c. Guidelines for fluoroscopy and portable units (NCRP, Code of Federal Regulations [CFR]-21)
C. Radiation exposure and monitoring—9 questions
1. Basic properties of radiation
2. Units of measurement
   a. Rad (gray)
   b. Rem (sievert)
   c. Roentgen (C/kg)
3. Dosimeters (types; proper use)
4. NCRP recommendations for personnel monitoring
   a. ALARA ("As Low As Reasonably Achievable") and dose equivalent limits
   b. Evaluation of cumulative dose records
   c. Maintenance of cumulative dose records

Equipment Operation and Maintenance—30 questions

A. Radiographic Equipment—21 questions
1. Components of basic radiographic unit
   a. Control panel
   b. X-ray tube
      (1) Tube construction
      (2) Warm-up procedures
      (3) Tube rating charts
   c. Automatic exposure controls
      (1) Radiation detectors (e.g., ionization chamber, photomultiplier tube)
      (2) Backup timer
2. X-ray generator, transformers, and rectification system
   a. Basic principles
   b. Phase and pulse
3. Fluoroscopic unit
   a. Image intensifier
   b. Viewing systems (e.g., TV monitor)
   c. Recording systems (e.g., videotape)
   d. Automatic brightness control
4. Types of units
   a. Stationary
   b. Portable (mobile)
   c. Specialized or dedicated units
B. Evaluation of radiographic equipment and accessories—9 questions
1. Equipment calibration
   a. kVp
   b. mAs
   c. Time
2. Beam restriction
   a. Light field to radiation field alignment
   b. Central ray alignment
3. Recognition of malfunctions

4. Screens and cassettes
   a. Construction
   b. Handling
   c. Artifacts
   d. Maintenance
5. Shielding accessories (e.g., lead apron testing)

Image Production and Evaluation—50 questions

A. Selection of technical factors—26 questions
   1. Density
      a. mAs
      b. kVp
      c. Distance
      d. Film-screen combinations
      e. Grids
      f. Filtration
      g. Beam restriction
      h. Anatomic and pathologic factors
      i. Anode heel effect
   2. Contrast
      a. kVp
      b. Beam restriction
      c. Grids
      d. Filtration
      e. Anatomic and pathologic factors
   3. Recorded detail
      a. OID (object-image distance)
      b. SID (source-image distance)
      c. Focal spot size
      d. Film-screen combinations
      e. Motion
   4. Distortion
      a. Size
      b. Shape
   5. Film, screen, and grid selection
      a. Film characteristics
         (1) Film contrast
         (2) Film latitude
         (3) Exposure latitude
      b. Film-screen combinations
         (1) Phosphor type
         (2) Relative speed
         (3) Single- versus double-emulsion film
         (4) Special applications (e.g., detail, latitude)
      c. Conversion factors for grids
   6. Technique charts
      a. Caliper measurement
      b. Fixed versus variable kVp
      c. Anatomical considerations
         (1) Tissue density
         (2) Part thickness
      d. Special considerations (e.g., casts, pathology, pediatrics, contrast media)

   e. Automatic exposure control
   7. Manual versus automatic exposure
      a. Effects of changing exposure factors on radiographic quality
      b. Selection of ionization chamber or photocell
      c. Alignment of part to ionization chamber or photocell
B. Film processing and quality assurance—12 questions
   1. Film storage
      a. Pressure artifacts
      b. Fog (e.g., age, chemical, radiation, temperature, safelight)
   2. Cassette loading
      a. Matching film and screens
      b. Film handling artifacts (e.g., static, crinkle, marks, fog)
   3. Radiographic identification
      a. Methods (e.g., photographic, radiographic)
      b. Legal considerations (e.g., patient data, examination data)
   4. Automatic film processor
      a. Processor chemistry
      b. Components and systems
         (1) Transport
         (2) Replenishment
         (3) Temperature regulation
         (4) Recirculation
         (5) Dryer
      c. Maintenance
         (1) Start-up and shutdown procedure
         (2) Removal and cleaning of crossover assembly
         (3) Sensitometric monitoring
      d. System malfunction
         (1) Observable effects (e.g., artifacts, fluctuations in density, contrast, fog)
         (2) Possible causes of malfunctions (e.g., improper temperature, contamination, roller alignment, replenishment, water flow)
C. Evaluation of radiographs—12 questions
   1. Criteria for diagnostic quality radiographs
      a. Radiographic density
      b. Radiographic contrast
      c. Recorded detail
      d. Distortion
      e. Artifacts
      f. Grid alignment
      g. Proper demonstration of anatomical structure
      h. Identification markers (e.g., anatomical, patient, date)
   2. Causes of poor radiographic quality
      a. Technical factors (e.g., kVp, mAs, distance, filtration, film-screen combination, grids)
      b. Positioning (e.g., OID, SID, tube-part-film alignment)
      c. Patient considerations (e.g., pathologic conditions, motion)
      d. Processing (e.g., fog, contamination, temperature)

e. Artifacts
3. Improvement of suboptimal image

Radiographic Procedures—60 questions

A. General procedural considerations—6 questions
1. Patient preparation (e.g., explaining procedures, removal of radiopaque objects)
2. Equipment capabilities
3. Positioning terminology
4. Patient respiration and motion control
   a. Instructions for the examination
   b. Effect on radiographic quality
   c. Adapting to patient's cooperative ability (e.g., mA and time adjustments)
   d. Immobilization devices and techniques
5. Technique and positioning variations (e.g., for trauma or pediatric patients; adapting to patient's body habitus)

B. Specific imaging procedures—54 questions (including positioning, technical factors, anatomy, physiology, and pathology)
1. Thorax—6 questions
   a. Chest
   b. Ribs
   c. Sternoclavicular joints
   d. Sternum
2. Abdomen and GI studies—10 questions
   a. Abdomen
   b. Esophagus
   c. Upper GI series
   d. Small bowel series
   e. Barium enema, single-contrast
   f. Barium enema, double-contrast
   g. Operative cholangiography
   h. T-tube cholangiography
   i. Cholecystography
   j. ERCP (endoscopic retrograde cholangiopancreatography)
3. Urological studies—4 questions
   a. Cystography
   b. Cystourethrography
   c. Intravenous urography
   d. Retrograde urography
   e. Retrograde urethrography
4. Extremities—16 questions
   a. Toes
   b. Foot
   c. Os calcis
   d. Ankle
   e. Tibia, fibula
   f. Knee
   g. Patella
   h. Femur
   i. Fingers
   j. Hand
   k. Wrist
   l. Forearm
   m. Elbow
   n. Humerus
   o. Shoulder
   p. Scapula
   q. Clavicle
   r. Acromioclavicular joints
   s. Bone survey
   t. Long bone measurement
   u. Bone age
   v. Soft tissue
5. Spine and pelvis—8 questions
   a. Cervical spine
   b. Thoracic spine
   c. Scoliosis series
   d. Lumbosacral spine
   e. Sacrum
   f. Sacroiliac joints
   g. Coccyx
   h. Pelvis
   i. Hip
6. Head and neck—7 questions
   a. Skull
   b. Mastoids, temporal bones
   c. Facial bones
   d. Mandible
   e. Zygomatic arch
   f. Temporomandibular joints
   g. Nasal bones
   h. Optic foramina
   i. Orbit
   j. Paranasal sinuses
   k. Soft tissue neck
7. Other
   a. Tomography
   b. Arthrography
   c. Myelography
   d. Venography
   e. Hysterosalpingography

Patient Care—30 questions

A. Legal and professional responsibilities—6 questions
1. Scheduling and sequencing examinations
2. Legal aspects of radiology
   a. Request to perform examination
   b. Patient rights (e.g., confidentiality, consent)
   c. Professional liability
3. Patient identification (e.g., wrist band, questioning)
4. Verification of requested examination
   a. Clarification of terminology
   b. Comparison of request to clinical indications (e.g., observations [left arm injured, but right arm requested])

c. Evaluation of need for additional projections
d. Modification of routine projection
B. Patient education, safety, and comfort—4 questions
   1. Communication with patients
      a. Review of patient history
      b. Explanation of current procedure
      c. Response to inquiries about other imaging procedures (basic concepts of mammography, CT, MRI, sonography, nuclear medicine)
   2. Assessment of patient condition (e.g., motor control, severity of injury, support equipment)
   3. Proper body mechanics for patient transfer
   4. Patient privacy, safety, and comfort
C. Prevention and control of infection—6 questions
   1. Transmission of infection
   2. Universal precautions
   3. Disinfection and sterilization; asepsis and sterile technique
   4. Handling of biohazardous materials
   5. Isolation procedures
      a. Types (e.g., respiratory, protective, reverse)
      b. Radiography of isolation patients
D. Patient monitoring—9 questions
   1. Routine monitoring
      a. Equipment (e.g., stethoscope, sphygmomanometer)
      b. Vital signs (e.g., blood pressure, pulse, respiration, temperature)
      c. Physical signs and symptoms
   2. Support equipment (e.g., IV tubes, chest tubes, catheters)
   3. Common medical emergencies (e.g., seizure, cardiac arrest, loss of consciousness, bleeding)
   4. Management of common medical emergencies (e.g., CPR, hemostasis)
E. Contrast media—5 questions
   1. Types and properties (e.g., iodinated, water soluble, barium, ionic versus nonionic)
   2. Appropriateness of contrast medium to exam and patient condition (e.g., perforated bowel, patient age, patient weight)
   3. Contraindications
   4. Patient education
   5. Administration
      a. Routes (e.g., venous, rectal, oral)
      b. Supplies (e.g., enema kits, needles)
      c. Venipuncture
   6. Complications/reactions
      a. Local effects (e.g., extravasation, phlebitis)
      b. Systemic effects
         (1) Mild (e.g., flushing, hives, nausea)
         (2) Severe (e.g., shock, hypotension)
      c. Radiographer's response (e.g., first aid, documentation)

▲ Conventions Used in the ARRT Radiography Examination

The American Registry of Radiologic Technologists employs a list of conventions in an attempt to standardize nomenclature used in the examination. The conventions include terminology, abbreviations, and formats specific to the field of radiography. Many of the conventions listed are already quite familiar to you and their exclusion from this chapter will have no impact on your understanding of the terminology. Other conventions involve terminology changes and additions or deletions with which the student may be unfamiliar.

If you find, as you examine the following list, that you have learned certain terminology in your educational program and the exam uses slightly different terminology, don't conclude that your educational program was in error. This list is an attempt to standardize terminology for the purpose of test construction. The primary conventions are listed below:

Absorbed dose—unit is the rad; energy absorbed per unit mass of the radiated material

Accumulated dose 5(N-18)—this formula is obsolete because of changes enacted by the NCRP

Anode/film distance—replaced by *SID (FFD)*

Apron thickness for fluoroscopy—minimum thickness required is 0.5 millimeters lead equivalent, according to NCRP Report #102

Automatic exposure control—term used instead of *photo timing*

Automatic positive beam limitation—replaced by the term *automatic collimation*

Blur—used in place of the term *recorded detail* when describing the effect of patient motion on the radiograph; blur is synonymous with motion

Caldwell—test uses the term *PA (Caldwell) projection*

Capitellum—term used is *capitulum*

Centigrade—abbreviated as C

#21 - CFR (1992)—21 Code of Federal Regulations; sections to be covered on the exam

Contrast—radiographic contrast is defined as the visible differences between any two selected areas of density levels within the radiographic image

Cycles per second—unit used is hertz (Hz)

Definition—term used is *recorded detail*

Density—radiographic density is the degree of blackening or opacity of an area in a radiograph caused by the accumulation of black metallic silver following exposure and processing of a film; density equals log incident light intensity divided by transmitted light intensity

Detail—term used is *recorded detail*

Distortion—the misrepresentation of the size or shape of a structure recorded in a radiographic image

Dose equivalent—unit is the rem; defined as absorbed dose multiplied by a quality factor that accounts for the difference in biological effectiveness of different types of radiation; used in questions involving radiation protection and personnel monitoring

Dose equivalent limits—used to refer to radiation exposure limits for radiation workers; replaces the term *maximum permissible dose (MPD)*

Edge gradient—term is not used

Entrance skin exposure—used in place of *skin exposure*

Exposure—amount of radiation; the unit is the roentgen (R)

Exposure in air—term found in questions involving use of ionization chambers

Exposure factors—refers to mA, time, kVp, and distance

Exposure latitude—defined as the range of exposure factors that will produce a diagnostic radiograph

Film—refers to unexposed film; otherwise, the term *radiograph* is used to refer to exposed film

Film contrast—defined as the inherent ability of the film emulsion to react to radiation and record a range of densities

Film latitude—defined as the inherent ability of the film to record a long range of density levels on the radiograph

Film latitude and film contrast—dependent upon the sensitometric properties of the film and the processing conditions; directly determined from the characteristic H and D curve

Focal film distance or FFD—replaced by *SID* (FFD)

Geometric sharpness—term used is *geometrically recorded detail*

Grid radius—term used is *grid focusing distance*

Grid technique conversion factors—because of variations in the many textbooks available, answers are given in ranges

Impulse timers—not tested

Ionic contrast media—included on exam

Law—term used is *modified lateral (Law) projection*

LD 50/30—not covered on exam

Lead glove thickness—minimum thickness required is .25 millimeters according to NCRP report #102

Long-scale contrast—used when there are slight differences between densities present (low contrast) but the total number of densities is increased

Loss of recorded detail—if caused by patient motion, the term used is *blur* or *motion*; if caused by large focal spot or intensifying screens, the term used is *unsharpness* or *poor recorded detail*

Lower or higher contrast—used instead of *decreased* or *increased contrast*

Manual processing—not on the exam

Mechanical timers—not on the exam

NCRP Report #91—included on exam

NCRP Report #102—included on exam; replaces NCRP Report #33

NCRP Report #105—included on exam; replaces NCRP Report #48

Nonionic contrast media—included on the exam

Nonscreen technique—not on the exam

Object-film distance or OFD—term used is *OID* (OFD)

Par speed screens—not included on the exam

Part-film distance—term used is *OID* (OFD)

Penumbra—term not used on the exam; terms used are *motion, blur,* or *unsharpness of recorded detail* depending upon the cause

Position (radiographic position)—used to describe a specific body position, such as supine or prone; only refers to the patient's physical position

Projection (radiographic projection)—only used to refer to the path of the central ray

Radiograph—film that has been exposed

Recorded detail—the sharpness of the structural lines as recorded in the radiographic image

Remnant radiation—term used is *exit radiation* or *image-forming radiation*

Rhese—term used is *parietoorbital oblique (Rhese) projection*

Scale of contrast—defined as the number of densities visible or the number of shades of gray

Screen speed—expressed using film screen system numbers rather than names

Sharpness—term used is *recorded detail*

Sharpness of detail—term used is *recorded detail*

Short-scale contrast—this term is used when considerable differences among densities are present (high contrast) but the total number of densities is reduced

SI units—sieverts, grays, becquerels; are not used on the examination

Size distortion (magnification)—the enlargement of the recorded image compared with the actual size of the structure

Shape distortion—the misrepresentation of the shape of the structure (elongated or foreshortened) of the recorded image compared with the actual shape of the structure

Spinning top test—only the principle of the test is covered on the exam

Stenvers—term used is *posterior profile (Stenvers) projection*

Subject contrast—defined as the difference in the amount of radiation transmitted by a particular part as a result of the different absorption characteristics of the tissues and structures that the part comprises

Submento vertical—term used is *submento vertical (full basal) projection*

Target-film distance—term used is *SID* (FFD)

Technique—term used is *exposure factors* or *technical factors*

Valve tubes—not used on the exam

View (radiographic view)—term used to refer to the body part as seen by the image recording medium such as film; only used in discussion of a radiograph or image

Waters—term used is *parietoacanthial (Waters) projection*

Wavelength—term used only in reference to comparisons of X rays, gamma rays, and other forms of radiation; in other situations the term used is *average photon energy*

▲ *You're on Your Way !*

Using this first chapter as a planner, you are now ready to work toward one of the crowning achievements of your educational career. Do all that is expected and use your time and talents wisely. Do not allow external distractions to send you off course. It is time to plan and work for what is yet to come . . . passing the radiography examination and moving on to the next phase of your career. You have numerous human and material resources available to assist you, one of which you are reading. Use them all and go for it!

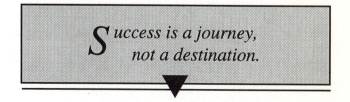

Success is a journey, not a destination.

Chapter 2

Review of Radiation Protection

> T*o be a winner, all you need*
> *to give is all you have.*

▼

▲ Basic Principles of Radiation Protection

Responsibility for Radiation Protection

A. Radiographer is primarily responsible for protecting the patient from unnecessary exposure
  1. Best accomplished by avoiding repeat exposures
  2. Should use smallest amount of radiation that will produce a diagnostic radiograph
B. Radiologist and referring physician assume shared responsibility for radiation safety of patient
  1. Best accomplished by consultation and not ordering unnecessary exams
C. Safe use of radiation in diagnostic imaging to determine extent of pathology or injury outweighs risk involved

Ionizing Radiation

A. X-radiation exposure involves a transfer of energy: photon-tissue interactions
  1. Possesses the ability to remove electrons from atoms by a process called ionization
  2. Ionization in human cells results in:
    a. Unstable atoms
    b. Free electrons
    c. Production of low-energy x rays
    d. Formation of new molecules harmful to the cell
    e. Cell damage may be exhibited as abnormal function or loss of function
B. General types of cell damage
  1. Somatic—damage to the cell itself
  2. Genetic—damage to cell's genetic code contained in the DNA
C. Sources of ionizing radiation
  1. Natural background radiation
    a. Contained in the environment
    b. Present since the formation of the universe
    c. Source of 82% of human exposure to radiation; annual effective dose equivalent per person of 295 mrem
    d. Greatest source of natural background radiation exposure to humans is radon, 55% (198 mrem annually)
    e. Next source of natural background radiation is the human body, radioactive nuclides in tissues (carbon-14, potassium-40, strontium-90, and hydrogen-3)
    f. Terrestrial radiation from radioactive minerals such as uranium and radium which varies by geographic region
    g. Cosmic rays from the stars, partially shielded by earth's magnetic fields and atmosphere; annual absorbed dose equivalent is approximately 30 mrem; dose is greater at higher elevations because of lower atmospheric shielding; dose equivalent during an airline flight is 1 mrem per hour (depending upon duration of flight and actual altitude achieved)
  2. Artificial radiation
    a. Made by humans
    b. Source of 18% of human exposure to radiation
    c. Annual effective dose equivalent of approximately 66 mrem : 54 mrem = diagnostic imaging procedures; 11 mrem = consumer products; 1 mrem = nuclear weapons testing and all other sources

▲ Photon-Tissue Interactions

Basic Definitions

A. Primary radiation—radiation exiting the x-ray tube
B. Exit radiation (image-producing radiation)—x rays that emerge from the patient
C. Attenuation—absorption and scatter (loss of intensity) of the x-ray beam as it passes through the patient
D. Heterogeneous beam—x-ray beam contains photons of many different energies
E. Most common photon-tissue interactions in diagnostic radiography are photoelectric and Compton's interactions
  1. Photoelectric interaction (Fig. 2-1)
    a. A photon absorption interaction

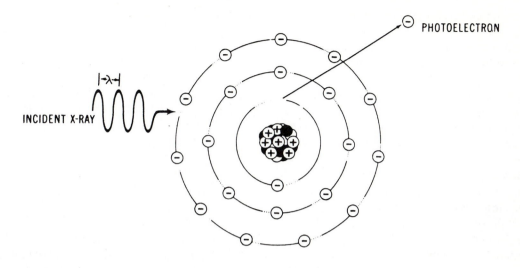

Figure 2-1 Photoelectric effect. From Bushong, SC: Radiologic science for technologists: physics, biology, and protection, ed 5, St. Louis, 1993, Mosby.

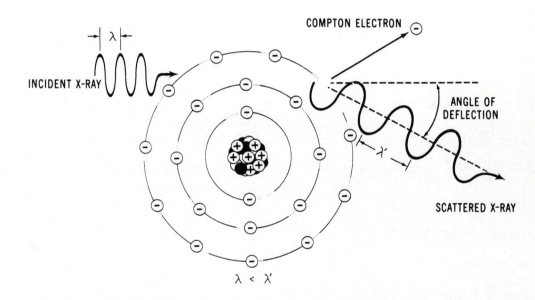

Figure 2-2 Compton effect. From Bushong, SC: Radiologic science for technologists: physics, biology, and protection, ed 5, St. Louis, 1993, Mosby.

b. Incoming x-ray photon strikes a *K*-shell electron
c. Energy of x-ray photon is transferred to electron
d. The electron is ejected from the *K* shell, now called a photoelectron
e. The x-ray photon has deposited all of its energy and ceases to exist
f. Photon has been completely absorbed
g. Photoelectron may ionize or excite other atoms until it has deposited all of its energy
h. Hole in *K* shell is filled by electrons from outer shells, releasing energy which creates low-energy characteristic photons that are locally absorbed
i. Photoelectric interaction results in increased dose to the patient

j. Photoelectric interaction produces contrast in the radiograph because of the differential absorption of the incoming x-ray photons in the tissues

2. Compton's interaction (Fig. 2-2)
a. Also called *Compton's scattering* or *modified scattering*
b. Incoming x-ray photon strikes a loosely bound, outer-shell electron
c. Photon transfers part of its energy to the electron
d. Electron is removed from orbit as a scattered electron, known as a recoil electron
e. Ejected electrons may ionize other atoms or recombine with an ion needing an electron
f. Photon scatters in another direction, with less en-

ergy than before because of its encounter with the electron

   g. Scattered photon may interact with other outer-shell electrons causing more ionization, or it may exit the patient

   h. Scattered photons emerging from the patient travel in very divergent paths

   i. Scatter photons may also be present in the room and expose the radiographer or radiologist

3. Coherent scatter (also known as *classical* or *Thompson's*)

   a. Produced by low-energy x-ray photons

   b. Atomic electrons are not removed, but vibrate because of the deposition of energy from the photon

   c. As the electrons vibrate, they emit energy equal to that of the original photon

   d. This energy travels in a path slightly different from the original photon

   e. Ionization has not occurred, though the photon has scattered

4. Pair production

   a. Does not occur in radiography

   b. Produced at photon energies above 1.02 million electron volts

   c. Involves an interaction between the incoming photon and the atomic nucleus

▲ Units of Radiation Measurement

Basic Information

A. Traditional units used are the roentgen, rad, rem, and curie

B. International System of Units (SI) used are the coulomb/kilogram, gray, sievert, and becquerel

  1. Adopted by the International Commission on Radiation Units and Measurements (ICRU) in 1989

  2. Not yet in widespread use in the United States

C. Radiation exposure in air

  1. Measurement of positive and negative particles created when radiation ionizes the atoms in air (x and gamma rays only, up to three million electron volts, in-air measurements only)

  2. This is the amount of radiation that may be expected to strike an object placed near the source of radiation

  3. Traditional unit is the roentgen (R)

    a. 1 roentgen equals 2.58×10^{-4} coulombs of positive and negative charges produced per kilogram of air

  4. SI unit is the coulomb/kilogram (C/kg)

  5. $1 \text{ R} = 2.58 \times 10^{-4} \text{ C/kg}$

  6. $1 \text{ C/kg} = \dfrac{1}{2.58 \times 10^{-4} \text{ R}}$

D. Unit of absorbed dose

  1. The amount of energy absorbed by the object

  2. Absorption of the energy may result in biological damage

  3. As the atomic number of the object increases, so does the absorbed dose

  4. Traditional unit is the rad (radiation absorbed dose)

    a. 1 rad is defined as 100 ergs of energy deposited per gram of tissue

  5. SI unit is the gray

    a. 1 gray = 1 joule of energy deposited per kilogram of tissue

  6. 1 gray = 100 rads

  7. 1 rad = $\frac{1}{100}$ gray

E. Unit of absorbed dose equivalent

  1. Used to take into account the different biological effects caused by different types of radiation

  2. A quality factor (QF) is used to modify the absorbed dose amount to account for the greater damage inflicted by some forms of ionizing radiation (rads × QF = rem)

    a. QF takes into account linear energy transfer (LET), the amount of energy transferred by ionizing radiation per unit length of tissue traveled

    b. LET varies for different types of radiation

    c. High-ionization radiations such as alpha particles and neutrons have high LET (cause more biological damage)

    d. Lower-ionization radiations such as x and gamma rays have lower LET (cause less biological damage)

    e. QF for x and gamma rays = 1

    f. Therefore, 100 rads of x rays = 100 rem

    g. QF for neutrons = 20

    h. Therefore, 100 rads of neutrons = 2000 rem (a higher dose equivalency)

    i. For x and gamma rays, with QF = 1, 1 roentgen = 1 rad = 1 rem (approximately)

  3. Traditional unit is the rem

    a. 1 rem = $\frac{1}{100}$ sievert

  4. SI unit is the sievert

    a. 1 sievert = 100 rem

▲ Absorbed Dose Equivalent Limits

Basic Information

A. Agencies involved in dose-response evaluations

  1. National Council on Radiation Protection and Measurements (NCRP)

  2. International Commission on Radiologic Protection (ICRP)

  3. Nuclear Regulatory Commission (NRC)

    a. Enforces standards at the federal level

B. Effective absorbed dose equivalent limit

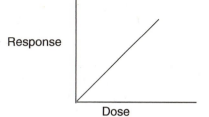

Figure 2-3 Linear-nonthreshold relationship.

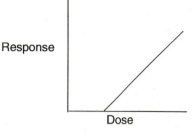

Figure 2-4 Linear-threshold relationship.

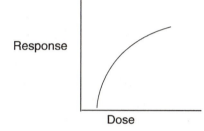

Figure 2-5 Nonlinear-threshold relationship.

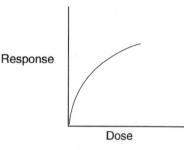

Figure 2-6 Nonlinear-nonthreshold relationship.

1. The upper boundary dose that can be absorbed, either in a single exposure or annually, that carries a negligible risk of somatic or genetic damage to the individual
2. ALARA—"As Low As Reasonably Achievable"
    a. A concept of radiologic practice which encourages radiation users to adopt measures that keep the dose to the patient and themselves at minimum levels
C. Dose-response relationship
    1. Linear-nonthreshold relationship (Fig. 2-3)
        a. States that there is no level of radiation that may be considered completely safe and that the degree of response is directly proportional to the amount of radiation received
    2. Linear-threshold relationship (Fig. 2-4)
        a. States that there is a dose of radiation below which a response does not occur; when that threshold is crossed, the response is directly proportional to the dose received (e.g., cataractogenesis does not occur at low levels of radiation exposure; therefore, there is a threshold, or safe, dose)
    3. Nonlinear-threshold relationship (Fig. 2-5)
        a. States that there is a safe (threshold) dose of radiation which, when crossed, results in responses that are not directly proportional to the dose received
    4. Nonlinear-nonthreshold relationship (Fig. 2-6)
        a. States that there is no level of radiation that may be considered completely safe and that the degree of the response is not directly proportional to the dose received
    5. Stochastic effects—effects of radiation that randomly occur where the probability of such effects is propor-

tional to the dose (increased dose equals increased probability, not severity, of effects)
    6. Nonstochastic effects—effects that become more severe at high levels of radiation exposure and are characterized by a threshold dose below which the effects do not occur
D. NCRP Report #91
    1. Recommends balance between the risk and benefit of using radiation for diagnostic imaging
    2. Recommends that somatic and genetic effects be kept to a minimum when using radiation for diagnostic imaging
    3. Takes into account all human organs that may be vulnerable to radiation damage
    4. Occupational exposure, annual effective absorbed dose equivalent limit for stochastic effects = 5 rem
    5. Occupational exposure, annual effective absorbed dose equivalent limits for nonstochastic effects
        a. Lens of the eye = 15 rem
        b. All other organs = 50 rem
    6. Occupational cumulative exposure = age in years times 1 rem
    7. Students (under age 18), annual effective absorbed dose equivalent limit = 0.1 rem
    8. Students (over age 18), annual effective absorbed dose equivalent limit for skin, extremities, and eye lens = 5 rem
    9. General public, annual effective absorbed dose equivalent limit for frequent exposure = 0.1 rem
    10. General public, annual effective absorbed dose equivalent limit for infrequent exposure = 0.5 rem
    11. General public, annual effective absorbed dose

equivalent limit for extremities, skin, and eye lens = 5 rem
12. Embryo-fetus, total dose equivalent for gestation = 0.5 rem
13. Embryo-fetus, dose equivalent limit per month = 0.05 rem
14. Level of negligible risk = 0.001 rem

▲ Review of the Cell

The Cell

A. Contains three main parts
  1. Cell membrane
  2. Cytoplasm
  3. Nucleus
B. Cell membrane
  1. Protects cell
  2. Holds in water and nucleus
  3. Allows water, nutrients, and waste products to pass into and out of the cell (semipermeable)
C. Cytoplasm
  1. Composed primarily of water
  2. Conducts all cellular metabolism
  3. Contains organelles
    a. Centrosomes—participate in cell division
    b. Ribosomes—synthesize protein
    c. Lysosomes—contain enzymes for intracellular digestive processes
    d. Mitochondria—produce energy
    e. Golgi apparatus—combines proteins with carbohydrates
    f. Endoplasmic reticulum—transportation system used for moving food and molecules within the cell
D. Nucleus
  1. Contains deoxyribonucleic acid (DNA, the master molecule) and the nucleolus (with RNA)
  2. DNA controls cell division
  3. DNA controls all cellular functions
E. Other cell components
  1. Proteins—15% of cell
  2. Carbohydrates—1% of cell
  3. Lipids—2% of cell
  4. Nucleic acids—1% of cell
  5. Water—80% of cell
  6. Acids, bases, salts (electrolytes)—1% of cell
F. Cellular life cycle
  1. Interphase
    a. Cell growth occurring before mitosis
    b. Consists of three phases: G_1, S, G_2
    c. G_1—pre-DNA synthesis
    d. S—DNA synthesis
    e. G_2—post-DNA synthesis, preparation for mitosis
  2. Mitosis—four stages
    a. Prophase
    b. Metaphase
    c. Anaphase
    d. Telophase—division complete, 46 chomosomes in each new somatic cell
  3. Meiosis
    a. Cell division of sperm or ovum (germ cells) that halves the number of chromosomes in each cell
    b. Sperm and ovum will unite to return the number of chromosomes in each cell of the new individual to 46

Biological Effects of Ionizing Radiation

A. As LET of radiation increases, so does biological damage
B. Relative biologic effectiveness (RBE)—ability to produce biological damage, which varies with the LET
C. The quality factor (QF) used to calculate rem is a measure of the RBE of the radiation being used
D. Ionizing radiation may change a cell's molecular structure, affecting its ability to function properly
E. Somatic cell exposure may result in a disruption in the ability of the organism to function
F. Reproductive (germ) cell exposure may result in changes called mutations to be passed on to the next generation
G. Basically, radiation striking a cell will deposit energy in either the DNA (direct effect) or water in the cytoplasm (indirect effect) if an interaction occurs
H. Most radiation passes through the body without interacting because matter is composed mainly of empty space

Direct Effect

A. Occurs when radiation transfers its energy directly to the DNA (the master molecule) or RNA
B. As these macromolecules are ionized, disruption in cell processes may occur
C. Some of this damage may be repaired
D. If sufficient damage to the DNA structure occurs, particularly to its nitrogenous bases, a mutation may result
E. Mutation—erroneous information passed to subsequent generations via cell division
F. Results of the direct effect:
  1. No effect—most common result of LET
  2. Disruption of chemical bonds causing alteration of structure and function of the cell
  3. Cell death
  4. Cell line death—the tissues or organs that would have been produced from continued cell division had the cell survived; particularly significant if it results in the failure of a major organ or system to develop
  5. Faulty information passed on in the next cell division—possible results include: mutations, cancers, abnormal formations

Indirect Effect

A. Because water is the largest constituent of the cell, the probability that it will be struck by radiation is greater

B. Radiolysis of water—radiation depositing its energy in the water of the cell

C. The result of radiolysis is an ion pair in the cell: a positively charged water molecule (HOH^+) and a free electron

D. Several possibilities exist for chemical reactions at this point, most of them creating further instability in the cell

E. Should the two recombine, no damage occurs

F. Positive and negative water molecules may be formed and then break into smaller molecules including free radicals

G. Free radicals—highly reactive ions which have an unpaired electron in the outer shell

H. Free radicals may cause biological damage by transferring their excess energy to surrounding molecules or by disrupting chemical reactions

I. Some free radicals may chemically combine to form hydrogen peroxide

J. Hydrogen peroxide is a poison that will cause further damage to the cell

K. The DNA in the cell may be affected by the free radicals or the hydrogen peroxide

L. Such action is called indirect, because the DNA itself was not struck by the radiation

M. Indirect effect results from ionization or excitation of water molecules

N. Results of the indirect effect:
1. No effect—most common response
2. Formation of free radicals
3. Formation of hydrogen peroxide (H_2O_2)

O. Most damage to the body occurs as a result of the indirect effect, because most of the body is water and free radicals are readily mobile in water

Target Theory

A. Each cell has a master molecule that directs cell activities

B. Research indicates that DNA is the master molecule

C. If the DNA is the target of radiation damage and is inactivated, the cell will die

D. DNA may be inactivated by either direct or indirect effects

E. All photon-cell interactions occur by chance

F. It cannot be determined if a given cell death was a result of direct or indirect effect

Radiosensitivity of Cells

A. Law of Bergonié and Tribondeau
1. States that cells are most sensitive to radiation when they are immature, undifferentiated, and rapidly dividing

B. If cells are more oxygenated, they are more sensitive to radiation damage (known as *oxygen enhancement ratio*)

C. As cells mature and become specialized, they are less sensitive

D. Blood cells—whole body dose of 25 rads depresses blood count
1. Results from irradiation of bone marrow
2. Lymphocytes are the most radiosensitive blood cells in the body
3. Stem cells in bone marrow are especially radiosensitive

E. Epithelial tissue—highly radiosensitive, rapidly dividing, lines body tissue

F. Muscle—relatively insensitive because of high specialization and lack of cell division

G. Adult nerve tissue—requires very high doses (beyond medical levels) to cause damage; very specialized, lack of cell division, relatively insensitive to radiation

H. Reproductive cells:
1. Immature sperm cells—very radiosensitive, rapidly dividing, unspecialized, need 10 rads or more (which is beyond most commonly used diagnostic levels) to increase chances of mutation
2. Ova in female fetus and child are very radiosensitive
3. Ova radiosensitivity decreases until near middle age, then increases again

Somatic Effects of Radiation

A. Somatic effects are evident in the organism being exposed

B. Such doses are far beyond the levels of radiation used in diagnostic radiography

C. Caused when a large dose of high-LET radiation is received by a large area of the body

D. Examples of early somatic effects of radiation are:
1. Hematopoietic syndrome—decreases total number of all blood cells; can result in death
2. Gastrointestinal syndrome—causes total disruption of GI tract structure and function, can result in death
3. Central nervous system syndrome—causes complete failure of nervous system and results in death

E. Examples of late somatic effects are:
1. Carcinogenesis—causes cancer
2. Cataractogenesis—causes cataracts to form, follows a nonlinear-threshold dose-response curve
3. Embryological effects—most sensitive during the first trimester of gestation
4. Thyroid is a very radiosensitive organ
5. Life span shortening—not present in modern radiation workers

Genetic Effects of Radiation

A. Caused by damage to DNA molecule, which is passed to the next generation
B. Follows a linear-nonthreshold dose-response curve; no such thing as a safe gonadal dose; any exposure can represent a genetic threat
C. Usually causes recessive mutations, so generally not manifested in the population
D. Doubling dose—amount of radiation that causes the number of mutations in a population to double (for humans, approximately 50 to 250 rads)
E. Genetic mutations will not cause defects that are not already present in the human race from other causes; that is, no defects are unique to radiation exposure

▲ *Patient Exposure and Protection*

The heart of radiation protection for the patient lies in the concept of ALARA—"As Low As Reasonably Achievable." It is primarily the radiographer's responsibility to see that ALARA is in practice so that patients are properly protected. Taking adequate histories, communicating clearly, using proper immobilization, and conducting radiographic and fluoroscopic examinations in a calm, professional manner add to the safety patients will experience while under your care. This section reviews the many technical aspects of the radiographer's practice that contribute to ALARA for the patient.

Beam Limitation

Beam limitation protects the patient by limiting the area of the body and the volume of tissue being irradiated.

A. Collimator
  1. Variable aperture device
  2. Contains two sets of lead shutters placed at right angles to one another
  3. Higher set of lead shutters is placed near the x-ray tube window to absorb off-stem (off-focus) radiation
  4. Lower set of lead shutters is placed near the bottom of the collimator box to further restrict the beam as it exits
  5. Accuracy of the collimator is subject to strict quality control standards (described in Chapter 3)
  6. Collimation should be no larger than the size of the image receptor being used
  7. Collimators that automatically restrict the beam to the size of the cassette have a feature called *positive beam limitation (PBL)*, also called *automatic collimation*
  8. PBL responds when a cassette is placed in the tray containing sensors that measure its size

B. Cylinder cones
  1. Metal cylinders that attach to the bottom of the collimator
  2. Used to tightly restrict the beam to a small circle
  3. Diameter of the far end of the cone determines field size
  4. Cones may be extended an additional 10 to 12 inches by a telescoping action for even tighter restriction of the beam
  5. Cones may be used for exams of the os calcis, various skull projections, and cone-down views of vertebral bodies
  6. Use of cones results in a restriction of the x-ray beam by cutting out a major portion of the beam
  7. mAs must always be increased when using cones to make up for the rays attenuated by the cone
  8. Cylinder cones do NOT work by focusing the x-ray beam down the cone; x rays cannot be focused

C. Aperture diaphragm
  1. A flat piece of lead with a circle or square opening in the middle
  2. Placed as near the x-ray tube window as possible
  3. Has no moving parts

Filtration

A filter is placed in the x-ray beam to remove long wavelength (low-energy) x rays. Low-energy x rays contribute nothing to the diagnostic image but increase patient dose through the photoelectric effect. As low-energy rays are removed, the beam becomes "harder" (predominantly short wavelength, high energy).

A. Two types of filtration—inherent and added
B. Inherent filtration
  1. Glass envelope of the x-ray tube
  2. Insulating oil around the tube
C. Added filtration
  1. Aluminum sheets placed in the path of the beam near the x-ray tube window
D. Total filtration
  1. Equals inherent plus added filtration
  2. Must equal 2.5 mm aluminum equivalent for x-ray tubes operating above 70 kVp
E. Half-value layer—amount of filtration that reduces the intensity of the x-ray beam to one-half its original value
  1. Measured, at least annually, by a qualified radiation physicist
F. Filtration is never adjusted by the radiographer
  1. If it is suspected that the filtration has been altered, the x-ray tube must not be used until checked by a radiation physicist

Gonadal Shields

Gonadal shields are used to protect male and female gonads from unnecessary radiation exposure. They should be used whenever they will not obstruct the area of clinical interest.

A. Gonadal shielding may reduce female gonad dose by up to 50%
B. Gonadal shielding may reduce male gonad dose by up to 95%
C. Proper collimation may also greatly reduce gonadal dose and should be used in conjunction with gonadal shields
D. Most commonly used gonadal shields
  1. Flat contact shield—flat piece of lead or a lead apron placed over the gonads
  2. Shadow shield—suspended from the x-ray tube housing and placed in the x-ray beam light field; requires no contact with the patient; especially useful during procedures requiring sterile technique

Exposure Factors

Exposure technique determines the quantity and quality of x-rays striking the patient.

A. Use optimum kVp for the part being radiographed
B. Use the lowest possible mAs to reduce the amount of radiation striking the patient
C. Part being radiographed should be measured using calipers
D. A reliable technique chart should be consulted in order to determine the proper exposure factors to use
E. Use of automatic exposure controls (AEC) reduces the number of repeat radiographs

Film-Screen Combinations

Faster film-screen combinations reduce patient dose by allowing for the use of fewer x-ray photons (lower mAs) to produce a diagnostic image. The efficient conversion of x-ray energy to light energy through the intensifying screens provides the same information with far less radiation exposure to the patient.

A. Use fastest practical film-screen combination for imaging a particular body part
B. Take into account region of the body being irradiated, age of the patient, and the requirements for recorded detail

Processing

The automatic processor should be a constant in the production of a visible radiographic image. Elimination of repeat films because of optimum processor performance reduces the dose to the patient and the radiographer.

A. Subject to strict quality control standards to eliminate retakes caused by processor malfunction (described in Chapter 3)
B. Exercise care in loading and unloading cassettes
C. Prevent unnecessary exposure of film to safelight

Grids

A. Result in an increase in patient dose because increased mAs required
B. May result in lower overall patient dose by eliminating retakes caused by poor radiographic contrast
C. Use appropriate type and ratio of grid for part being radiographed and exam being performed

Repeat Radiographs

A. Always result in an increase in radiation dose to the patient
B. Must be kept to a minimum
C. Should be tracked via a departmental discard film analysis
D. Reasons for repeat films should be documented
E. In-service education for areas of frequent repeat films should be conducted by qualified radiographers or radiologists

Technical Standards for Patient Protection

A. Minimum source-to-skin distance for portable radiography—at least 12 inches
B. Fluoroscopy
  1. Use of intermittent fluoroscopy (as opposed to a constant beam-on condition)
  2. Tight collimation of the beam
  3. High kVp
  4. Source-to-tabletop distance for fixed fluoroscopes—not less than 15 inches
  5. Source-to-tabletop distance for portable fluoroscopes—not less than 12 inches, 15 inches preferred
  6. Proper filtration of the beam
  7. Fluoro timer that sounds alarm after 5 minutes (300 seconds) of beam-on time
  8. Fluoro timer should NOT be reset before alarm goes off; fluoroscopist must be made aware of length of time of exposure to patient and those in the room
  9. Limit dose at the tabletop to no more than 10 R per minute

Other Factors Relating to Patient Dose

A. Measuring patient dose
1. Skin entrance dose
2. Mean marrow dose (MMD)—average dose to active bone marrow; indicator of somatic effects on population
B. Genetically significant dose (GSD)—radiation dose which, if received by the entire population, would cause the same genetic injury as the total of doses received by the members actually being exposed; the average gonadal dose to the childbearing age population
C. Pediatrics—children need to be carefully protected from unnecessary exposure; high-speed film-screen combinations should be used along with adequate immobilization
D. Pregnant patients
1. Consideration of the 10-day rule—abdominal radiographic examinations should be performed during the first 10 days following the onset of menstruation
2. 10-day rule is based on the probability that most females are not pregnant during that time
3. The position of the American College of Radiology is that such exams should be carried out any time they are clinically indicated
4. Radiation doses to the embryo-fetus below 15 to 20 rads are considered low risk

▲ *Radiation Worker Exposure and Protection*

The ALARA concept applies to radiographers as well as to the general public. Many of the steps taken to reduce the dose to the patient will also reduce the dose to the radiographer. However, additional steps may be taken to further protect the radiation worker. Agency standards also apply to the equipment used by radiographers. This section reviews practices and standards used to protect occupationally exposed individuals. As you study the factors involved in protecting the radiation worker, reexamine the annual effective absorbed dose equivalent limits covered previously.

Cardinal Principles of Radiation Protection

A. Time—amount of exposure is directly proportional to the duration of exposure
B. Distance—the most effective protection from ionizing radiation
1. Dose is governed by the inverse square law
2. The greater the distance from the radiation, the lower the dose
3. Dose decreases inversely according to the square of the distance

4. Example: if the dose of radiation is 5 R at a distance of 3 feet, by stepping back to a distance of 6 feet the dose will drop to 1.25 R
5. Inverse square law should always be used during fluoroscopy when close contact with the patient is not required and during mobile radiography and fluoroscopy
C. Shielding—lead-equivalent shielding will absorb most of the energy of the scatter radiation striking it
1. A lead apron of at least 0.5 mm lead equivalent should be worn when being exposed to scatter radiation; use of a thyroid shield of at least 0.50 mm lead equivalent should be used for fluoroscopy
2. The radiographer must NEVER be exposed to the primary beam
3. If radiographer exposure to the primary beam is unavoidable, then the exam should not be performed
4. Family, nonradiology employees, or radiology personnel not routinely exposed should be the first choices to assist with immobilization of the patient for an exam, only after all other types of immobilization have proven inadequate
5. The radiographer should be the last person chosen to assist with immobilization during an exposure
6. Radiographers and student radiographers should not be viewed as quick and easy-to-use immobilization devices

Radiographer's Source of Radiation Exposure

A. Radiographer's source of radiation exposure is scatter radiation produced by Compton's interactions in the patient
B. Radiographer's greatest exposure occurs during fluoroscopy, portable radiography, and surgical radiography
C. Photons lose considerable energy after scattering
D. Scattered beam intensity is about $1/1000$ the intensity of the primary beam at a 90-degree angle and a distance of 1 meter away from the patient
E. Beam collimation helps to reduce the incidence of Compton's interactions resulting in decreased scatter from the patient
F. The use of high-speed image receptors may reduce further the amount of scatter produced

Structural Protective Barriers

A. Primary protective barriers
1. Consist of $1/16$ inch lead equivalent
2. Located where the primary beam may strike the wall or floor
3. If in the wall, extends from the floor to a height of 7 feet
B. Secondary protective barriers
1. Consist of $1/32$ inch lead equivalent

2. Extends from where primary protective barrier ends to the ceiling with ½ inch overlap
3. Located wherever leakage or scatter radiation may strike
4. X-ray control booth is also a secondary protective barrier
   a. Exposure switch must have cord short enough so that the radiographer has to be behind the secondary protective barrier to operate the switch
5. Lead window by control booth is usually 1.5 mm lead equivalent
C. Determinants of barrier thickness
   1. Distance—between the source of radiation and the barrier
   2. Occupancy—who occupies a given area
      a. Uncontrolled area—general public areas such as waiting rooms and stairways; shielded to keep exposure under the annual effective absorbed dose equivalent limit for infrequent exposure of 0.5 rem
      b. Controlled area—occupied by persons trained in radiation safety and wearing personnel monitoring devices; shielded to keep exposure under the annual effective absorbed dose equivalent limit of 5 rem
   3. Workload—measured in mA minutes per week (mA min/wk); takes into account the volume and types of exams performed in the room
   4. Use factor—amount of time the beam is on and directed at a particular barrier

X-ray Tube Housing

A. X rays may leak through the housing during an exposure
B. The patient and all others present in the room must be protected from excess leakage radiation
C. Leakage radiation may not exceed 100 mR per hour at a distance of 1 meter from the housing

Fluoroscopic Equipment

A. Exposure switch—must be dead-man type
B. Protective curtain—minimum 0.25 mm lead equivalent
C. Bucky slot shield—minimum 0.25 mm lead equivalent
D. Five-minute timer

Portable Radiographic Equipment and Procedure

A. Exposure switch must be on a cord at least 6 feet long
B. Lead aprons should be worn if mobile barriers are unavailable
C. Least scatter is at a 90-degree angle from the patient
D. Apply the inverse square law to reduce dose by using exposure cord at full length
E. Radiographer should NEVER hold the cassette in place for a portable exam, risking exposure to the primary beam

F. Commercial cassette holders, pillows, sponges, etc. should be used to hold the cassette in place

▲ Monitoring Radiation Exposure

Monitoring Personnel Exposure

A. Film badges
   1. Consist of plastic case, film, and filters
   2. Plastic case holds film and filters and provides a clip for attaching to clothing
   3. Film used is similar to dental x-ray film and measures doses as low as 10 mrem
   4. Film is sensitive to extremes in temperature and humidity
   5. Filters made of aluminum and copper measure intensity of radiation striking the film badge
   6. Film badges are usually developed monthly with readings returned to the institution via a film badge report
   7. Film badge report indicates wearer's name, ID number, and radiation dose (expressed in millirem for deep and shallow doses)
   8. Badge reading of "M" indicates exposure below film's sensitivity
B. Thermoluminescent dosimeters (TLD)
   1. Use lithium fluoride crystals instead of film to record dose
   2. Crystals' electrons are excited by radiation exposure and release this energy upon heating
   3. Energy released is visible light, which is measured by a photomultiplier tube
   4. Light is in direct proportion to the amount of radiation received
   5. TLDs are used mainly in ring badges worn by nuclear medicine technologists
   6. Sensitive to exposures as low as 5 mrem
   7. Relatively unaffected by temperature and humidity
   8. Can be worn for longer periods of time than film badges
   9. TLDs and equipment used to read them are expensive
C. Pocket ionization chambers
   1. Small cylinder, a few inches long, containing gas
   2. Gas is ionized by radiation striking it
   3. Small scale, reading from 0 to 200 mR, contained inside
   4. After exposure, chamber is held up to the light and viewed through one end
   5. Exposure scale may be seen indicating exposure
   6. Limited to 200 mR, so dose above that level cannot be ascertained
   7. Must be reset to zero on a special charging device after each use
   8. Very expensive device, susceptible to breakage if dropped
   9. Not routinely used for personnel monitoring

Monitoring Area Exposure

A. Cutie pie meter (ionization chamber)
   1. Used to measure radiation in an area, such as a fluoroscopic room, storage areas for radioisotopes, doses traveling through barriers, and patients who have radioactive sources within them
   2. Not used to monitor short exposure times
   3. Measures exposure rates as low as 1 mR per hour
   4. Operates on principle similar to pocket ionization chamber, with internal gas being ionized when struck by radiation
B. Geiger-Mueller detector
   1. Used to detect radioactive particles in nuclear medicine facilities
   2. Sounds audible alarm when struck by radiation, with sound increasing as radiation becomes more intense
   3. Meter reads in counts per minute

▲ *Review Questions*

Read the following paragraph. Determine the accuracy of each underlined word or phrase. Then refer to items 1–8 below the paragraph and choose the one statement that best corrects and completes it.

Background Radiation

Humans' exposure to ionizing radiation comes from two sources, natural background and artificial radiation. Natural background radiation represents (1) 18% to 20% of this exposure. It includes cosmic radiation from space, exposure from radioactive minerals, and the human body itself. Of these, the greatest source is (2) cosmic radiation. (3) Cosmic radiation tends to concentrate over land masses and in low-lying areas. Of recent discovery, but (4) in extremely low doses, is exposure to radon gas. (5) Also included in this category are gamma rays, which are naturally occurring in radioisotopes that are used in nuclear medicine procedures. Artificial sources of radiation include (6) fallout from nuclear weapons testing, consumer products, and medical and dental procedures not included in natural background radiation. Exposure to artificial background radiation constitutes the other (7) 80% to 82% of humans' exposure. Most exposure to artificial radiation comes from (8) fallout from the nuclear bombings in World War II which remains in the upper atmosphere.

1.
   a. The underlined word or phrase is accurate as written
   b. 20% to 25%
   c. 82%
   d. 92%
   e. 8%

2.
   a. The underlined word or phrase is accurate as written
   b. Radon gas
   c. Radioactive materials
   d. The body itself
   e. All of the above are equal in dose

3.
   a. The underlined word or phrase is accurate as written
   b. Cosmic radiation is present only in space
   c. Cosmic radiation is a source of exposure only to those who lie in the sun
   d. Cosmic radiation is greater at higher altitudes
   e. Cosmic radiation is greater at higher altitudes because of a thinner atmospheric shield

4.
   a. The underlined word or phrase is accurate as written
   b. In extremely high doses
   c. In doses proportional to other sources
   d. Exposure to radon gas is the greatest source of natural background radiation, 55% percent of annual background dose
   e. Radon gas is only present in homes in the mountains

5.
   a. The underlined word or phrase is accurate as written
   b. False; gamma rays are not used in nuclear medicine procedures
   c. False; gamma rays used in nuclear medicine procedures are part of artificial background radiation
   d. Statement should also include natural x rays
   e. None of the above

6.
   a. The underlined word or phrase is accurate as written
   b. d and e
   c. Should also include microwave ovens
   d. There are no medical or dental procedures included in natural background radiation
   e. Nuclear weapons testing fallout, consumer products, and medical and dental procedures

7.
   a. The underlined word or phrase is accurate as written
   b. 18 %
   c. 8 %
   d. 75 %
   e. 92 %

8.
   a. The underlined word or phrase is accurate as written
   b. Microwave ovens
   c. Smoke alarms
   d. Color television sets
   e. Medical and dental procedures using ionizing radiation

Use the listing below to answer questions 9–22. Items may be used more than once. Choose the one best answer for each question.

A. Photoelectric interaction
B. Compton's interaction
C. Coherent scatter
D. Pair production
E. Primary radiation; exit radiation

9. Occurs above 1.02 million electron volts

10. Also called *incoherent scattering*

11. Radiation coming from the anode; radiation exiting the patient

12. Photon-tissue interaction that never occurs in diagnostic radiography

13. Responsible for producing contrast on the radiograph

14. Produces scatter radiation that exits the patient and may fog the radiograph

15. Produces scatter energy as a result of vibration of orbital electrons

16. Radiation striking the patient; image-forming radiation

17. Results in total absorption of incident photon

18. Only photon-tissue interaction that does not result in ionization

19. Only photon-tissue interaction that involves an incident photon and atomic nucleus

20. Photon-tissue interaction that primarily involves *K*-shell electrons

21. Photon-tissue interaction that primarily involves loosely bound outer-shell electrons

22. Results in the production of a photoelectron that is ejected from the atom

For questions 23–25 regarding radiation units, determine whether or not the statement is correct or complete. If incorrect, choose the answer that best corrects it. If incomplete, choose the answer that provides a more complete and accurate description. If accurate as written, choose "a."

23. The unit of absorbed dose is the rad

a. This statement is correct, complete, and accurate as written; no choices below correct or complete it
b. The unit of absorbed dose is the rad, which equals rem × a quality factor
c. The unit of absorbed dose is the rad, which is the amount of energy absorbed by an object
d. The unit of absorbed dose is the rad, which equals 100 ergs of energy deposited per gram of tissue; the SI unit of absorbed dose is the gray
e. The unit of absorbed dose is the rad, which equals 100 ergs of energy deposited per gram of tissue

24. The unit of radiation exposure in air is the roentgen; this unit in the SI system is the coulomb/kilogram

a. This statement is correct, complete, and accurate as written; no choices below correct or complete it
b. The unit of radiation exposure in air is the roentgen; this unit in the SI system is the coulomb/kilogram; the roentgen is equal to 2.58×10^{-4} coulombs per kilogram
c. The unit of radiation exposure in air is the roentgen; this unit in the SI system is the coulomb/kilogram; the roentgen is equal to 2.58×10^{-4} coulombs per kilogram; it measures positive and negative charges produced in air
d. The unit of radiation exposure in air is the roentgen; this unit in the SI system is the coulomb/kilogram; the roentgen is equal to 2.58×10^{-4} coulombs per kilogram; it measures positive and negative charges produced in air; the roentgen measures the amount of radiation received by the patient during fluoroscopy and is reported on film badge reports

25. The unit of dose equivalency is the rem; it is calculated using the equation: rads times quality factor; the SI unit of absorbed dose equivalent is the sievert

    a. This statement is correct, complete, and accurate as written; no choices below correct or complete it
    b. The unit of dose equivalency is the rem; it is calculated using the equation: rads times quality factor; the SI unit of absorbed dose equivalent is the sievert; the rem takes into account different biological effects caused by various sources of radiation; the rem is the unit reported on film badge reports
    c. The unit of dose equivalency is the rem; it is calculated using the equation: rads times quality factor; the SI unit of absorbed dose equivalent is the sievert; the rem takes into account different biological effects caused by various sources of radiation
    d. The unit of dose equivalency is the rem; it is calculated using the equation: rads times quality factor; the SI unit of absorbed dose equivalent is the sievert; the rem is the unit reported on film badge reports

For each of the following questions, choose the single best answer.

26. The amount of energy deposited by radiation per unit length of tissue being traversed is:

    a. LET, which determines the use of a QF when calculating the absorbed dose equivalent
    b. Linear energy transfer
    c. Higher for wave radiations than for particulate radiations
    d. LET, which is expressed as a QF when calculating absorbed dose

27. The agency that publishes radiation protection standards based on scientific research is the:

    a. Nuclear Regulatory Commission (NRC)
    b. International Commission on Radiation Protection (ICRP)
    c. National Council on Radiation Protection and Measurements (NCRP)
    d. Bureau of Radiological Health (BRH)
    e. None of the above

28. The agency that enforces radiation protection standards at the federal level is the:

    a. Nuclear Regulatory Commission (NRC)
    b. International Commission on Radiation Protection (ICRP)
    c. National Council on Radiation Protection and Measurements (NCRP)
    d. Bureau of Radiological Health (BRH)
    e. None of the above

29. Effective absorbed dose equivalent limit is defined as:

    a. The upper boundary dose that can be absorbed annually that carries a negligible risk of somatic or genetic damage to the individual
    b. The upper boundary dose that can be absorbed, either in a single exposure or annually, that carries no risk of damage to the individual
    c. The upper boundary dose that can be absorbed, either in a single exposure or annually, that carries no risk of somatic or genetic damage to the individual
    d. The upper boundary dose that can be absorbed, either in a single exposure or annually, that carries a negligible risk of somatic or genetic damage to the individual

30. ALARA is an acronym for:

    a. "As Long As Reasonably Achievable"
    b. "As Little As Reasonably Achievable"
    c. "As Long As Radiologist Allows"
    d. A radiation protection concept which encourages radiation users to keep the dose to the patient "As Low As Reasonably Achievable"

Use the listing below to answer questions 31–36. Items may be used more than once.

    A. Nonlinear-nonthreshold effect
    B. Linear-nonthreshold effect
    C. Linear-threshold effect
    D. Nonlinear-threshold effect
    E. Dose-response curves

31. Graphs that show the relationship between dose of radiation received and incidence of effects

32. Basis for all radiation protection standards

33. No safe level of radiation and the response to the radiation is not directly proportional to the dose received

34. No safe level of radiation and the response to the radiation is directly proportional to the dose received

35. There is a safe level of radiation for certain effects; those effects are directly proportional to the dose received when the safe level is exceeded

36. There is a safe level of radiation for certain effects; those effects are not directly proportional to the dose received when the safe level is exceeded

For each of the following questions, choose the single best answer.

37. Effects of radiation that occur randomly, where the probability of such effects is proportional to the dose received are called:

    a. Dose-response curves
    b. Stochastic effects
    c. Genetic effects
    d. Somatic effects
    e. Nonstochastic effects

38. Effects of radiation which, once the threshold dose is exceeded, become more severe at higher levels of exposure are called:

    a. Dose-response curves
    b. Stochastic effects
    c. Genetic effects
    d. Somatic effects
    e. Nonstochastic effects

Use the listing below to answer questions 39–46. Items may be used more than once.

    A. 5 rem
    B. 0.1 rem
    C. 0.5 rem
    D. 0.05 rem
    E. 1 rem

39. Embryo-fetus dose equivalent limit per month

40. Occupational cumulative exposure = age in years multiplied by this dose

41. Annual occupational effective absorbed dose equivalent limit for stochastic effects

42. Annual effective absorbed dose equivalent limit for students age 18 or below

43. Annual effective absorbed dose equivalent limit for general public, infrequent exposure

44. Embryo-fetus dose equivalent limit for gestation

45. Annual effective absorbed dose equivalent limit for general public, frequent exposure

46. Annual effective absorbed dose equivalent limit for general public for extremities, skin, and lens of eye

For each of the following questions, choose the single best answer.

47. The quality factor used in calculating rem takes into account:

    a. Duration of exposure
    b. Source of exposure
    c. LET
    d. Dose
    e. b and c

48. LET and biological damage are:

    a. Directly proportional
    b. Indirectly proportional
    c. Inversely proportional
    d. Unrelated

49. The ability of different types of radiation to produce the same biological response in an organism is called:

    a. LET
    b. QF
    c. RBE
    d. Doubling dose
    e. Mutant dose

50. The phases of the cellular life cycle, in order, are:

    a. Prophase, metaphase, anaphase, telophase
    b. Interphase, prophase, metaphase, anaphase, telophase
    c. G_1, S, G_2, telophase
    d. Interphase (G_1, S, G_2), prophase, metaphase, anaphase, telophase
    e. Interphase (G_1, G_2, S), prophase, metaphase, anaphase, telophase

51. The process of cell division for germ cells is called:

    a. Mitosis
    b. Spermatogenesis
    c. Organogenesis
    d. Cytogenesis
    e. Meiosis

Use the listing below to answer questions 52–60. Items may be used more than once.

    A. Indirect effect
    B. Target theory
    C. Direct effect
    D. Doubling dose
    E. Mutations

52. Occurs when radiation transfers its energy to DNA

53. States each cell has a master molecule that directs all cellular activities and which, if inactivated, will result in cellular death

54. Amount of radiation required to increase number of mutations in a population by a factor of two

55. Occurs when radiation transfers its energy to the cellular cytoplasm

56. Induces radiolysis

57. Changes in genetic code passed on to next generation

58. Responsible for producing free radicals

59. Occurs when master molecule is struck by radiation

60. Poisons the cell with H_2O_2

For the following question, choose the single best answer.

61. Most of the damage to a cell occurs as a result of:

    a. Direct effect
    b. Mutations
    c. Law of Bergonié and Tribondeau
    d. Indirect effect
    e. None of the above is primarily responsible for damage

Read the following paragraph. Determine the accuracy of each underlined word or phrase. Then refer to questions 62–68 below the paragraph and choose the one statement that best corrects and completes it.

Cell Radiosensitivity

Cell radiosensitivity is described by the (62) Law of Bergonié and Tribondeau, (63) which states that cells are most sensitive to radiation when they are specialized and rapidly dividing. Further, it is believed that (64) cells are more radiosensitive when fully oxygenated.(65) Blood count can be depressed with a whole body dose of 25 rem, which is a result of irradiation of the bone marrow. However, (66) the most radiosensitive cells in the body are lymphocytes. Other highly radiosensitive cells are (67) epithelial cells, nerve cells, sperm, and muscle cells. Less radiosensitive are (68) ova in women of reproductive age.

62.
  a. The underlined word or phrase is accurate as written
  b. There is no law used by these scientists
  c. Bergonié and Tribondeau described dose-response relationships
  d. This law is really just a hypothesis

63.
  a. The underlined word or phrase is accurate as written
  b. False; cells are equally radiosensitive at all times
  c. False; cells are most sensitive to radiation when they are nonspecialized, immature, and dividing rapidly
  d. False; cells are most radiosensitive when they are specialized, mature, and rapidly dividing

64.
  a. The underlined word or phrase is accurate as written
  b. False; cells are most radiosensitive when least oxygenated, such as when the patient has cancer
  c. False; cells are equally radiosensitive regardless of state of oxygenation
  d. False; cells are most radiosensitive when in a state of high concentration of CO_2

65.
  a. The underlined word or phrase is accurate as written
  b. False; whole body dose required is at least 125 rem
  c. False; dose does not need to be whole body
  d. False; absorbed dose is expressed in rads

66.
  a. The underlined word or phrase is accurate as written
  b. False; the most radiosensitive cells are sperm
  c. False; the most radiosensitive cells are ova
  d. False; the most radiosensitive cells are epithelial cells
  e. False; the most radiosensitive cells are red and white blood cells

67.
  a. The underlined word or phrase is accurate as written
  b. False; nerve cells and muscle cells are relatively insensitive
  c. False; epithelial cells and sperm are relatively insensitive, especially in adults
  d. False; all cells listed are relatively insensitive to radiation effects

68.
  a. The underlined word or phrase is accurate as written
  b. False; this is why gonadal shielding must be used whenever possible
  c. False; this is why the 10-day rule must be followed, as recommended by the ACR
  d. False; this is a common misconception

Read the following paragraph. Determine the accuracy of each underlined word or phrase. Then refer to questions 69–71 below the paragraph and choose the one statement that best corrects and completes it.

Somatic and Genetic Effects of Radiation

Most somatic effects occur at (69) <u>doses delivered during diagnostic radiography</u>. Somatic effects manifest themselves (70) <u>in the person who has been irradiated</u>. Examples of early somatic effects are gastrointestinal syndrome, CNS syndrome, and hematopoietic syndrome. Examples of late somatic effects are (71) <u>carcinogenesis, genetic effects, embryological effects, and life span shortening</u>.

69.
    a. The underlined word or phrase is accurate as written
    b. True; this is the basis for radiation protection standards; this is a more complete answer than choice "a"
    c. False; most somatic effects occur at doses far beyond diagnostic levels
    d. False; all somatic effects occur during radiation therapy, which is what makes it so effective

70.
    a. The underlined word or phrase is accurate as written
    b. False; because the gonads are also irradiated, these effects are also manifested in the next generation
    c. False; genetic effects are manifested in the person irradiated, if it is a child
    d. False; both somatic and genetic effects are manifested in the person being irradiated; this is the basis for the formation of mutations

71.
    a. The underlined word or phrase is accurate as written
    b. False; genetic effects are considered early somatic effects
    c. False; these are all the result of genetic effects because the genes in the cells have been irradiated causing the effect
    d. False; genetic effects are not considered somatic effects

For each of the following questions, choose the single best answer.

72. Methods of limiting the area of the patient being irradiated include the use of:

    a. Cylinder cones
    b. Aperture diaphragms
    c. Collimators
    d. Gonadal shields
    e. All of the above

73. Which of the following statements concerning gonadal shields is (are) accurate?

    a. Gonadal shields should be used on all patients
    b. Gonadal shields may reduce male gonad dose by up to 50%
    c. Gonadal shields may reduce female gonad dose by up to 95%
    d. All of the above
    e. None of the above

74. Which of the following sets of exposure factors would result in the lowest dose to the patient?

    a. High mAs, low kVp, 400 speed film-screen combination
    b. Low mAs, high kVp, 400 speed film-screen combination
    c. Low mAs, high kVp, small focal spot, 100 speed filmscreen combination
    d. Low mAs, high kVp, large focal spot, 100 speed filmscreen combination
    e. Low mAs, high kVp, small focal spot, 50 speed filmscreen combination

75. Which of the following are used as part of an effort to observe the ALARA concept?

    a. More than one but not all of the below
    b. Collimation
    c. High speed film-screen combinations
    d. Grids
    e. b, c, and d

76. The cardinal rules of radiation protection include:

    a. Collimation, gonadal shielding, no repeats
    b. Collimation, short exposure time, no repeats
    c. Shielding, distance, time
    d. Time, distance, collimation
    e. ALARA, ACR, NCRP

Use the listing below to answer questions 77–85. Items may be used more than once.

A. TLD
B. Film badge
C. Pocket ionization chamber
D. Cutie pie monitor
E. Geiger-Mueller detector

77. Used to survey an area for radiation detection and measurement

78. Accurate as low as 10 mrem

79. Includes filters for measurement of radiation energy

80. Measures in-air exposures from 0 to 200 mR

81. Detection device that sounds alarm to indicate presence of radioactivity

82. Accurate as low as 5 mrem

83. Must be reset for each use

84. May be used up to three months at a time

85. Sensitive to extremes in environment

For each of the following questions, choose the single best answer.

86. An indicator of somatic effects to the population as a whole which is the average dose to active bone marrow is called:

  a. GSD
  b. ALARA
  c. MMD
  d. MPD
  e. None of the above

87. The radiation dose that would cause the same genetic injury to the population as the sum of doses received by individuals actually being exposed is called:

  a. GSD
  b. ALARA
  c. MMD
  d. MPD
  e. None of the above

88. The timer used in fluoroscopy:

  a. Must be 3 minutes
  b. Should always be reset before going off so as not to annoy the radiologist
  c. Sounds an alarm after 3 minutes
  d. Sounds an alarm after 5 minutes of the procedure
  e. Is used to alert the fluoroscopist after 5 minutes of fluoroscopy have elapsed

89. The most effective protection against radiation exposure for the radiographer is:

  a. Lead aprons
  b. Lead gloves
  c. Lead glasses
  d. Short exposure times
  e. Distance

90. If the dose of scatter radiation in fluoroscopy to the radiographer is 10 mR at a distance of 2 feet from the table, where should the radiographer stand to reduce the dose to 2.5 mR?

  a. 8 feet from the table
  b. 4 feet from the table
  c. At the foot of the table
  d. Directly behind the fluoroscopist
  e. 1 foot from the table

91. Lead aprons used in fluoroscopy must be at least:

  a. 0.50 mm lead
  b. 0.25 mm lead
  c. 0.10 mm lead
  d. 0.25 mm lead equivalent
  e. 2.5 mm lead equivalent

92. Which of the following statements is true concerning the holding of patients for radiographic examinations?

  a. May be performed routinely in order to obtain a diagnostic examination
  b. Should only be done when absolutely necessary and then the holding should be done by a competent radiographer so that a repeat will not be needed
  c. Should only be done when absolutely necessary and then the holding should be done by a nonpregnant member of the patient's family
  d. May be performed using a student radiographer to hold because students are not exposed as often as staff radiographers
  e. Should only be done when absolutely necessary and then the holding should be done by a member of the patient's family

93. The factor(s) that must be considered when designing structural shielding for a radiology room or department include:

    a. Use factor
    b. Occupancy
    c. Distance
    d. Workload
    e. All of the above

94. The lowest intensity of scatter radiation from the patient is located:

    a. At the head of the table
    b. At a 90-degree angle from the patient
    c. At a 180-degree angle from the patient
    d. At the foot of the table
    e. At a 45-degree angle from the patient

95. A film badge reading of "M" means:

    a. Dose below 10 mrem has been received
    b. Maximum dose has been received
    c. Mean (average) dose has been received
    d. Much radiation has been received
    e. None of the above

96. A reading of 200 mR with a pocket ionization chamber means:

    a. 200 roentgens have been received
    b. 200 milliroentgens have been received
    c. 200 millirads have been received
    d. 2 roentgens have been received
    e. At least 200 milliroentgens have been received

97. Which of the following doses are considered low risk to the embryo-fetus?

    a. < 100 rads
    b. < 50 rads
    c. < 15 to 20 rads
    d. < 30 rads
    e. Any dose above 5 rads should be considered extremely dangerous to the embryo-fetus

98. Minimum source-to-skin distance for mobile radiography must be at least:

    a. 15 inches
    b. 12 inches
    c. 36 inches
    d. 55 inches
    e. 10 inches

99. Positive beam limitation is also known as:

    a. Use of collimators
    b. Beam limitation used for all exams
    c. Use of beam restrictors
    d. Automatic collimation
    e. Collimation

100. Filtration should be adjusted by the radiographer:

    a. To "harden" the x-ray beam
    b. To remove the soft rays from the x-ray beam
    c. To exercise radiation protection
    d. Never
    e. If it is suspected that it has been changed

Chapter 3

Review of Equipment Operation and Maintenance

Persistence prevails when all else fails.

▲ Basic Physics Terminology

Matter—has form or shape and occupies space
Mass—the amount of matter in an object; generally considered the same as weight
Energy—the ability to do work
Potential energy—the energy of position
Kinetic energy—the energy of motion
Chemical energy—energy from a chemical reaction
Electrical energy—a result of the movement of electrons
Thermal energy—heat energy resulting from the movement of atoms or molecules
Nuclear energy—energy from the nucleus of an atom
Electromagnetic energy—energy that is emitted and transferred through matter
Ionizing radiation—electromagnetic radiation that is able to remove an electron from an atom
Ionization—the removal of an electron from an atom

▲ Measurement Standards

Length—meter
Mass—kilogram
Time—second
SI system—meter, kilogram, second
MKS system—meter, kilogram, second
CGS system—centimeter, gram, second
British system—foot, pound, second
Velocity (speed)—how fast an object is moving
Acceleration—the rate of change of speed per unit of time
Work—force applied on an object over a distance
Power—the rate of doing work (the unit is the watt)

▲ Atomic Structure

Atomic nucleus—contains protons (positive charges) and neutrons (no charge); contains most of the mass of an atom
Atomic mass—number of protons plus number of neutrons; represented by the letter A
Electron shells—contain orbital electrons (negative charges); electron shells represented by the letters K, L, M, N, O, P, Q; in a stable atom, the number of electrons and protons is equal
Atomic number of an atom—equals the number of protons in the nucleus; represented by the letter Z; the atomic number determines the chemical element; all chemical elements are represented in the periodic table of the elements
Isotopes—atoms with the same number of protons but with a different number of neutrons
Electron-binding energy—force that holds electrons in orbit around the nucleus
Octet rule—the outer shell of an atom may not contain more than eight electrons
Particulate radiation—alpha particles (helium nucleus: two protons and two neutrons); beta particles (electron-like particles emitted from the nucleus of a radioactive atom)

▲ Characteristics of Electromagnetic Radiation

Photon—the smallest amount of any type of electromagnetic radiation; also considered a bundle of energy called a *quantum*; travel at the speed of light; travel in waves in a straight path
Sine waves—waves of electromagnetic radiation; sine waves have height (*amplitude*); distance between the peaks (*wavelength*); as photon wavelength decreases, photon energy increases
Frequency—number of wavelengths passing a given point per unit time; unit of frequency is the hertz (Hz)

Speed of travel—electromagnetic radiation travels at the speed of light (186,000 miles per second); travel at the speed of light is constant regardless of wavelength or frequency; wavelength and frequency of electromagnetic radiation are inversely proportional to one another

Gamma rays—electromagnetic rays produced in the nucleus of radioactive atoms; x rays and gamma rays differ only in their origin

Wave-particle duality—the concept that x-ray photons, while existing as waves, exhibit properties of particles

Attenuation—partial absorption of the energy of an x-ray beam as it traverses an object

Inverse square law—law that governs the intensity of x radiation; states that the intensity of the x-ray beam is inversely proportional to the square of the distance between the source of the x rays and the object

Law of conservation of matter—matter can neither be created nor destroyed

Law of conservation of energy—energy can neither be created nor destroyed

▲ *Principles of Electricity and Magnetism*

Electrostatics—stationary electric charges (static electricity)

Electrification—movement of electrons between objects

Laws of electrostatics—unlike charges attract; like charges repel; electrostatic charges reside on the outer surface of a conductor; concentrate at the area of greatest curvature of a conductor; only negative charges move; inverse square law

Methods of electrification—friction, contact, and induction

Conductor—material that allows the free flow of electrons

Insulator—object that prohibits the flow of electrons

Electric current—the movement of electrons along a conductor or pathway (electric circuit); unit of measurement is the ampere

Electromotive force (emf)—unit is the volt; the force with which electrons move in an electric circuit

Electrodynamics—electric charges in motion

Semiconductor—material that may act as an insulator or conductor under different conditions

Electric resistance—unit of measurement is the ohm

Ohm's law—voltage in the circuit is equal to the current times resistance

Electric circuits—path along which electrons flow; may be wired as series circuits or parallel circuits

Alternating current—electric circuit in which the current of electrons oscillates back and forth

Direct current—unidirectional flow of electrons in an electric conductor

Sine wave—representation of electron flow as alternating current

Magnetic field—energy field surrounding an electric charge in motion; can magnetize a ferromagnetic material such as iron, if the material is placed in the magnetic field

Magnetic poles—every magnet has a north pole and a south pole

Laws of magnetics—like poles repel, unlike poles attract; the force of attraction between poles is governed by the inverse square law

Electromagnetism—movement of electrons in a conductor produces a magnetic field around the conductor; a coiled conductor (i.e., a wire), through which an electric current is flowing, will have overlapping magnetic fields

Solenoid—stacks of wire coil through which electric current flows, creating overlapping force field lines; a magnetic field is concentrated through the center of the coil

Electromagnet—a solenoid with an iron core which concentrates the magnetic field

Electromagnetic induction—the process of causing an electric current to flow in a conductor when it is placed within the force field of another conductor; two types of electromagnetic induction are self-induction and mutual induction

Self-induction—opposing voltage created in a conductor by passing alternating current through it

Mutual induction—inducing current flow in a secondary coil by varying the current flow through a primary coil

Electric generator—device that converts mechanical energy to electrical energy; usual output of an electric generator is alternating current

Single-phase, two-pulse alternating current—is the simplest type of current; voltage (and accompanying current) flows as a sine wave (~); voltage begins at zero, peaks at full value at the crest of the wave, returns to zero, reverses and again peaks on the inverse portion of the cycle at the trough

Three-phase alternating current—special wiring patterns (wye, star, delta) are used to create voltage wave forms that are placed 120 degrees out of phase with one another; these voltage wave forms are called three-phase; three-phase may have six pulses per cycle or twelve pulses per cycle; three-phase, six-pulse wave forms contain 360 pulses per second; three-phase, twelve-pulse contain 720 pulses per second; high-frequency generators produce high-frequency electricity (thousands of hertz)

Electric motor—device that converts electrical to mechanical energy

Transformer—changes electric voltage and current into higher or lower values; transformer operates on the principle of mutual induction; therefore, it requires alternating current

Step-up transformer—transformer that increases voltage from the primary to the secondary coil and decreases current in the same proportion; a step-up transformer has more turns in the secondary than in the primary coil; a step-up transformer is used in the x-ray circuit to increase voltage to the kilovoltage level for x-ray production

Step-down transformer—transformer that decreases voltage from the primary to the secondary coil and increases current in the same proportion; a step-down transformer has more turns in the primary than in the secondary coil; a step-down transformer is used in the filament portion of the x-ray circuit to increase current flow to the cathode

Autotransformer—a transformer that contains an iron core and a single winding of wire; an autotransformer is used in the x-ray circuit to provide a small increase in voltage in advance of the step-up transformer; it is at the autotransformer that the kVp settings are made

Rectification—the process of changing alternating current to direct current

Line voltage compensation—x-ray circuit depends on a constant source of power; power coming into radiology department may vary; line voltage compensator keeps incoming voltage adjusted to proper value; usually operates automatically, may be manually adjusted on older equipment

▲ Conditions Necessary for the Production of X-rays

A. Source of electrons
B. Acceleration of electrons
C. Sudden stoppage of electrons against target material

Equipment Used in the Production of X-rays (Fig. 3-1)

A. Autotransformer
 1. Also known as a variable transformer
 2. Provides for the variation of voltage flowing in the x-ray circuit
 3. Single coil of wire with an iron core
 4. Source for selecting kVp
 5. Operates on the principle of self-induction
    a. The single winding of wire incorporates both the primary and secondary coils of the transformer
 6. Primary turns (primary taps) are fed 220 volts from the radiology department's incoming line
 7. Secondary turns (secondary taps) are selected by the radiographer using the kVp select control
 8. Voltage is then stepped up or stepped down by only a small amount and sent to the primary side of the high-voltage step-up transformer
 9. The high-voltage step-up transformer then boosts the voltage to the kVp that was selected

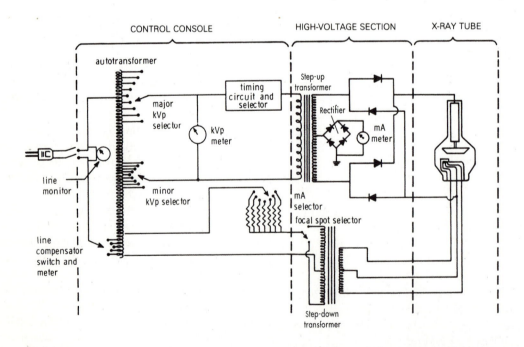

Figure 3-1 Simplified electric circuit diagram for x-ray machine. From Bushong, SC: Radiologic science for technologists: physics, biology, and protection, ed 5, St. Louis, 1993, Mosby.

B. Prereading voltmeter
  1. The voltmeter in the x-ray circuit indicates the voltage that is selected
  2. Called prereading because it indicates the kilovoltage that will be flowing through the tube once the exposure is made
  3. Placed in the circuit between the autotransformer and the high-voltage transformer
C. Timer
  1. Used to regulate the duration of the x-ray exposure
  2. Wired in the circuit between the autotransformer and the high-voltage transformer
  3. Synchronous timer
    a. Operates from a motor with a frequency of 60 Hz turning at 60 rotations per second
    b. Timer increments are in multiples of $\frac{1}{60}$ (i.e., $\frac{1}{30}$, $\frac{1}{15}$, etc.)
    c. Shortest time possible is $\frac{1}{60}$ second
  4. Impulse timer
    a. Counts voltage pulses
    b. In a 60 Hz, full-wave rectified current there are 120 pulses per second; therefore, a setting of one pulse would yield an exposure of $\frac{1}{120}$ second
  5. mAs timer
    a. Provides the safest tube current in the shortest time possible
    b. Measures total tube current
    c. Located after the secondary coil of the high-voltage transformer
  6. Electronic timer
    a. Microprocessor-controlled
    b. Contained in most radiographic equipment
    c. Allows exposure times as low as 1 millisecond (.001 second)
  7. Automatic exposure control (AEC)
    a. AEC is used to provide consistency of radiographic quality
    b. Relies on excellent positioning skills and extensive knowledge of surface and internal anatomy, because the part being radiographed must be accurately positioned over ionization sensors
    c. Consists of a flat ionization chamber which is located between the patient and the image receptor (some units use a photomultiplier tube placed behind the film that senses the brightness produced by a fluorescent screen)
    d. As radiation passes through the ionization chamber, it ionizes the gas contained inside
    e. The level of ionization is directly proportional to the density that will appear on the film
    f. When a predetermined level of ionization is reached (allowing time for a sufficient amount of radiation to pass through to strike the film), an electronic switch terminates the exposure
    g. Backup timer must be set to terminate the exposure in the event of a malfunction
    h. Backup timer protects the patient from overexposure and the x-ray tube from overheating
    i. Minimum response time—shortest time possible with an AEC because of the time it takes to operate
    j. Shortest time with an AEC is 1 millisecond (.001 second)
  8. Falling load generator
    a. Modern generator that takes advantage of extremely short time capabilities and tube heat loading potential
    b. Radiographer sets mAs and kVp
    c. Falling load generator calculates the most efficient method of obtaining the required mAs
    d. X-ray tube current starts at highest level possible for first portion of the exposure
    e. When the tube's maximum heat load has been reached for that mA, the generator drops the mA to the next lower level that the tube can handle
    f. The exposure continues at succeedingly lower levels of mA, for the shortest times possible, until the desired mAs has been reached
    g. Falling load generator always uses the shortest times possible to obtain a given mAs
    h. Disadvantages: exams where long exposure times are used (e.g., breathing techniques for lateral thoracic spine); rapid sequence exposures where heat buildup in the tube may cause exposure times to increase
D. Step-up transformer (high-voltage transformer)
  1. Consists of primary coils and secondary coils
  2. Requires alternating current to operate
  3. Primary coil receives voltage from the autotransformer
  4. Operates on principle of mutual induction
    a. Force field surrounding a wire with electricity flowing through it will induce (cause) electricity to flow in a second wire placed within the force field
  5. Voltage in the primary coil is boosted to the kilovoltage level (thousands of volts) in the secondary coil
    a. Number of turns of wire in the primary coil compared with the number of wire turns in the secondary coil is called the *turns ratio*
    b. Turns ratio determines how much the voltage is stepped up
    c. The greater the turns ratio, the higher the resulting kilovoltage
    d. Voltage is being induced in the secondary coil, which has many more wire turns compared with the number of turns in the primary coil
  6. Turns ratio may be 500 to 1000, depending on the machine
  7. Voltage is varied at the autotransformer
  8. Turns ratio in the step-up transformer is not varied

E. Rectifier
  1. X-ray tube requires direct current to operate properly
  2. Rectifier changes alternating current (AC) coming from the step-up transformer to direct current (DC)
  3. Rectifiers are solid-state semiconductor diodes
     a. Consist of silicon-based n-type and p-type semiconductors
  4. Located between the step-up transformer and the x-ray tube
  5. Unit with four diodes provides full-wave rectification for single-phase generator
     a. Full-wave rectification produces pulsating DC
     b. Resultant wave form contains two pulses per cycle (120 pulses per second)
     c. Uses both portions of rectified AC
     d. Results in 100% ripple, with voltage dropping to zero 120 times per second
     e. X-ray production ceases 120 times per second
  6. Unit with six or twelve diodes provides full-wave rectification for three-phase equipment
     a. Because three-phase current is used, voltage never drops to zero during the exposure
     b. Voltage ripple for three-phase, six-pulse is approximately 13%; therefore, the voltage actually used is about 87% of the kVp set
     c. Voltage ripple for three-phase, twelve-pulse is approximately 4%; therefore, the voltage actually used is about 96% of the kVp set
     d. Voltage ripple for high-frequency generators is approximately 1%; therefore, the voltage actually used is about 99% of the kVp set
     e. High-frequency units result in lower patient dose
     f. Three-phase, full-wave rectified wave forms produce higher average photon energy (35% higher for three-phase, six-pulse; 41% higher for three-phase, twelve-pulse)
     g. Three-phase and high-frequency units result in 12% to 16% more x rays produced than single-phase
     h. kVp values used with single-phase equipment may be decreased 12% to 16% when performing the same exam on three-phase or high-frequency equipment

F. Milliammeter (mA meter)
  1. Measures tube current in milliamperes
  2. Wired between the rectifier and x-ray tube

G. mA control (filament circuit)
  1. Regulates the number of electrons available at the filament to produce x rays
  2. Voltage is provided by tapping windings of the autotransformer and varying the voltage being sent to the step-down transformer
     a. Step-down transformer reduces voltage and increases current in response to the use of variable resistors (rheostats) manipulated by the radiographer via the mA stations on the control panel

  b. Resultant high current is sent on to heat the filament
  c. A filament ammeter may also be connected at this point

H. X-ray tube
  1. Cathode assembly—negative electrode in the x-ray tube
     a. Contains two filaments, a small and a large
     b. Filaments are made of tungsten (because of its high melting point), with a small amount of thorium added to reduce vaporization and prolong tube life
     c. Filaments are heated slightly when x-ray machine is turned on; no electrons are ejected at this low level of heating
     d. During x-ray exposure, one filament will be heated to a level whereby electrons will be "boiled off" in preparation for x-ray production (thermionic emission)
     e. Over time, filaments will vaporize and coat the inner surface of the x-ray tube with tungsten, leading to tube failure
     f. Cathode assembly also includes the focusing cup
     g. Focusing cup surrounds the filaments on three sides
     h. Focusing cup has negative charge applied, which tends to concentrate electrons boiling off the filaments into a narrower stream and repels them toward the anode
     i. Electron concentration keeps the electrons aimed at a smaller area of the anode
     j. Some x-ray tubes use the focusing cup as an electronic grid that can turn the current on and off rapidly, allowing for very short and precise exposure times such as those needed for rapid serial exposures (this is called a *grid-controlled tube*)
  2. Anode—positive electrode in the x-ray tube
     a. Consists of a metal target made of a tungsten-rhenium alloy (because of its high melting point and high atomic number) embedded in a disk (or base) of molybdenum with a motor to rotate the target
     b. Must be able to tolerate extremely high levels of heat produced during x-ray production
     c. Anode rotates from 3300 rpm to 10,000 rpm depending upon tube design
     d. Rotation is achieved by the use of an induction motor located outside of the x-ray tube, which turns a rotor located inside the x-ray tube (the target is attached at the end of the rotor)
     e. Rotation of the target allows greater heat dissipation
     f. Rotation of the target is stopped by a braking action provided by the induction motor
     g. The x-ray machine should never be shut off immediately after an exposure until the target has stopped rotating

h. Without the braking action, the target may spin for up to one-half hour, causing great strain on the bearings

i. Electrons strike the target on the focal track (sometimes called the focal spot)

j. Focal track is beveled, producing the target angle

k. The target angle allows for a larger actual focal spot (area bombarded by electrons) while producing a smaller effective focal spot (area seen by the image receptor)

l. The larger the actual focal spot, the greater heat capacity it has; the smaller the effective focal spot, the greater the sharpness of the radiographic image

m. This effect is called the *line-focus principle*

n. Target angle may be from 7 degrees to 20 degrees, depending upon tube design

o. The exposure switch should be activated in one continuous motion, activating the rotor and then the exposure button

p. The equipment allows the rotor to come up to speed before making the exposure

q. The radiographer does not control this by activating the rotor and waiting to press the exposure button

r. Activating the rotor and allowing it to operate by itself only results in unnecessary heating of the filament and wear on the induction motor, shortening tube life

3. Glass envelope with window

a. Cathode and target are contained inside the glass envelope (some models use a partial metal envelope)

b. Glass envelope also contains a vacuum, so electrons from the filament do not collide with atoms of gas

c. Tube window—thinner section of glass envelope allowing x rays to escape

4. Tube housing—encases x-ray tube

a. Made of aluminum with lead lining

b. Functions to support and protect the tube, restrict leakage radiation during exposure, and provide electrical insulation

c. Also contains oil in which the x-ray tube is immersed to assist with cooling and additional electrical insulation

▲ X-ray Production

A. Overview of the x-ray production circuit

1. The x-ray machine is turned on, a small amount of current is sent to the filament to warm it and ready it for much higher current

2. Radiographer takes equipment through warm-up exposures to further warm the filament and the anode

3. Radiographer chooses exposure factors on control console for the examination to be performed

4. Electricity coming into the radiology department is adjusted by the line voltage compensator in the x-ray equipment to maintain it at a constant level

5. When making the exposure, the radiographer presses the rotor switch and exposure switch in one continuous motion

6. The induction motor begins spinning the anode as the filament gets hotter

7. When the exposure switch is closed, the voltage selected by the mA control flows from the autotransformer, through the variable resistors, and into the step-down transformer in the filament circuit

8. The filament heats considerably, boils off electrons (thermionic emission), and creates a space charge or electron cloud around the filament

9. At the same time, the alternating current and voltage selected by choosing taps off the autotransformer is sent to the primary coils of the high-voltage step-up transformer where it is boosted to kilovoltage levels

10. After leaving the secondary coils of the step-up transformer, the voltage and alternating current are sent through the rectifier, which changes the alternating current to pulsating direct current

11. The kilovoltage creates a high potential difference in the x-ray circuit, making the anode less negative (relatively positive) and the cathode highly negative

12. This high potential difference causes the electrons to move at very high speed (approximately one-half the speed of light) from the cathode to the anode

13. The collision of these projectile electrons with the atoms of the target material causes a conversion of the electrons' kinetic energy (100%) to heat (99%) and x rays (1%)

14. Heat is produced by the projectile electrons striking the outer-shell electrons of the target material and placing them in an excited state, as a result of which they emit infrared radiation

15. The production of x rays comes from two interactions with the anode

B. Brems radiation (Fig. 3-2)

1. A projectile electron misses outer-shell electrons in the target and moves in close to the nucleus

2. Because the nucleus is positive and the electron is negative, it is slowed or braked

3. The reduction in kinetic energy causes the electron to slow and release energy as an x-ray photon

4. The resultant x rays are called bremsstrahlung (braking) x rays, because they are produced by the slowing (braking) of projectile electrons

5. At diagnostic levels, most x rays produced are from brems interaction

C. Characteristic radiation (Fig. 3-3)
1. A projectile electron collides with an inner-shell electron of a target atom
2. It removes that electron from orbit and ionizes the atom
3. A hole exists in the inner shell from the vacated electron
4. An electron from the next outer shell falls in to fill the hole
5. As the electron falls in, energy is given off in the form of an x-ray photon
6. This creates a hole in its shell of origin, and an electron from the next outer shell falls in to fill this vacancy; this continues until the atom is once again stable
7. Each time an electron falls in to fill a hole, an x-ray photon is given off

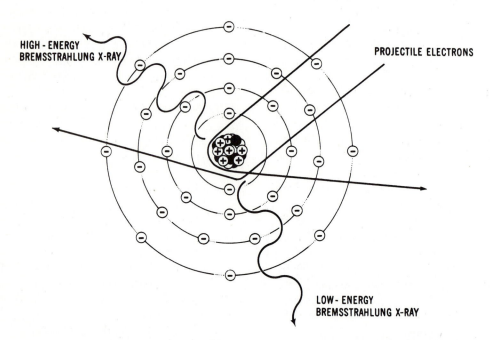

Figure 3-2 Production of bremsstrahlung x rays. From Bushong, SC: Radiologic science for technologists: physics, biology, and protection, ed 5, St. Louis, 1993, Mosby.

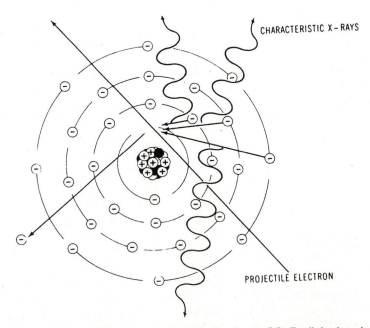

Figure 3-3 Production of characteristic x rays. From Bushong, SC: Radiologic science for technologists: physics, biology, and protection, ed 5, St. Louis, 1993, Mosby.

8. Each x-ray photon has a specific energy, equal to the difference in the binding energies of the two shells involved

9. Only x rays produced at the *K* shell are of sufficient energy to be used in diagnostic radiography

10. Because the x rays possess energy characteristic of the specific binding energies of the atom involved, they are called characteristic x rays

11. Characteristic x rays are produced at kVp levels above 70, but only in small numbers

D. X-ray properties

1. Part of the electromagnetic radiation spectrum
2. Highly penetrating
3. Invisible
4. Travel at the speed of light, 186,000 miles per second
5. Travel in straight lines, as waves
   a. Wavelength of diagnostic x rays: 0.1 to 0.5 angstroms (1 angstrom equals 10^{-10} meters, which is one ten-billionth of a meter)
   b. Wavelength is the distance from crest to crest or trough to trough or the distance covered by one complete sine wave
   c. Frequency: the number of waves passing a given point per unit time
   d. Wavelength and frequency are inversely proportional to one another: as wavelength increases, frequency decreases; as wavelength decreases, frequency increases
   e. Short wavelength rays are more penetrating, long wavelength rays are less penetrating
6. Invisible to the human eye
7. Have characteristics of waves and particles; travel in bundles or packets of energy called *photons*
8. Exist in a wide range of wavelengths and energies
9. Can ionize matter and gases
10. Cause fluorescence of phosphors
11. Unable to be focused by a lens
12. Liberate a small amount of heat when passing through matter
13. Electrically neutral
14. Affect photographic film
15. Cause biologic and chemical changes through excitation and ionization
16. Scatter and produce secondary radiation

E. X-ray beam characteristics

1. Because x rays are produced by brems and characteristic interactions at the anode, the resultant x-ray beam contains many different energies
2. An x-ray beam containing many different energies is called heterogeneous
3. The collection of all different energies (wavelengths) of x rays is called the x-ray emission spectrum
4. Discrete x-ray spectrum—produced by characteristic x rays, because energies involved are specific to the target atom and are predictable
5. Continuous x-ray spectrum—produced by brems radiation, because these energies are all different (from the peak electron energy down to zero energy)
6. The maximum energy an x-ray photon can have corresponds to the kVp that was used
7. Beam characteristics may be altered by using filtration
   a. A filter is usually a sheet of aluminum placed in the primary beam just as it exits the x-ray tube before it reaches the collimator
   b. The tube housing and glass envelope of the x-ray tube offer inherent filtration
   c. Total beam filtration equals inherent filtration plus added filtration
   d. Total filtration must be at least 2.5 mm aluminum equivalent
   e. Filtration removes the low energy (long wavelength, "soft") rays from the beam
   f. The result of removing soft rays from the beam is lower patient skin dose
   g. Other types of filters may be used that directly affect the radiographic image: trough filter; wedge filter
   h. Half-value layer: amount of filtration that reduces the beam intensity by one-half

F. Heat units and their management

1. Heat units are a calculation of the total heat produced during an x-ray exposure
2. Heat units are calculated using the following equations:
   a. Single-phase, full-wave rectified equipment— kVp × mAs
   b. Three-phase, six-pulse, full-wave rectified equipment—kVp x mAs x 1.35 (Remember: this equipment produces x-ray photons with 35% higher average photon energy)
   c. Three-phase, twelve-pulse, full-wave rectified equipment—kVp x mAs x 1.41 (Remember: this equipment produces x-ray photons with 41% higher average photon energy)
3. X-ray tubes and tube housing are constructed to absorb certain levels of heat units
4. A tube rating chart indicates the amount of heat that can be tolerated by a specific x-ray tube and housing
5. A tube rating chart takes the following factors into account that are to be used for an exposure:
   a. kVp
   b. mAs
   c. Focal spot size
   d. Anode rotation speed
   e. Voltage wave form
   f. Ability to conduct heat away from the unit
   g. The specific design of the unit
6. When consulting a tube rating chart, follow these steps to determine the safety of an exposure:
   a. On the x-axis, find the time to be used

b. On the y-axis, find the mA to be used
c. Find their intersecting point on the graph
d. If the intersecting point is below the kVp to be used, the exposure will be safe in terms of heat units produced
e. If the intersecting point is above the kVp to be used, the exposure will be unsafe in terms of heat units produced
f. If a series of exposures is to be made, the heat unit equations must be multiplied by the number of exposures

7. Most modern x-ray equipment will automatically prevent the user from making an exposure capable of producing too much heat to the tube (this is indicated on some control panels by the warning "technique over-load," by a red light, or by a failure to get a green light indicating that the anode is ready)
8. An anode cooling curve may be used to determine how many exposures can be made in a given period of time or how much time must elapse, after a series of exposures, for the tube to cool to a level at which additional exposures may be made
9. To use an anode cooling curve, first calculate the heat units produced times the number of exposures made
10. The anode cooling curve will show cooling time on the x-axis and heat units stored on the y-axis
11. The cooling curve will be a descending arc extending from the maximum heat storage capacity value to the maximum time needed to cool
12. Most modern x-ray equipment will prevent overloading the tube during a series of exposures and will not allow additional exposures until the tube has cooled sufficiently

▲ Other Imaging Equipment

A. Fluoroscopy
1. Provides dynamic visualization of internal structures
2. Consists of x-ray table to hold patient, with x-ray tube inside the table, the spot film device and image intensifier (image receptors) over the table, and a television monitor nearby
3. Spot film device allows the fluoroscopist to take radiographs of an area of interest as it is seen "live" on the television monitor
4. X-ray tube and image receptor(s) are connected with a C arm so as to keep them the appropriate distance apart, regardless of the movement of the equipment
5. X-ray tube for fluoroscopy is operated at 3 to 5 mA
6. Regulation of kVp and mA for fluoroscopy depends upon the part being examined
7. kVp and mA determine the brightness level of the fluoroscopic image
   a. kVp and mA are automatically adjusted during fluoroscopy by a process known as *automatic brightness control* (also called *automatic brightness stabilization* and *automatic gain control*)
8. Visible image on the television monitor is a result of image intensification
9. Image-intensifier tube converts x-ray energy into visible light and then into an electronic signal which is displayed as an image on the monitor
10. Image-intensifier tube consists of the following parts (Fig. 3-4):
    a. Input phosphor—made of cesium iodide; receives exit rays from patient and converts them into

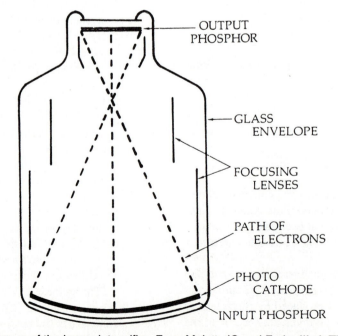

OUTPUT PHOSPHOR

GLASS ENVELOPE

FOCUSING LENSES

PATH OF ELECTRONS

PHOTO CATHODE

INPUT PHOSPHOR

Figure 3-4 Diagram of the image intensifier. From Malott, JC and Fodor III, J: The art and science of medical radiography, ed 7, St. Louis, 1993, Mosby—Year Book.

visible light

    b. Visible light from input phosphor strikes photocathode, a thin layer next to the input phosphor; it releases electrons in amounts directly proportional to the visible light striking it

    c. The electrons are attracted toward the other end of the image-intensifier tube (anode) by a series of electrostatic lenses carrying positive charges and by 25 kVp applied through the tube

    d. The electrons strike the output phosphor made of zinc cadmium sulfide

    e. The energy of the electrons is converted by the phosphors to visible light, in amounts 50 to 75 times greater than at the photocathode

    f. This increase in brightness caused by acceleration of the electrons is called *flux gain*

    g. The output phosphor is smaller than the input phosphor resulting in an increase in brightness called *minification gain*

    h. Total brightness gain is a product of minification gain and flux gain

    i. Total brightness gain ranges from 5000 to 20,000, decreasing as the tube ages

    j. By varying the voltage flowing through the image-intensifier tube, different areas of the input phosphor/photocathode assembly are tapped for electrons; this results in the ability to perform magnification during fluoroscopy

    k. Magnification is possible only with dual-focus or trifocus tubes at a cost of increased patient dose

  11. Viewing and recording of fluoroscopic image

    a. Image may be sent to various viewing and recording devices using an image distributor located near the output phosphor

    b. By using vidicon or plumbicon video tubes or a charge-coupled device (CCD), the signal may be sent to a television monitor for viewing

    c. The signal may be sent to a spot film camera (using 70, 90, or 105 mm cut film) or a cine camera (using 16 mm or 35 mm movie film)

    d. The fluoroscopic image may be recorded on videotape or on magnetic disk

    e. Digital fluoroscopy provides computerized images from the output phosphor

B. Mobile radiographic and fluoroscopic units

  1. Mobile fluoroscopic units are usually called *C arms*

    a. X-ray tube and image intensifier are located on opposite cusps of the "C" just as in stationary fluoroscopy

    b. Mobile units are capable of providing stationary images (using a last-image-hold feature) and dynamic images

    c. They are used primarily in surgery

  2. Mobile radiographic units allow for radiography under almost any conditions

    a. Most common mobile radiographic units operate on nickel-cadmium batteries

    b. These batteries are recharged by plugging the machine into an outlet

    c. The batteries provide power to propel the unit and operate the x-ray tube

    d. Capacitor—discharge mobile radiographic units must be plugged into a wall outlet for power; must have capacitor charged before each exposure

    e. High-frequency mobile radiographic units are smaller and provide ripple-free output

C. Other dedicated x-ray equipment

  1. Mammographic equipment

  2. Head (skull) units

  3. Tomographic equipment

D. Maintenance of x-ray producing equipment

  1. Quality assurance—a complete program in a radiology department that addresses all aspects of quality, including customer service, image interpretation, accuracy of diagnosis, and distribution of radiologist's reports

  2. Quality control—a program that specifically addresses the safe and reliable operation of equipment

  3. Quality control program is required by the Joint Commission on Accreditation of Healthcare Organizations (JCAHO)

  4. Responsibility for quality control program: radiologist, radiology manager, radiation physicist, quality control technologist (sometimes a separate position, sometimes a staff radiographer's duties, depending upon size of the radiology department)

  5. Many different tests may be performed as part of a quality control program

  6. Filtration-beam quality—tested using a digital dosimeter; half-value layer measurement is required

  7. Collimator—must be accurate to within 2% of the SID

  8. Effective focal spot size—measured using the slit camera, pinhole camera, or star test pattern; should be within 50% of size stated in equipment specifications

  9. kVp—tested using the Wisconsin kVp test cassette or similar devices or digital kVp meter; kVp must be accurate to within 4 kVp of that chosen

  10. Timer

    a. Timer on single-phase equipment may be tested using a spinning top test; one dot appears on radiograph for each $\frac{1}{120}$ second exposure (assuming full-wave rectification)

    b. Timer on three-phase equipment may be tested using a motorized spinning top, which indicates an arc on the finished radiograph; amount of arc in degrees (fractions of 360 degrees) indicates exposure time

    c. Timer on three-phase equipment may also be tested using a digital testing device

11. Exposure linearity—tested using a digital dosimeter; various mA-time combinations for a given mAs are checked; adjacent mA stations should be within 10% of one another

12. Exposure reproducibility—tested using digital dosimeter; tests kVp, mA, and time in successive exposures; variation in measured radiation intensity should not be more than 5%

13. Automatic exposure controls—tested to verify reproducibility of exposure using phantoms to simulate variations in patient thickness

14. Fluoroscopy exposure rate—tested using digital dosimeter; entrance skin dose should not be more than 5 rads per minute

15. Patient dose using cassette spot films and spot film cameras

16. Automatic brightness control on image intensifier—checked to ensure that radiation dose hitting the input phosphor is constant

17. Resolution of television system—tested using resolution test patterns

18. Other equipment used affecting the recorded image must also be part of a quality control program (these tests are described in Chapter 4)

▲ Review Questions

For the following question, choose the single best answer.

1. Which of the following definitions are accurate?

(1) Ionization is the removal of an electron from an atomic nucleus
(2) Matter has form and occupies space
(3) Kinetic energy is the energy of position
(4) Mass is the amount of matter in an object
(5) Electrical energy results from the heat produced when electrons are in motion
(6) The radiations in the electromagnetic spectrum are all ionizing

 a. All are accurate
 b. 1, 3, 5, 7
 c. 2, 4
 d. 1, 2, 4
 e. None are accurate

Read the following paragraph describing atomic structure. Determine the accuracy of each numbered underlined word or phrase. Then refer to questions 2-10 below the paragraph and choose the answer that best corrects the word or phrase so as to make the sentence accurate.

Atomic Structure

The atom consists of a (2) <u>positively charged</u> nucleus and electrons in orbital shells. The orbital shells are designated by the letters (3) <u>A, B, C, D, etc.</u> Most of the mass of the atom is contained in the (4) <u>electrons</u>. The atomic number of an atom is the (5) <u>number of protons in the nucleus and is represented by the letter Z</u>. Atomic mass is (6) <u>the number of electrons in the atom and is represented by the letter A</u>. In a stable atom, (7) <u>the number of electrons and protons is equal</u>. Atoms with the same number of protons but with a different number of neutrons are called (8) <u>ionized</u>. Electrons are held in orbit around the nucleus by a force called (9) <u>electromagnetic induction</u>. The law that states that the outer shell of an electron must always contain eight electrons is called the (10) <u>octet rule</u>.

2.
 a. The underlined word or phrase is accurate as written
 b. Negatively charged
 c. Neutral

3.
 a. The underlined word or phrase is accurate as written
 b. *Z, Y, X,* etc.
 c. *K, L, M,* etc.
 d. 1, 2, 3, 4, etc.

4.
 a. The underlined word or phrase is accurate as written
 b. Protons
 c. Neutrons
 d. Nucleus

5.
 a. The underlined word or phrase is accurate as written
 b. Number of electrons in the orbital shells and is represented by the letter *A*
 c. Number of electrons in the orbital shells and is represented by the letter *Z*
 d. Number of protons in the nucleus and is represented by the letter *A*

6.
 a. The underlined word or phrase is accurate as written
 b. Number of protons and neutrons in the nucleus and is represented by the letter *A*
 c. Number of protons in the nucleus and is represented by the letter *Z*
 d. Number of electrons in the nucleus and is represented by the letter *Z*

7.
 a. The underlined word or phrase is accurate as written
 b. The number of electrons is greater than the number of protons
 c. The number of protons is greater than the number of electrons
 d. The number of protons and electrons is equal, but there is a different number of neutrons

8.
 a. The underlined word or phrase is accurate as written
 b. Electrified
 c. Antimatter
 d. Isotopes

9.
 a. The underlined word or phrase is accurate as written
 b. Mutual induction
 c. Electron-binding energy
 d. Gravity

10.
 a. The underlined word or phrase is accurate as written
 b. Outer shell rule
 c. Eight electron rule
 d. There is no such rule

For the following question, choose the single best answer.

11. Examples of particulate radiation are:

   a. X-rays, gamma rays, and cosmic rays
   √b. Helium nuclei and beta particles
   c. Electrons, protons, and meteorites
   d. X-rays and quarks

Read the following paragraph describing electromagnetic radiation. Determine the accuracy of each numbered underlined word or phrase. Then refer to questions 12-22 below the paragraph and choose the answer that best corrects the word or phrase so as to make the sentence accurate.

Electromagnetic Radiation

Electromagnetic radiation travels (12) in waves along a straight path. (13) It travels as bundles of energy called protons. The speed of electromagnetic radiation is equal to the speed of (14) light. (15) The waves of radiation are called sign waves, each of which has wavelength and frequency. Wavelength is the distance from the (16) source of radiation to the object it strikes. (17) Frequency is the number of times the radiation strikes an object. As wavelength increases and frequency decreases, (18) the speed of the radiation also decreases. Generally speaking, wavelength and frequency (19) are proportional to one another. (20) As radiation strikes and travels through matter, a process called attenuation occurs which results in partial or full transfer of the radiation's energy to the atoms. Radiation is governed by the inverse square law which states that (21) the intensity of radiation is directly proportional to the square of the distance between the source of radiation and the point at which it is measured. Finally, (22) as the radiation strikes matter, the energy of the rays is destroyed as are the atoms with which it interacts.

12.
   √a. The underlined word or phrase is accurate as written
   b. In straight lines along a straight path
   c. As electrons in waves along a straight path
   d. Radiation only travels through a vacuum

13.
   a. The underlined word or phrase is accurate as written
   b. It travels as bundles of energy called electrons
   √c. It travels as bundles of energy called photons
   d. It travels as bundles of energy called phasers

14.
   a. The underlined word or phrase is accurate as written
   b. Sound
   √c. One-half the speed of light
   d. One-half the speed of sound

15.
   a. The underlined word or phrase is accurate as written
   b. The waves of radiation are called current
   c. The waves of radiation are called signal waves
   √d. The waves of radiation are called sine waves

16.
   a. The underlined word or phrase is accurate as written
   √b. Crest of a wave to the crest of the next wave
   c. Trough of a wave to the trough of the next wave
   d. b and c

17.
   a. The underlined word or phrase is accurate as written
   b. Electrons that are transferred by radiation to the object
   √c. Waves that pass a given point per unit time
   d. Seconds it takes for waves to pass a given point per unit time

18.
   a. The underlined word or phrase is accurate as written
   b. The speed of radiation increases
   √c. The speed of radiation remains constant
   d. The speed of radiation depends upon the presence or absence of a vacuum

19.
   a. The underlined word or phrase is accurate as written
   √b. Are inversely proportional to one another
   c. Are directly proportional to one another
   d. Are inversely proportional to the square of their values

20.
   √a. The underlined word or phrase is accurate as written
   b. As radiation strikes and travels through matter, a process called electrification occurs which results in partial or full transfer of energy
   c. As radiation strikes matter, all energy is surrendered by a process known as attenuation
   d. As radiation strikes matter, its energy is destroyed and the photons cease to exist

21.

    a. The underlined word or phrase is accurate as written

    b. The intensity of radiation is inversely proportional to the distance between the source of radiation and the point at which it is measured

    c. The intensity of radiation is inversely proportional to the square of the distance between the source of radiation and the point at which it is measured

    d. The intensity of radiation is inversely proportional to the square of the distance between the source of radiation and the point at which it is measured and is calculated using the equation:
Old R/New R = Old D^2/New D^2

22.

    a. The underlined word or phrase is accurate as written

    b. As the radiation strikes matter, the energy of the rays is increased from acquiring the energy of the atoms

    c. As the radiation strikes matter, the energy of the rays is not destroyed but converted to matter

    d. As the radiation strikes matter, the energy of the rays is transferred to the atoms according to the law of conservation of energy

For the following questions, choose the single best answer.

23. Which of the following statements are true regarding electrostatic charges?

    (1) Electrostatics is the study of electric charges at rest

    (2) The movement of electrons from one object to another is called ionization

    (3) Like charges attract, unlike charges repel

    (4) Electrostatic charges concentrate on a conductor in the area of greatest curvature

    (5) Friction, contact, and induction are methods of ionization

    a. 2, 3, 5

    b. 1, 4

    c. All above statements are true

    d. None of the above statements are true

    e. 1, 2, 4

24. Which of the following statements are false?

    (1) A magnetic field always surrounds an electrical charge in motion

    (2) Current flows back and forth in AC

    (3) Current flows in one direction in DC

    (4) The volt is the unit of electric current

    (5) A conductor allows the free flow of electrons

    (6) The ampere is the unit of electromotive force

    (7) The volt is the unit of potential difference

    (8) The path of electric current is called the circuit

    (9) Ohm's Law is calculated using the equation: VI=R

    (10) A semiconductor is a material that may act as a conductor under some conditions and an insulator under other conditions

    a. 4, 6, 9

    b. 1, 2, 3, 5, 7, 8, 10

    c. 1, 7, 10

    d. 4, 6, 9, 10

    e. All statements are true

Read the following paragraph. Determine the accuracy of each numbered underlined word or phrase. Then refer to questions 25-33 below the paragraph and choose the answer that best corrects the word or phrase so as to make the sentence accurate.

Electromagnetic induction is the process of causing an electric current to flow in a conductor (25) when it is placed in contact with another conductor. The two types of electromagnetic induction are (26) autoinduction and mutual induction. (27) Autoinduction is used in the operation of the autotransformer. Mutual induction is used in the operation of the step-up and step-down transformers. Because the wires in the transformers are coiled, (28) their magnetic fields lie next to one another, thereby increasing the strength of the fields. Electricity is provided by a device known as a (29) motor. The electricity provided to the radiology department is (30) 120 Hz AC. This current is single-phase, two-pulse current, providing (31) 120 pulses per second. By using special wiring patterns called wye, star, or delta the current is converted to three-phase. Three-phase power uses three wave forms placed 120 degrees out of phase with one another. (32) Three-phase, six-pulse power has 240 pulses per second while three-phase, twelve-pulse power has 360 pulses per second. The primary advantage of three-phase power is that (33) voltage only drops to zero three times per second.

25.
a. The underlined word or phrase is accurate as written
b. When is placed near a generator
c. When it is placed in the electromagnetic field of another conductor
d. When it is placed in the electromagnetic field created by the x-ray beam

26.
a. The underlined word or phrase is accurate as written
b. Solenoid induction and mutual induction
c. Generated induction and self-induction
d. Self-induction and mutual induction

27.
a. The underlined word or phrase is accurate as written
b. Self-induction is used in the operation of the autotransformer
c. Mutual induction is used in the operation of the autotransformer
d. Direct current is used in the operation of the autotransformer

28.
a. The underlined word or phrase is accurate as written
b. Their magnetic fields overlap, thereby decreasing the strength of the fields and making them less effective
c. Their magnetic fields overlap, thereby increasing the strength of the fields
d. Their magnetic fields remain separate around each turn of the wire

29.
a. The underlined word or phrase is accurate as written
b. Solenoid
c. An induction motor
d. Generator

30.
a. The underlined word or phrase is accurate as written
b. 60-hertz alternating current
c. 60 Hz DC
d. 120 Hz DC

31.
a. The underlined word or phrase is accurate as written
b. 60
c. 30
d. 2

32.
a. The underlined word or phrase is accurate as written
b. Three-phase, six-pulse power has 120 pulses per second, while three-phase, twelve-pulse power has 360 pulses per second
c. Three-phase, six-pulse power has 360 pulses per second, while three-phase, twelve-pulse power has 720 pulses per second.
d. Three-phase, six-pulse power has 6 pulses per second while three-phase, twelve-pulse power has 12 pulses per second

33.
a. The underlined word or phrase is accurate as written
b. Voltage only drops to zero six times per second
c. Voltage only drops to zero twelve times per second
d. Voltage never drops to zero

For questions 34–38, choose the single best answer.

34. A variable transformer that is used to select kVp for the x-ray circuit is the:

    a. Step-up transformer
    ✓b. Autotransformer
    c. Step-down transformer
    d. Rectifier
    e. Selective transformer

35. A transformer that has more turns in the secondary than in the primary coil is called a:

    ✓a. Step-up transformer
    b. Solenoid
    c. Step-down transformer
    d. Filament transformer
    e. Low-voltage transformer

36. The transformer used to boost voltage to kilovoltage levels is called a (an):

    a. Autotransformer
    b. Step-down transformer
    c. Step-up transformer
    d. High-voltage transformer
    ✓e. More than one but not all of the above

37. Voltage coming to the x-ray machine is kept constant through the use of a (an):

    a. Autotransformer
    b. Step-down transformer
    c. Rectifier
    d. Line voltage compensator
    e. Step-up transformer

38. A step-down transformer:

    a. Steps down voltage
    b. Steps down current
    c. Steps up voltage
    d. Steps up current
    ✓e. a and d

Use the listing below to answer questions 39-47. Items may be used more than once.

    a. Step-down transformer
    b. Rectifier
    c. Cathode
    d. Timer
    e. kVp meter

39. The site of the process of thermionic emission C

40. Prereading device e

41. Reduces voltage and provides current to produce electron cloud or space charge A

42. Usually electronic, with increments as low as .001 seconds D

43. Changes AC to DC b

44. Surrounded by negatively charged focusing cup C

45. Composed of solid state, silicon-based diodes B

46. Regulates the duration of x-ray production D

47. Located in x-ray circuit between high voltage transformer and x-ray tube b

Use the listing below to answer questions 48-56. Items may be used more than once.

    a. Anode
    b. mA meter
    c. Ionization chamber
    d. Falling load generator
    e. Step-up transformer

48. Measures tube current b

49. Spins at 3300 to 10,000 rpm A

50. Uses maximum heat storage ability of tube to deliver mAs D

51. Source of bremsstrahlung and characteristic rays A

52. Increases voltage approximately 500 times e

53. Most commonly used AEC C

54. Always delivers shortest exposure time possible D

55. Turned by a rotor A

56. Located between the patient and the image receptor C

Read the following paragraph. Determine the accuracy of each numbered underlined word or phrase. Then refer to questions 57-66 below the paragraph and choose the one complete statement that best corrects and completes it.

▲ The Production of X-radiation

(57) The filament is kept warmed with a standby current from the time the x-ray machine is turned on. (58) The machine is immediately ready for use. The proper exposure factors are selected and the patient is accurately positioned. If a student radiographer is performing the positioning, (59) activating the rotor will accelerate the process. (60) When ready to make the exposure, the rotor switch is activated for several seconds to bring the rotor up to speed and to heat the filament. At this time the exposure switch is depressed. Electrons are boiled off the filament and the electron stream is aimed at the target with the assistance of a (61) positively-charged focusing cup. The electron stream moves toward the anode because of the kilovoltage being passed through the tube, which creates a high potential difference between the two electrodes. (62) As the electrons strike the anode, they break apart and a great amount of heat is liberated. However, (63) most of the energy is converted to x rays. (64) Some electrons strike and remove K-shell (outer-shell) electrons from the target material. (65) As these vacancies are filled by L-shell electrons, energy is given off in the form of x rays. (66) Other incident electrons miss hitting orbital electrons and instead are slowed as they near the nucleus of the target material. This braking action produces heat and x rays.

57.
   a. False; turning on the machine activates the control panel only
   b. This statement is true
   c. This statement is true only if the machine has a three-phase generator
   d. False; because the exposure switch has not been activated, the filament cannot be heated

58.
   a. True; modern x-ray equipment is all electronic so it needs no preparation for use
   b. False; a high kVp, high mAs technique must first be used to warm up the generator
   c. False; modern x-ray equipment requires time to warm up before making the first exposure of the day
   d. False; x-ray equipment must first be put through a series of low heat unit warm-up exposures designed to heat the filament and anode before making diagnostic exposures

59.
   a. This always works and should be used to build confidence in students
   b. Activating the rotor begins a series of events which results in unnecessary exposure to the student and patient
   c. Because thermionic emission begins each time the rotor switch is activated, all this accomplishes is to reduce the life of the x-ray tube by burning up the filament
   d. This action prolongs the life of the x-ray tube by keeping current flowing as often as possible

60.
   a. False; the rotor and exposure switch should be activated in one fluid motion, as prescribed by most equipment manufacturers
   b. True; the equipment must be ready to make the exposure and the radiographer has full control of the process
   c. False; the filament is already heated to incandescence when the mA station is selected
   d. True; because x rays are produced along the focal track, the anode does not need to be at full speed before the exposure begins, as long as it is spinning at full speed by the termination of the exposure

61.
   a. False; focusing cup has a neutral charge
   b. False; focusing cup has a negative charge
   c. False; focusing cup has a positive charge, but it becomes negative from the thermionic emission
   d. False; focusing cup is negative so as to repel the electron cloud

62.
   a. True; most of the energy is converted to heat rather than x rays
   b. False; the electrons do not break apart; however, the process of x-ray production yields a great amount of heat
   c. True; it is the breaking of electron bonds that produces the heat
   d. False: the electrons do not break apart

63.
   a. True; of all the energy involved, 99.8% is converted to x rays and .2% is converted to heat
   b. True; this is how a sufficient number of x rays are produced for diagnostic imaging
   c. False; of all the energy involved, 99.8% is converted to heat and .2% is converted to x rays
   d. False; more than 99% of the energy is converted to heat which, in turn, converts to x rays at the anode

64.
    a. Statement is false
    b. False; *K*-shell electrons are not removed, just caused to vibrate
    c. False; electrons cannot be removed from the *K* shell because of its extremely high binding energy
    ✓d. False; *K* shell is the inner shell

65.
    a. True
    b. True; such x rays are called brems rays
    ✓c. True; such x rays are called characteristic x rays
    d. True; but such x rays are long wavelength and not considered diagnostic

66.
    ✓a. True; these rays are called brems rays
    b. True; these rays are called characteristic rays
    c. False; all incident electrons strike orbital electrons; the target atoms are so large they cannot be missed
    d. False; only characteristic x-ray production produces heat

For the following questions, choose the single best answer.

67. Which of the following are properties of x rays?

    (1) Electrically negative
    (2) Affect film emulsion
    (3) Scatter and produce secondary radiation
    (4) Invisible to the human eye
    (5) Travel at the speed of light (186,000 miles per hour)
    (6) Possess wavelengths between 1 and 5 angstroms
    (7) Travel in bundles of energy called photons
    (8) Can ionize matter and gases
    (9) Can be focused by collimators
    (10) Cause phosphors to fluoresce

    a. 1, 2, 3, 4, 5, 6, 7, 8, 9, 10
    ✓b. 2, 3, 4, 7, 8, 10
    c. 1, 5, 6, 9
    d. 2, 3, 4, 6, 8, 9, 10
    e. 2, 3, 4, 5, 7, 8, 9, 10

68. The x-ray beam is:

    a. Heterogeneous, all rays possess the same energy
    b. Homogeneous, all rays possess the same energy
    c. Monoenergetic, all energies correspond to the kVp
    ✓d. Heterogeneous or polyenergetic, consisting of many different energies (wavelengths)

69. The x-ray emission spectrum consists of:

    a. Brems and characteristic rays
    b. Discrete spectrum (produced by brems rays) and continuous spectrum (produced by characteristic rays)
    ✓c. Discrete spectrum (produced by characteristic rays) and continuous spectrum (produced by brems rays)
    d. X rays and electrons, both part of the electromagnetic spectrum
    e. Only x rays that have been filtered using aluminum

70. The primary purpose of filtration is:

    a. Radiation protection
    b. Removal of short wavelength (soft) rays
    c. To harden the beam for imaging
    d. Removal of long wavelength (hard) rays
    e. Primary purpose is not listed here

71. The amount of material needed to reduce the intensity of the beam by $1/10$ is called:

    a. Half-value layer
    ✓b. Tenth-value layer
    c. Total filtration
    d. Inherent filtration
    e. Wedge filtration

72. Which of the following statements regarding filtration is true?

    a. Total filtration must not be less than 2.0 mm Al equivalent
    b. Total filtration must remove all soft rays from the beam
    c. Total filtration (added+compensating) must not be less than 2.5 mm Al equivalent
    d. Compensating filtration should be used for all exams to reduce exposure to parts not being radiographed
    ✓e. Total filtration (not less than 2.5 mm Al equivalent) = inherent filtration (glass envelope, tube housing, oil) + added filtration (aluminum)

73. Calculating heat units for three-phase, twelve-pulse equipment requires the use of _____ as a constant; calculating heat units for single-phase equipment requires the use of _____ as a constant; calculating heat units for three-phase, six-pulse equipment requires the use of _____ as a constant.

    a. 1.0, 1.35, 1.41
    b. 1.35, 1.0, 1.41
    c. Calculating heat units does not require the use of a constant because all x rays possess the same ionizing potential
    d. 1.41, 1.0, 1.35
    e. 1.41, 1.0, 1.35—because average photon energy is different with each type of equipment

74. Which of the following charts may be consulted to determine the safety of a single x-ray exposure?

    a. Anode cooling curve
    b. H & D curve
    c. Characteristic tube chart
    d. Tube rating chart
    e. mA-time calculator

75. Which of the following charts may be consulted to determine the safety of a series of x-ray exposures?

    a. Anode cooling curve
    b. H & D curve
    c. Characteristic tube chart
    d. Tube rating chart
    e. mA-time calculator

76. The portion of the image-intensifier tube that converts electron energy to visible light is the:

    a. Output phosphor
    b. Photocathode
    c. Input phosphor
    d. Brightness gain
    e. Electrostatic lenses

77. The portion of the image-intensifier tube that converts visible light to an electronic image is the:

    a. Output phosphor
    b. Photocathode
    c. Input phosphor
    d. Brightness gain
    e. Electrostatic lenses

78. The input phosphor of the image-intensifier tube converts:

    a. Electron energy to x-ray energy
    b. X rays and heat to visible light
    c. X-ray energy to visible light
    d. X-ray energy to an electronic image
    e. X-ray energy to a visible image, which is transmitted directly to the TV monitor

79. Total brightness gain achieved using an image intensifier equals:

    a. Flux gain times minification gain
    b. Diameter of input phosphor times diameter of output phosphor
    c. Intensification factor: brightness without an image intensifier divided by brightness with an image intensifier
    d. Total light emitted at photocathode
    e. Flux gain (increase in brightness caused by the acceleration of the electronic image) plus minification gain (increase in brightness)

80. Single-phase, full-wave rectification produces

    a. Direct current
    b. Pulsating direct current
    c. Pulsating direct current with 60 pulses per second
    d. Pulsating direct current with 120 pulses per second
    e. Pulsating direct current with 120 pulses per second and 100% ripple

81. Three-phase, six-pulse full-wave rectification produces

    a. Direct current with 13% ripple
    b. Direct current with 4% ripple
    c. Direct current with 100% ripple
    d. Alternating current with 13% ripple
    e. Alternating current with 87% ripple

82. Three-phase, twelve-pulse full-wave rectification produces

    a. Direct current with 13% ripple
    b. Direct current with 4% ripple
    c. Direct current with 100% ripple
    d. Alternating current with 13% ripple
    e. Alternating current with 96% ripple

83. The increase in average photon energy when using three-phase, six-pulse equipment compared with single-phase equipment is

    a. 1.35%
    b. 41%
    c. 1.41%
    √d. 35%
    e. Average photon energy is the same

84. The increase in average photon energy when using three-phase, twelve-pulse equipment compared with single-phase equipment is

    a. 1.35%
    √b. 41%
    c. 1.41%
    d. 35%
    e. Average photon energy is the same as three-phase, six-pulse

85. Programs that deal with the safe and reliable operation of equipment and those which address all aspects of the delivery of radiology services are called, respectively:

    a. Quality assurance and quality control
    b. Total quality improvement
    √c. Quality control (QC) and quality assurance (QA)
    d. Total quality management
    e. Continuous quality improvement

86. Examples of dedicated x-ray equipment include:

    a. Mammography units
    b. Tomography units
    c. General x-ray rooms
    d. Mobile x-ray machines
    √e. More than one but not all of the above

For each of the following quality checks in items 87–90, choose the parameters that must be met from the list below:

    a. 4
    b. 5 %
    c. 2 % of SID
    d. 10 %
    e. 4 %

87. Collimator C

88. kVp A

89. Exposure linearity D

90. Exposure reproducibility B

91. When performing a spinning top test on single-phase equipment, a radiograph exhibiting <u>4</u> dots would indicate:

    a. An accurate timer, if set on $1/20$ second
    b. A malfunctioning timer, if set on $1/30$ second
    √c. A malfunctioning timer, if set on $1/3$ second
    √d. An accurate timer, if set on $1/30$ second
    √e. c and d

92. When performing a spinning top test on three-phase equipment, a timer setting of $1/60$ second should indicate the following on the resultant radiograph:

    a. 2 dots
    b. 60 dots
    √c. A 6-degree arc
    d. A 90-degree arc
    e. Unable to use spinning top on three-phase equipment

93. The test that measures the accuracy of adjacent mA stations is:

    a. Exposure reproducibility
    b. Spinning top test
    c. Pinhole camera
    √d. Exposure linearity
    e. Wire mesh test

94. The test that measures the accuracy of successive exposures is:

    √a. Exposure reproducibility
    b. Spinning top test
    c. Pinhole camera
    d. Exposure linearity
    e. Wire mesh test

95. Effective focal spot size may be measured using the following tool(s):

    a. Slit camera
    b. Star test pattern
    c. Pinhole camera
    √d. All of the above
    e. b and c

96. Resolution of the television system may be measured using the following tool(s):

    a. Wire mesh test
    b. Line pairs per millimeter resolution tool
    √c. Resolution test pattern
    d. All of the above
    e. Wisconsin kVp test cassette

97. The fluoroscopic image may be viewed or recorded using which of the following devices?

   a. TV system
   b. Cine camera
   c. Spot film camera
   √ d. All of the above
   e. b and c

98. The amount of mA used for fluoroscopy is:

   a. 300 to 500
   b. 3 to 5
   c. 10 to 12
   d. 100 to 300
   e. 200 to 500

99. Marks on the focal track of the anode resulting from bombardment of electrons are called:

   a. Melts
   b. Bullet marks
   c. Pitting
   d. Cracks
   e. Electron craters

100. Effective quality control and quality assurance programs are required for accreditation by:

   a. Joint Commission on Accreditation of Healthcare Organizations
   b. Joint Review Committee on Education in Radiologic Technology
   c. American Healthcare Radiology Administrators
   d. Starfleet Academy
   e. All of the above

Chapter 4

Review of Image Production and Evaluation

> *Accept the challenges so that you may feel the exhilaration of victory.*

▲ Density

A. Amount of blackness on a given area of a radiograph
B. Also known as the *logarithm of opacity* or *optical density*
C. Defined as the ratio of the amount of light incident on the film to the amount of light transmitted through the film
  1. Light incident may be thought of as the light striking the radiograph from the back, coming from the view box
  2. Light transmitted may be thought of as the light which is seen coming through the radiograph while being viewed either by the human eye or by a densitometer
  3. $OD = LOG_{10} \dfrac{\text{light incident}}{\text{light transmitted}}$
D. A result of exit x rays and light rays from intensifying screens striking the film's emulsion
E. Made visible when the crystals in the film's emulsion are converted to black metallic silver in the developer solution
F. Controlled by:
  1. The number of exit rays striking the film-screen combination
  2. The speed of the film-screen combination
  3. Processing

Factors That Control and Influence Density

A. mAs
  1. Controls the number of electrons passing from cathode to anode in the x-ray tube
  2. Controls the quantity of x rays produced at the anode
  3. mAs controls the amount of radiation exiting the x-ray tube
    a. This is a directly proportional relationship
    b. As mAs is increased, density increases in the same amount
    c. As mAs is decreased, density decreases in the same amount
  4. mAs directly controls the number of x-ray photons that will emerge from the patient as exit rays
  5. mAs directly controls the number of x rays that eventually strike the film-screen system as exit rays
  6. Governed by the reciprocity law
    a. Any combinations of mA and time that produce the same mAs value will result in the same density on the radiograph
    b. Sometimes expressed by the equation: mAs = mAs
B. kVp
  1. Directly controls the energy or quality of the x rays produced
    a. As the kVp increases, a greater potential difference exists between the cathode and the anode
    b. As the potential difference increases, the electrons from the cathode strike the anode in greater numbers and with greater energy
    c. This results in an increased level of production of short wavelength, high-energy radiation
  2. Directly affects density, though not in a directly proportional relationship
    a. As kVp increases, density increases
    b. As kVp decreases, density decreases
    c. Governed by the 15% rule (an increase in kVp of 15% will double density; a decrease in kVp of 15% will halve density)
  3. Determines the penetrating ability of the x-ray beam
    a. As kVp is increased, wavelength decreases, x rays become more penetrating
    b. As kVp is decreased, wavelength increases, x rays become less penetrating
  4. Penetrating ability of the x rays also determines the number of x rays exiting the patient to strike the film

C. Distance
  1. Density is inversely proportional to the square of the distance
  2. Governed by the inverse square law
    a. The intensity of the x-ray beam is inversely proportional to the square of the distance
    b. Density is expressed by the equation:

$$\frac{\text{old mAs}}{\text{new mAs}} = \frac{\text{new distance squared}}{\text{old distance squared}} \; \left(\frac{mAs_o}{mAs_n} = \frac{D_n{}^2}{D_o{}^2} \right)$$

    c. If distance is doubled, density decreases four times
    d. If distance is halved, density increases four times
    e. Any other combinations can be calculated using the inverse square law equation above
    f. Variation in density is the result of the divergence of the x-ray beam as it travels through space
D. Film-screen combination
  1. Directly proportional relationship with density
    a. As speed (sensitivity) increases, density increases
    b. As speed (sensitivity) decreases, density decreases
E. Grids
  1. Decrease the amount of scatter radiation striking the film
  2. Density decreases when using grids unless mAs is increased to compensate for the loss of scatter fog
F. Beam restriction
  1. Decreases density by limiting the size of the x-ray beam unless mAs is increased to compensate
  2. Decreases density by limiting the area of the patient being struck by x rays
  3. Reduces the amount of scatter radiation being produced, which adds density to the film in the form of fog
G. Anatomy and pathology
  1. Anatomy affects density through its variation of atomic number, tissue thickness, and tissue density
  2. Pathology affects density by altering tissue integrity, atomic number, tissue density, tissue thickness (see Chapter 5 for specific pathologies and their effect on radiographic technique)
H. Anode heel effect
  1. X-ray intensity varies along the longitudinal axis of the x-ray beam
    a. Density is greater near the cathode end of the x-ray beam
    b. Density is less near the anode end of the x-ray beam, because of absorption of x rays by the "heel" of the anode
  2. Thicker anatomy should be placed under the cathode side of the x-ray tube to take advantage of the anode heel effect
I. Filtration
  1. Negligible effect on density; largely a radiation protection accessory
  2. Some reduction in the number of soft, long wavelength rays striking the patient, most of which would not have exited the patient to strike the film

  3. Compensating filters even out density of irregular anatomy

▲ *Contrast*

A. Differences in adjacent densities on the radiograph
B. Primary function is to make the detail visible
C. High contrast = few gray tones, mainly black and white image; may also be referred to as short-scale contrast
D. Low contrast = many gray tones on image; may also be referred to as long-scale contrast

Factors That Control and Influence Contrast

A. kVp
  1. Directly controls contrast
  2. Controls differential absorption of the x-ray beam by the body because of its control of x-ray beam energy
    a. As kVp is increased, contrast decreases (becomes lower or longer scale) because there is more uniform penetration of anatomic parts by the shorter wave-length rays
    b. As kVp is decreased, contrast increases (becomes higher or shorter scale) as a result of greater absorption of lower energy rays by the anatomic parts (increased photoelectric interaction)
  3. High kVp = low contrast = long-scale contrast = many gray tones
  4. Low kVp = high contrast = short-scale contrast = few gray tones (mainly black and white tones)
B. Grids
  1. Reduce the amount of scatter reaching the film
  2. Less scatter fog results in fewer gray tones, which increases contrast
C. Beam restriction
  1. Limits area being irradiated
  2. Produces less scatter by reducing number of Compton's interactions taking place
  3. Less scatter fog reduces the number of gray tones on the radiograph, thereby increasing contrast
D. Filtration
  1. As filtration is increased, beam becomes harder (average photon striking the patient has shorter wavelength)
  2. Contrast decreases as filtration increases
E. Anatomy and pathology
  1. Also known as *subject contrast*
  2. Control contrast with variations in:
    a. Atomic number
    b. Tissue density
    c. Tissue thickness
  3. Cause differential absorption of x-ray photons, which results in contrast

▲ Recorded Detail

A. Sharpness with which anatomical structures are displayed on an image receptor
B. May be described as the geometric representation of part being radiographed
C. May also be referred to as *detail sharpness*, *definition*, or *image resolution*

Factors That Control and Influence Recorded Detail

A. Object-image distance (OID)
  1. Distance from the anatomical part being imaged to the image receptor (usually film)
  2. Shortest possible OID should be used
  3. Increased OID causes magnification of the image, resulting in loss of recorded detail
B. Source-image distance (SID)
  1. Distance from the source of radiation (usually anode in the x-ray tube) to the image receptor (usually film)
  2. Longest practical SID should be used
  3. Shorter SID causes magnification of the image resulting in loss of recorded detail
C. Focal spot size
  1. Use small focal spot whenever possible
  2. Use of large focal spot causes unsharpness of recorded detail
  3. Unsharpness is caused by x rays emanating from a larger area of the anode; accentuates beam divergence
D. Film-screen combination
  1. Use of slower speed film-screen system results in greater sharpness of recorded detail
  2. Use of faster speed film-screen system results in less sharpness of recorded detail
  3. Film-screen system speed primarily affected by size of phosphor crystals in the active layer of the intensifying screen and, to a lesser degree, the size of the silver bromide crystals in the emulsion of the film
    a. The larger the crystals, the poorer the recorded detail *(resolution)*
    b. The smaller the crystals, the greater the recorded detail *(resolution)*
E. Motion
  1. Any motion results in image blur and subsequent loss of recorded detail
  2. Motion may be caused by:
    a. Patient motion
    b. X-ray tube motion
    c. Excessive motion from reciprocating grid

▲ Distortion

A. Any misrepresentation of an anatomic structure on an image receptor that alters its size and/or shape
B. Two types of distortion: size and shape

Factors Controlling Distortion

A. Size
  1. Magnification
  2. Caused by excessive OID
  3. Caused by insufficient SID
  4. Causes anatomic structure to appear larger on film than in reality
B. Shape
  1. Elongation
    a. Causes anatomic structure to appear longer than in reality
    b. Caused by improper tube, part, or film angulation or alignment
    c. Caused by angulation along the long axis of the part
  2. Foreshortening
    a. Causes anatomic structure to appear shorter than in reality
    b. Caused by improper tube, part, or film angulation
    c. Caused by angulation against the main axis of the part

▲ Radiographic Film

A. Base
  1. Made of polyester
  2. Approximately .008 inch thick
  3. Blue dye added
    a. To enhance contrast
    b. To reduce glare
B. Emulsion
  1. Double-emulsion film (also called *duplitized film*)—coated on both sides of base
  2. Single-emulsion film—coated on one side of base
  3. Consists of silver halide crystals suspended in gelatin
    a. Gelatin—easily suspends crystals and expands and contracts in processing solutions
    b. Silver halide crystals—primarily silver bromide, most of which have sensitivity specks on the surface
    c. Sensitivity specks serve as centers for making the latent image visible; made of an impurity (silver sulfite)
    d. Latent image—image contained in the silver halide crystals after exposure but before development
  4. Approximately .0003 inch thick per coating

C. Film characteristics
1. Speed (sensitivity)
   a. Determined by the size and/or number of the silver halide crystals and the thickness of the emulsion
   b. The larger the crystals and/or the thicker the emulsion, the faster the film
2. Contrast
   a. Determined by the size of the silver halide crystals and the thickness of the emulsion
   b. A function of speed
   c. The faster the film, the higher the contrast (shorter scale, more black and white image)
   d. The slower the film, the lower the contrast (longer scale, grayer image)
3. Latitude
   a. Determined by the inherent contrast of the film
   b. The lower the inherent contrast, the wider the latitude of the film
   c. The higher the inherent contrast, the narrower the latitude of the film
   d. Latitude may be thought of as the range of exposures over which the film will produce diagnostically useful densities
4. Exposure latitude
   a. Wider exposure latitude at higher kVp levels
   b. Narrower exposure latitude at lower kVp levels

Sensitometry

A. H & D curves
1. Also called *sensitometric curves*, *characteristic curves*, *D log E curves*
2. Compare exposure (plotted on x-axis) with density (plotted on y-axis)
3. Curve always assumes some form of 'S' or sigmoid shape
4. Toe
   a. Portion of curve representing low exposure and density
   b. Portion of curve from 0.0 to 0.25 density
5. Body
   a. Also called *straight line portion*, *gamma*, or *slope*
   b. Portion of curve from 0.25 to 2.5 density
   c. Measures usable densities
   d. Indicates overall gray scale (contrast) of the film
6. Shoulder
   a. Portion of curve from 2.5 to maximum density (also called *D-max*)
   b. Measures unusable densities on the radiograph (blackest portion)
7. Use of H & D curves
   a. May be used to determine the characteristics of a certain film

b. May be used to compare the characteristics of several films
8. Film characteristics as plotted on H & D curves
   a. Speed (sensitivity)—the closer the curve to the y-axis, the faster the film
   b. Contrast—the steeper the curve, the higher the contrast; the more shallow the curve, the lower the contrast
   c. Latitude—the steeper the curve, the more narrow the latitude; the more shallow the curve, the wider the latitude
   d. Recorded detail (based on film speed)—the steeper the curve, the poorer the recorded detail; the more shallow the curve, the better the recorded detail
   e. When comparing several films, the curves to the left are faster with higher contrast and more narrow latitude
   f. When comparing several films, the curves to the right are slower with lower contrast and wider latitude

Film Storage and Handling

A. Storage
1. Temperature no greater than 68° to 70° F
2. Humidity from 40% to 60%
3. Protected from the following to prevent increased density and fog:
   a. Radiation
   b. Fumes
   c. Outdating
   d. Light
4. Boxes stored on end, never flat
   a. Pressure mark artifacts (areas of increased density) if stored flat
B. Handling
1. Pressure marks
   a. Area of increased density caused by excessive pressure applied to the film
2. Static
   a. Caused by static electricity discharge on film
   b. Static buildup on loading tray
   c. Static buildup on loading bench
   d. Rapidly pulling film from cassette as it rubs against intensifying screens
   e. Low humidity in film-handling area
3. Crinkle or half-moon marks
   a. Bending film over fingernail during handling
   b. Other rough handling

▲ *Intensifying Screens*

A. Base or backing
1. Made of polyester
2. Mounted inside the cassette, in pairs, for use with double-emulsion film

B. Reflective layer
1. Between base and active layer
2. Reflects light from crystals toward film, increasing the speed of the system

C. Active layer
1. Also called the *phosphor layer*
2. Adheres to the base
3. Contains phosphors—crystals that glow with visible light when struck by radiation
4. As phosphor size or active layer thickness decreases, the resolution of the screen increases
   a. Resolution is measured in line pairs per millimeter
   b. Resolution quality control test uses device called *resolution grid* which is radiographed and the image evaluated

D. Protective layer
1. Thin coating placed on top of active layer to provide protection from scratching or other damage

E. Screen speed (sensitivity)
1. Primarily controlled by:
   a. Phosphor used
   b. Phosphor size (larger phosphors are faster)
   c. Active layer thickness (thicker layer is faster)
   d. Efficiency of reflective layer (higher efficiency makes screen faster)
   e. kVp used (higher kVp increases screen speed)
   f. Presence of yellow dye in active layer (yellow dye absorbs some of the phosphors' light and reduces speed)
   g. Conversion efficiency—ability of phosphors to absorb x-ray energy and convert it to visible light rays

F. Film-screen combination summary (speed primarily controlled by screens; contrast primarily controlled by film)
1. Faster speed system
   a. Higher contrast
   b. Narrower latitude
   c. Less recorded detail
   d. Increased density
2. Slower speed system
   a. Lower contrast
   b. Wider latitude
   c. Greater recorded detail
   d. Decreased density
3. Single-emulsion films
   a. Used with one intensifying screen
   b. Slower
   c. Lower contrast
   d. Wider latitude

e. Better recorded detail
f. Decreased density
4. Double-emulsion films
   a. Used with two intensifying screens
   b. Faster
   c. Higher contrast
   d. Narrower latitude
   e. Poorer recorded detail
5. Identified by relative speed numbers—100 speed is the "base speed"
   a. Based on intensification factor—ratio of exposure in mAs needed to produce image without screens to exposure in mAs needed to produce image with screens:

$$IF = \frac{\text{exposure without screens}}{\text{exposure with screens}}$$

   b. Example: 200 speed system is twice as fast as a 100 speed system, so ½ the mAs would be needed to produce the same density
   c. Relative speed numbers allow for exposure calculations and modifications when moving from one film-screen system to another, eliminating guesswork
   d. Generally, slower systems used for extremity radiography; faster systems used for spine, abdomen, trauma, pediatrics
6. Spectral matching
   a. Wavelength of light emitted by screens must be matched with wavelengths to which film is most sensitive
   b. Example: green-emitting screens must be used with green-sensitive film
7. Film-screen contact
   a. Must be perfect
   b. Poor contact results in localized loss of recorded detail
   c. Tested by radiographing a wide mesh screen

▲ *Grids*

A. Use
1. Reduces the amount of scatter radiation reaching the film
   a. Scatter travels in divergent paths compared with image producing rays
   b. More likely to be absorbed in the grid
2. Generally used when part thickness is 10 centimeters or greater

B. Construction
1. Lead strips separated by aluminum interspacers
2. Grid ratio
   a. Grid ratio is the height of the lead strips divided by the distance between the lead strips: grid ratio = H/D
   b. Ratios range from 4:1 to 16:1
3. Grid frequency
   a. Number of lead strips per inch (or centimeter)

b. As grid frequency increases, lead strip thickness decreases and becomes less visible

c. Ranges from 60 to 150 lines per inch

C. Grid types

1. Linear

a. Lead strips are parallel to one another

b. X-ray tube may be angled along the length of the grid without cutoff

c. Grid cutoff—decreased density along the periphery of the film caused by absorption of image-forming rays

d. Used primarily with large SID or small field

2. Focused grids

a. Lead strips are angled to coincide with divergence of the x-ray beam

b. Used within specific ranges of SID

c. Grid radius—distance at which focused grid may be used (also called *focal distance* or *focal range*)

d. Focal range is high for low ratio grids

e. Focal range is low for high ratio grids

f. Focal range is stated on the front of the grid

3. Crossed grids

a. Also called *crosshatch grids*

b. Consist of two linear grids placed perpendicular to one another

c. Superior scatter cleanup

d. Allow for no angulation of x-ray beam

e. Require perfect positioning and centering

f. Primary use is biplane cerebral angiography

D. Grid characteristics

1. Contrast improvement factor

a. Measure of a grid's ability to enhance contrast

b. Expressed as the ratio of the contrast with a grid to the contrast without a grid

2. Grid selectivity

a. Expressed as the ratio of primary radiation transmitted through the grid to secondary radiation transmitted through the grid

b. The higher the grid frequency and grid ratio, the more selective it will be

c. High selectivity indicates high efficiency of scatter cleanup

3. Grid conversion factor

a. Also called *Bucky factor*

b. Amount of exposure increase necessary to compensate for the absorption of image-forming rays and scatter in the cleanup process

c. Used to indicate the increase in mAs needed when converting from nongrid status to grid

d. When converting from grid to nongrid status, use reciprocal of grid conversion factor

e. Grid conversion factors increase with higher kVp because there is an increase in Compton's interactions, which produce more scatter

f. Factors used at 120 kVp: 5:1 grid—3x; 8:1—4x; 12:1—5x; 16:1—6x

E. Grid motion

1. Stationary grids

a. Do not move during the exposure

b. Grid lines may be seen

2. Moving grids

a. Reciprocate (move back and forth) during exposure

b. Eliminate the visibility of grid lines

F. Grid errors-focused grids

1. Upside down

a. Result will be normal density in the middle of the radiograph with decreased density on the sides

b. Focused grid must be placed with labeled tube side facing x-ray tube

2. Off-level

a. Result will be image-forming rays absorbed all across the radiographic field, with cutoff (decreased density) visible over the entire radiograph

b. Grid must be perpendicular to the central ray

3. Lateral decentering

a. Central ray does not strike the grid in the center

b. Cutoff visible, more to one side of the radiograph

4. Grid-focus decentering

a. Violation of the grid radius when using a focused grid

b. Normal density in the middle of the radiograph with cutoff visible on the sides

G. Air gap technique

1. Uses increased OID

2. Increased OID allows scatter (which travels in widely divergent paths) to exit the patient and miss the film

3. Example: lateral cervical spine

a. Distance from spine to shoulder causes gap

b. Eliminates need for grid (gap is similar to using a 10:1 grid)

c. Use of grid only serves to increase patient dose

4. Example: cerebral angiography

a. Distance to the rapid film changers allows for gap

b. Biplane angiography produces large amount of scatter

c. Air gap usually used along with grids in rapid film changers

H. Radiographic quality and grids

1. Produce higher contrast by absorbing Compton's scatter rays, which produce fog if they strike the film

2. Decrease recorded detail, if used in a Potter-Bucky diaphragm because of increased OID

▲ Technique Charts

A. Measurement
   1. Part thickness should always be measured using calipers
   2. Caliper measurement is then used to consult the technique chart
B. Types of technique charts
   1. Fixed kVp-variable mAs
      a. Assumes optimum kVp for the part being radiographed
      b. Except for exceptionally large patients, kVp never changes for a given projection
      c. mAs is varied according to the part thickness as measured with the calipers
      d. Based on the assumption that thicker parts will absorb more rays, therefore, more rays must be placed in the primary beam
   2. Variable kVp
      a. kVp is varied according to part thickness as measured with the calipers
      b. Based on the assumption that thicker parts require a beam with shorter wavelength rays that are more penetrating
   3. Variable technique
      a. Provides for alteration of routine techniques because of pathology, patient age, ability to cooperate, casts, contrast media

▲ Automatic Exposure Controls

A. Use fixed kVp while machine controls mAs
B. Require proper ionization chambers to be selected for part being radiographed
C. Part being radiographed must be placed exactly over ionization chamber
D. Varying kVp when using AEC does not alter density, though contrast will change
E. Varying kVp serves to alter penetrating ability of the beam, resulting in faster or shorter exposure time
F. Changing density controls on AEC allows density to be increased or decreased
   1. Each step represents a change of æ 25% in density

▲ Automatic Processing and Quality Assurance

Chemistry

A. Developer
   1. Converts exposed silver bromide crystals (latent image) to black metallic silver (visible image)

   2. Reducing agents
      a. Hydroquinone—works slowly to build black tones
      b. Phenidone—works quickly to build gray tones
   3. Activator
      a. Sodium carbonate
      b. Softens and swells film emulsion
   4. Hardener
      a. Glutaraldehyde
      b. Controls swelling of film emulsion to allow for safe transport through the processor
   5. Restrainer
      a. Potassium bromide
      b. Prevents reducing agents from producing fog, which is created when unexposed silver bromide crystals develop
   6. Preservative
      a. Sodium sulfite
      b. Slows oxidation of reducing agents by room air
   7. Solvent
      a. Water
      b. Medium in which chemicals are dissolved
B. Fixer
   1. Fixing agent
      a. Also called *hypo*
      b. Ammonium thiosulfate
      c. Clears and removes unexposed silver bromide crystals
   2. Acidifier
      a. Acetic acid
      b. Provides acid medium in which fixing agent operates
      c. Stops action of alkaline developer solution on contact
   3. Hardener
      a. Aluminum chloride
      b. Shrinks and hardens emulsion in preparation for viewing and storage
   4. Preservative
      a. Sodium sulfite
      b. Slows oxidation of solution by room air
      c. Chemical component common to both developer and fixer
   5. Solvent
      a. Water
      b. Medium in which chemicals are dissolved
C. Washing solution
   1. Water
      a. Removes chemicals remaining on film

Systems

Transport

A. Moves film through the processor
B. Agitates chemistry
C. Consists of series of one-inch diameter rollers with three-inch rollers at the bottom of racks
  1. Entrance roller or detector roller
    a. Rubber serated edges grab film as it enters the processor and moves it into the developer tank
    b. Activates microswitch that turns on replenishment pump
  2. Deep racks (transport racks)
    a. Move film into and through solutions in developer, fixer, and wash tanks and between drying tubes in dryer section
    b. Use turnaround assembly (with metal guide shoes) at bottom of rack to change direction of film transport upward toward top of tank
  3. Crossover assembly
    a. Moves film from developer tank to fixer tank and from fixer tank to wash tank
    b. Rollers also help to force solution from film back into tank it is exiting
  4. Squeegee assembly
    a. Multiple roller assembly that moves film from wash tank to dryer section
    b. Uses extensive squeegee action to remove as much water as possible from film
    c. Shortens drying time and reduces humidity buildup in dryer section
D. Drive system
  1. Motor driven gears that mesh with gears at the end of top rollers on racks

Replenishment

A. Adds fresh developer and fixer solution for each film fed into the processor
B. Replenishment occurs as film is being fed into processor; activated by microswitch at end of entrance roller
  1. Motorized pumps send solution to the processor
  2. Films should always be fed into processor by the short length to prevent overreplenishment
C. Solution is pumped from holding tanks through tubing into processor
D. Replenishment rates based upon average number of 14- x17-inch films fed through the processor in a typical work day

Recirculation

A. Agitates developer solution
B. Helps to stabilize developer temperature

  1. Constant agitation and circulation of developer keeps temperature constant throughout the tank
  2. Agitation also keeps solution in contact with heater element in bottom of tank and prevents stratification of chemicals
  3. Developer temperature maintained in the range of 90° to 95° F, depending upon brand of chemicals used
  4. Heating element controlled by thermostat
C. Removes reaction particles by use of a filtration system

Dryer

A. Dries film after it leaves wash tank
B. Consists of thermostatically controlled heating element with blower fan
C. Film passes between tubes through which hot air is blowing
D. Film is dried at approximately 120° F

Maintenance

A. Start-up procedure
  1. Close wash tank valve
  2. Turn on water source
  3. Turn on processor
  4. Wash crossover racks
  5. Put lid in place
  6. Run several 14- x17- inch films through processor
  7. Check replenishment rates (also check several times throughout the day)
  8. Check developer temperature after warm-up
B. Shutdown procedure
  1. Turn off water source
  2. Turn off processor
  3. Open wash tank valve and drain tank
  4. Wash crossover racks
  5. Leave lid ajar several inches to prevent contamination of solutions resulting from condensation
C. Cleaning
  1. Daily
    a. Wash crossover racks
    b. Drain wash tank
  2. Weekly
    a. Clean deep racks
    b. Change water filters
  3. Monthly
    a. Drain and clean by hand all tanks and dryer
    b. Put in fresh developer and fixer
    c. Add starter solution to developer chemicals
    d. Change developer filter
D. Sensitometric testing
  1. Performed daily on every processor
  2. Assures consistent processing of films by monitoring speed, contrast, and base plus fog (routine may also include measuring developer temperature)

3. Film from control box is exposed using a sensitometer
4. Film is processed
5. Speed step on film is measured using densitometer
6. Contrast step on film is measured using densitometer and subtracted from speed step
7. Speed and contrast are plotted on sensitometric graph
8. Values must not fluctuate more than ± 0.10 from base-line
9. Unexposed region of film is measured using densitometer
10. Value given is base plus fog
11. Value must not fluctuate more than 0.05 from baseline
12. Speed and contrast steps are chosen from the H & D curve for the control film
    a. Speed step is the step closest to density reading of 1.0
    b. Contrast step is the step near the top of the straight line portion of the curve, just below the shoulder

Processor Malfunctions

A. Artifacts
  1. Unwanted, irregular mark or density on the radiograph
  2. Guide shoe scratches
     a. Straight line scratches, at regular intervals, running in direction of film travel
     b. Caused by guides shoes being out of adjustment
     c. Guide shoes must be readjusted
  3. Pi lines
     a. Small marks on radiograph 3.1416 inches apart on one inch rollers
     b. Caused by raised nick on roller scratching film as it passes by
     c. Also caused by chemical stain or dirt on roller
     d. Roller must either be replaced or carefully cleaned
B. Temperature fluctuations
  1. Increased developer temperature causes chemical fog, increased density
     a. Temperature must be adjusted
     b. Thermostat must be examined for possible malfunction
  2. Decreased developer temperature causes decreased density
     a. Temperature must be adjusted
     b. Thermostat must be examined for possible malfunction
  3. Damp films emerge from processor
     a. Dryer temperature must be increased
     b. Dryer thermostat must be examined for possible malfunction
  4. Damp films may also exist during times of high humidity when air within dryer compartment is saturated
     a. Dryer temperature may be increased
     b. Front of the processor may be temporarily removed to allow humidity to escape
C. Contamination
  1. Fixer solution splashing into developer tank in amount as small as one milliliter will cause contamination
  2. Verified by checking for odor of ammonia in developer solution
  3. Will cause increased density on films
  4. May occur when fixer deep rack is put back in place too rapidly and chemicals pour over divider
  5. May occur secondary to film jam if films splash around and spray fixer back into developer
  6. Processor must be immediately shut down; developer tank must be drained, completely cleaned, and refilled with fresh solution
D. Jamming
  1. Films caught during transport
  2. Rollers out of alignment
     a. May be caused by tension springs on the end of the racks breaking which releases rollers from proper position
     b. May be caused by inadequate replenishment rate, depriving the film of hardener which allows the emulsion to swell to the point where it will not pass between the rollers
E. Photographic anomalies: causes and corrections
  1. Dark films
     a. Developer temperature too high—adjust
     b. Developer overreplenishment—correct
     c. Fixer contamination of developer—clean and replace
     d. White light leak—find and correct
     e. Crack in safelight filter—replace
  2. Light films
     a. Developer temperature too low—adjust
     b. Underreplenishment—correct
  3. Films appear milky
     a. Poor fixer replenishment—correct
  4. Films appear greasy
     a. Inadequate washing—check water flow rate and level of water in tank
  5. Dark flakes
     a. Algae from wash water—drain tank, clean rollers
  6. Film fog
     a. Developer contamination—drain and clean tank, add fresh solution
     b. Developer overreplenishment—correct
     c. White light leak—find and correct
     d. Crack in safelight filter-replace
     e. Developer temperature too high—correct
     f. Outdated film—verify with date on box, discard if outdated

▲ Review Questions

For each of the following questions, choose the single best answer.

1. Density may be defined as:

   a. Differences in opacities on a radiograph
   b. The logarithm of opacity
   c. The darkness on a radiograph
   d. Light incident/light transmitted
   e. More than one but not all of the above

2. Most of the latent image is formed by:

   a. Exit rays striking the film's emulsion
   b. Light from intensifying screen phosphors responding to scatter radiation
   c. Cosmic rays
   d. Light from intensifying screen phosphors produced in response to exit rays
   e. Characteristic radiation

3. The primary controlling factor of density is:

   a. kVp
   b. mAs
   c. SID
   d. OID
   e. Focal spot size

4. Which of the following describes the relationship between mAs and density?

   (1) Density is directly proportional to mAs
   (2) Density is inversely proportional to mAs
   (3) Density is directly proportional to mAs^2
   (4) mAs controls the number of electrons boiled off the anode and, therefore, the number of x-rays produced
   (5) The number of electrons boiled off the cathode and, consequently, the number of x rays produced is controlled by mAs

   a. all of the above
   b. 1, 4
   c. 2, 5
   d. 1, 5
   e. 3, 5

5. The law stating that any combinations of mA and time that produce the same mAs value will produce the same radiographic density is the:

   a. Inverse square law
   b. mAs-density law
   c. Reciprocity law
   d. 15% law
   e. Technique law

6. Light incident/light transmitted is best described as:

   a. The ratio of light being seen from the radiograph divided by the light from the viewbox striking the radiograph
   b. Radiographic contrast
   c. The latent image
   d. The ratio of the light striking the radiograph from the viewbox divided by the light transmitted through the radiograph
   e. None of the above

7. mAs directly controls:

   a. The energy of the x-ray emission spectrum
   b. The quality and quantity of x rays produced at the cathode
   c. The quality and quantity of x rays produced at the anode
   d. The quantity of x rays produced and the resultant radiographic contrast
   e. The quantity of x rays produced

8. Differences in densities on a radiograph describes:

   a. Density
   b. Recorded detail
   c. Log relative exposure
   d. Contrast
   e. 15% rule

9. The primary controlling factor of contrast is:

   a. mAs, which controls the energy of the x rays produced
   b. kVp, which controls the quantity of x rays produced at the target
   c. Focal spot size, which controls the quantity and quality of x rays produced
   d. kVp, which controls the quality of x rays produced at the cathode and the quantity of x rays striking the patient
   e. kVp, which controls the quality of x rays produced at the anode

10. The relationship between kVp and density may be described as:

    a. Directly proportional
    b. Direct, though not proportional
    c. Governed by the 15-50 rule
    d. Controlled by x-ray tube current
    e. None of the above

11. The 15% rule states that:

    a. Density may be halved by decreasing kVp by 15%
    b. kVp should be 15% of the mAs selected
    c. Density may be doubled by increasing kVp by 15%
    d. kVp must always be 15% of the total exposure technique
    e. More than one but not all of the above

12. Which of the following is (are) true concerning the role of kVp in radiograph production?

    (1) As kVp is increased, penetrating ability of the x rays increases
    (2) As kVp is increased, more x rays exit the patient to strike the film-screen system
    (3) As kVp is decreased, wavelength and density decrease
    (4) As kVp increases, radiographic density increases
    (5) As kVp decreases, radiographic density remains constant because mAs controls density

    a. 1, 2, 4
    b. 1, 2, 3
    c. 1, 3, 4
    d. 5
    e. All are true

13. Given an original technique of 30 mAs and 80 kVp, which of the following will produce a radiograph with double the density?

    a. 60 mAs, 90 kVp
    b. 30 mAs, 92 kVp
    c. 60 mAs, 80 kVp
    d. 15 mAs, 92 kVp
    e. More than one but not all of the above

14. Which of the following describes the relationship between SID and density?

    a. Reciprocity law
    b. 15% rule
    c. Inverse square law
    d. Old mAs/new mAs = new distance/old distance
    e. More than one but not all of the above

15. If SID is doubled, what may be said about radiographic density?

    a. Density doubles
    b. Density is reduced by half
    c. Density is reduced by new mAs^2
    d. Density is reduced to ¼
    e. Density is unaffected because mAs is always doubled

16. If SID is reduced by one-half, what must be done to mAs to maintain a constant density?

    a. Reduce mAs to ¼ its original value
    b. Reduce mAs to ½ its original value
    c. Increase mAs by 4 times its original value
    d. Increase mAs by 2 times its original value
    e. Reduce mAs by a step in time

17. Which of the following describes the relationship between film-screen system speed and density?

    a. System speed is inversely proportional to density
    b. Density is inversely proportional to system speed
    c. Density is directly proportional to system speed
    d. There is no relationship between system speed and density
    e. System speed only affects contrast and recorded detail

18. As film-screen system sensitivity decreases,

    a. Radiographic density decreases
    b. Radiographic density increases
    c. Radiographic contrast increases
    d. Recorded detail decreases
    e. More than one but not all of the above

19. As film-screen system speed increases,

    a. Radiographic density decreases
    b. Radiographic contrast decreases
    c. Radiographic density increases
    d. a and b
    e. b and c

20. Which of the following describes the relationship between radiographic density and the use of grids?

    a. Grids always reduce density
    b. Grids reduce density unless mAs is increased to compensate
    c. Grids reduce density by absorbing scatter radiation
    d. Density increases as grid ratio increases
    e. None of the above are true

21. The use of filtration:

    a. Greatly reduces radiographic density because of the absorption of short wavelength x rays
    b. Greatly reduces radiographic density because of the absorption of high energy x rays
    c. Increases radiographic density by removing long wavelength x rays
    d. Has little effect on density because x rays removed from beam are not image-producing rays
    e. Increases the average wavelength of the beam

22. As beam restriction increases (tighter),

    a. Density increases
    b. Density increases as a result of focusing of x rays
    c. Density decreases
    d. Density is not affected
    e. Changes in density are negligible

23. Which of the following impact radiographic density?

    a. Atomic number of anatomical structures
    b. Tissue density of anatomical structures altered by pathology
    c. Tissue thickness
    d. Tissue integrity, intact or altered by pathology
    e. All of the above

24. The variation of x-ray intensity along the longitudinal axis of the x-ray beam describes:

    a. Beam collimation
    b. Positive beam limitation
    c. Anode heel effect
    d. X-ray emission spectrum
    e. Heterogeneous beam

25. The thicker part of anatomy should be placed under which aspect of the x-ray tube?

    a. Central ray
    b. Cathode
    c. Anode
    d. Collimator
    e. Part placement does not matter

26. Contrast may be defined as:

    a. The slope of the characteristic curve of a film
    b. Difference in densities on a radiograph
    c. The radiographic quality that makes detail visible
    d. All of the above
    e. More than one but not all of the above

27. A radiograph with few gray tones, primarily exhibiting black and white, would be described as having what type of contrast?

    (1) Long scale
    (2) Short scale
    (3) Low
    (4) High

    a. 2 and 4
    b. 1 and 3
    c. 1 and 4
    d. 2
    e. 2 and 3

28. The primary controlling factor of contrast is:

    a. mAs
    b. Focal spot size
    c. OID
    d. kVp
    e. SID

29. High kVp produces which of the following?

    (1) High contrast
    (2) Few gray tones
    (3) Long-scale contrast
    (4) Short-scale contrast
    (5) Low contrast
    (6) Many gray tones

    a. 1, 2, 4
    b. 3, 5, 6
    c. 5
    d. 1
    e. 3 and 5

30. Low kVp produces which of the following?

    (1) High contrast
    (2) Few gray tones
    (3) Long-scale contrast
    (4) Short-scale contrast
    (5) Low contrast
    (6) Many gray tones

    a. 1, 2, 4
    b. 3, 5, 6
    c. 5
    d. 1
    e. 3 and 5

31. More uniform penetration of anatomical structures occurs when using what level of kVp?

    a. Low
    b. High
    c. kVp does not affect penetration
    d. Level at which photoelectric interaction predominates
    e. None of the above

32. Differential absorption of the x-ray beam is a function of:

    a. Photoelectric interaction
    b. mAs
    c. kVp
    d. Atomic number of anatomical structures
    e. More than one but not all of the above

33. Beam restriction has the following effect on contrast:

    a. Decreases contrast by focusing x-ray beam
    b. Decreases contrast because of higher kVp level used
    c. Increases contrast because of reduction in the number of Compton's interactions that occur
    d. All of the above
    e. a and b above

34. The adjustment in technical factors required when using beam restriction is:

    a. Increase kVp
    b. Decrease kVp to reduce the number of Compton's interactions taking place
    c. Decrease mAs to reduce the number of Compton's interactions taking place
    d. Increase mAs to compensate for the number of rays removed from the primary beam
    e. No adjustment necessary

35. The use of radiographic grids has the following effect on contrast:

    a. Decreases contrast
    b. Increases contrast
    c. No effect on contrast
    d. Increases contrast by absorbing scatter radiation
    e. Decreases contrast because of higher kVp used

36. As the amount of beam filtration is increased:

    a. Contrast increases
    b. There is no effect on contrast
    c. Contrast decreases
    d. Contrast increases because beam is harder
    e. None of the above

37. That portion of contrast that is caused by variations in the anatomy or is secondary to pathological changes is called:

    a. Radiographic contrast
    b. Anatomical contrast
    c. Pathological contrast
    d. Photoelectric effect
    e. Subject contrast

38. Recorded detail is:

    a. Definition of the image
    b. Sharpness with which structures are imaged
    c. Geometric representation of the part being radiographed
    d. All of the above
    e. More than one but not all of the above

39. Poor recorded detail may be caused by which of the following factors?

    (1) Long SID
    (2) Long OID
    (3) Short SID
    (4) Short OID
    (5) Large focal spot
    (6) Small focal spot
    (7) Patient motion
    (8) Magnification
    (9) High speed film-screen combination
    (10) Low speed film-screen combination
    (11) X-ray tube motion

    a. 2, 3, 5, 7, 8, 9, 11
    b. 1, 4, 6, 8, 10
    c. 1, 4, 6, 10
    d. 2, 3, 6, 9
    e. 3, 5, 9

40. Optimum recorded detail may be caused by which of the following factors?

    (1) Long SID
    (2) Long OID
    (3) Short SID
    (4) Short OID
    (5) Large focal spot
    (6) Small focal spot
    (7) Patient motion
    (8) Magnification
    (9) High speed film-screen combination
    (10) Low speed film-screen combination
    (11) X-ray tube motion

    a. 2, 3, 5, 7, 8, 9, 11
    b. 1, 4, 6, 8, 10
    c. 1, 4, 6, 10
    d. 2, 3, 6, 9
    e. 3, 5, 9

41. Film-screen system effect on recorded detail is controlled by:

    a. Size of the screen's phosphors
    b. Size of the film's silver halide crystals
    c. Thickness of the screen's active layer
    d. Film's emulsion thickness
    e. All of the above

42. Distortion may be described as:

    a. Misrepresentation of an anatomical structure on film
    b. Foreshortening
    c. Elongation
    d. Magnification
    e. Minification

43. Elongation and foreshortening are examples of:

    a. Size distortion
    b. Shape distortion
    c. Motion
    d. Distortion caused by short SID and long OID
    e. Distortion that only occurs during mobile radiography

44. Magnification is caused by:

    (1) Short SID
    (2) Long SID
    (3) Short OID
    (4) Long OID
    (5) Long SOD
    (6) Short SOD

    a. 2, 3, 5
    b. 1, 4, 5
    c. 1, 3, 6
    d. 1, 4, 6
    e. 2, 4, 6

45. Distortion that occurs when the x-ray beam is angled against the long axis of a part is:

    a. Elongation
    b. Magnification
    c. Minification
    d. Misrepresentation
    e. Foreshortening

46. Distortion that occurs when the x-ray beam is angled along the long axis of a part is:

    a. Elongation
    b. Magnification
    c. Minification
    d. Misrepresentation
    e. Foreshortening

47. The purpose of adding blue dye to the base of radiographic film is to:

    a. Reduce glare when viewing the image
    b. Enhance radiographic contrast
    c. Reduce exposure to the patient
    d. b and c
    e. a and b

48. The emulsion of radiographic film consists of:

    a. Silver halide crystals suspended in plastic
    b. Sensitivity specks attached to silver halide crystals
    c. Gelatin in which silver halide crystals are suspended
    d. All of the above
    e. b and c

49. Sensitivity specks on silver halide crystals serve as:

    a. Focus centers for x rays
    b. Development centers for building the manifest image
    c. Crystals that allow the gelatin to expand and contract
    d. Gatekeepers for photon-crystal interactions
    e. None of the above

50. Characteristics associated with high speed film are:

    (1) Small silver halide crystals
    (2) Thick emulsion layer
    (3) Low film contrast
    (4) Large silver halide crystals
    (5) High film contrast
    (6) Thin emulsion layer
    (7) Wide latitude
    (8) Long-scale contrast
    (9) Narrow latitude
    (10) Short-scale contrast

    a. 1, 3, 6, 7, 8
    b. 1, 2, 5, 7, 10
    c. 2, 4, 5, 9, 10
    d. 3, 4, 6, 7, 8
    e. 4, 5, 6, 9, 10

51. Characteristics associated with slow speed film are:

    (1) Small silver halide crystals
    (2) Thick emulsion layer
    (3) Low film contrast
    (4) Large silver halide crystals
    (5) High film contrast
    (6) Thin emulsion layer
    (7) Wide latitude
    (8) Long-scale contrast
    (9) Narrow latitude
    (10) Short-scale contrast

    a. 1, 3, 6, 7, 8
    b. 1, 2, 5, 7, 10
    c. 2, 4, 5, 9, 10
    d. 3, 4, 6, 7, 8
    e. 4, 5, 6, 9, 10

52. A film's response to radiation exposure may be plotted using a graph known as:

    a. H & D curve
    b. D log E curve
    c. Characteristic curve
    d. Sensitometric curve
    e. All of the above

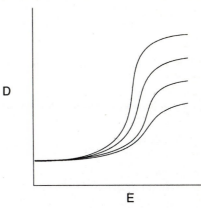

Figure 4-1

Use Fig. 4-1 to answer questions 53–63:

53. Which film is slowest?

54. Which film has the highest contrast?

55. Which film has the thinnest emulsion?

56. Which film has the narrowest latitude?

57. Which film has the lowest contrast?

58. Which film is fastest?

59. Which film has the thickest emulsion?

60. Which film provides the best recorded detail?

61. Which film has the widest latitude?

62. Which film has the poorest recorded detail?

63. Which film would most student radiographers prefer to use because of latitude?

For each of the following questions, choose the single best answer.

64. Which of the following best describes ideal storage conditions for x-ray film?

    a. Protected from radiation, fumes, outdating
    b. 68% to 70% humidity, 40° to 60° F
    c. 68° to 70° F, 40% to 60% humidity
    d. a and b
    e. a and c

65. Characteristics associated with high speed intensifying screens are:

(1) Poor contrast
(2) Poor recorded detail
(3) Thin active layer
(4) Good contrast
(5) Yellow dye incorporated into phosphor layer
(6) Small phosphors
(7) Good recorded detail
(8) Thick active layer
(9) Large phosphors
(10) Lower conversion efficiency
(11) Higher relative speed number
(12) Lower relative speed number
(13) Low intensification factor
(14) High intensification factor
(15) Higher conversion efficiency

  a. 2, 4, 5, 8, 9, 10, 11, 15
  b. 1, 3, 5, 6, 7, 10, 12, 13
  c. 2, 8, 9, 11, 14, 15
  d. 1, 2, 3, 6, 11, 14
  e. 4, 7, 8, 9, 11, 14

66. Characteristics associated with slower speed intensifying screens are:

(1) Poor contrast
(2) Poor recorded detail
(3) Thin active layer
(4) Good contrast
(5) Yellow dye incorporated into phosphor layer
(6) Small phosphors
(7) Good recorded detail
(8) Thick active layer
(9) Large phosphors
(10) Lower conversion efficiency
(11) Higher relative speed number
(12) Lower relative speed number
(13) Low intensification factor
(14) High intensification factor
(15) Higher conversion efficiency

  a. 2, 4, 5, 8, 9, 10, 11, 15
  b. 3, 5, 6, 7, 10, 12, 13
  c. 2, 4, 8, 9, 11, 14, 15
  d. 1, 2, 3, 6, 11, 14
  e. 4, 7, 8, 9, 11, 14

67. Grid ratio is defined as:

a. The ratio of the lead strips to the space between them
b. The thickness of the lead strips divided by the thickness of the aluminum interspacers
c. The ratio of the height of the lead strips over the distance between the lead strips
d. The ratio of the distance between the lead strips over the height of the lead strips
e. The amount of lead in the grid

68. Grid frequency is defined as:

a. The same as grid ratio
b. The amount of lead in the grid (expressed in terms of focusing distance)
c. How often a grid is used
d. The amount of lead in the grid (expressed as the number of lead strips per inch)
e. The amount of grid cut-off that occurs with a given grid

69. Which of the following statements concerning grids are true?

(1) Contrast improvement factor is the measure of a grid's ability to enhance contrast
(2) Grid selectivity is the ratio of primary radiation transmitted through the grid to secondary radiation transmitted through the grid
(3) Grids are used when part thickness is less than 10 centimeters
(4) Grid conversion factor is the amount of increase in kVp necessary when converting from nongrid to grid technique
(5) Their primary purpose is radiation protection
(6) Their main function is to prevent Compton's scatter from reaching the film
(7) Grids prevent the production of scatter

  a. 1, 2, 6
  b. 1, 2, 4, 6
  c. 1, 2, 3, 7
  d. 1, 2, 6, 7
  e. 1, 2, 5

70. A grid that has lead strips and aluminum interspacers which are angled to coincide with the divergence of the x-ray beam is called a:

a. Parallel grid
b. Focused grid
c. Crosshatch grid
d. Rhombic grid
e. Stationary grid

71. The range of SIDs that may be used with a focused grid is called:

    a. Grid ratio
    b. Objective plane
    c. Anti-cutoff distances
    d. Grid factor
    e. Grid radius

72. The best scatter cleanup is achieved with the use of:

    a. Air gap technique
    b. Focused grids
    c. Crosshatch grids
    d. Parallel grids
    e. 12:1 focused grids

73. Grid cutoff may be described as:

    a. Decreased density in the middle of the radiograph caused by the use of a parallel grid inserted upside down
    b. Decreased density on a radiograph as a result of absorption of image-forming rays
    c. Increased density in the center of a radiograph caused by the use of a focused grid inserted upside down
    d. Decreased density on the edges of a radiograph only
    e. Decreased density caused by using a focused grid at the proper grid radius

74. When changing from a nongrid technique using 10 mAs and 75 kVp to a 12:1 grid using 75 kVp, what new mAs must be used to maintain the same density as the original film?

    a. 50 mAs
    b. 2 mAs
    c. 40 mAs
    d. 120 mAs
    e. mAs is not altered; kVp should be increased

75. The use of air gap technique:

    a. Works because x rays are absorbed in the air between the patient and the film
    b. Should occur whenever possible
    c. May cause some magnification because of decreased OID
    d. Works only at short SID
    e. Works because scatter radiation travels in divergent paths and misses the film as a result of increased OID

76. The use of technique charts:

    a. Is unnecessary for any exam because of AECs
    b. Requires the part thickness to be measured using calipers
    c. Is usually based on fixed kVp, variable mAs
    d. All of the above
    e. Some of the above

77. When using automatic exposure controls (AEC), increasing the kVp will:

    a. Increase density proportionately
    b. Increase radiographic contrast
    c. Increase exposure time
    d. Have no effect on density
    e. Always be the best way to correct an unacceptable radiograph

78. The function of automatic processing is to:

    a. Make the latent image visible
    b. Convert exposed silver halide crystals to black metallic silver
    c. Prepare radiograph for viewing and storage
    d. All of the above
    e. More than one but not all of the above

79. Which of the following are contained in the developer solution?

    (1) Activator
    (2) Hypo
    (3) Hardener
    (4) Preservative
    (5) Reducing agents
    (6) Water
    (7) Acidifier
    (8) Restrainer

    a. 2, 3, 4, 6, 7
    b. 5, 6, 8
    c. 1, 3, 4, 5, 6, 8
    d. 1, 2, 5, 6
    e. None of the above combinations

80. Which of the following are contained in the fixer solution?

(1) Activator
(2) Hypo
(3) Hardener
(4) Preservative
(5) Reducing agents
(6) Water
(7) Acidifier
(8) Restrainer

a. 2, 3, 4, 6, 7
b. 5, 6, 8
c. 1, 3, 4, 5, 6, 8
d. 1, 2, 5, 6
e. none of the above combinations

81. Which of the following statements are true concerning developer solution?

(1) The reducing agents convert all silver halide crystals to black metallic silver
(2) A hardener is added to the developer to control the swelling of the emulsion
(3) The activator keeps the chemicals at full strength
(4) The reducing agents convert all silver halide crystals with sensitivity specks to black metallic silver
(5) Rapid oxidation of the reducing agents is prevented by mixing them in water
(6) The preservative keeps the finished radiograph from yellowing while in storage

a. All of the above statements are true
b. 2
c. None of the above statements are true
d. 4, 5, 6
e. 1, 2, 6

82. Which of the following statements are false concerning the fixer solution?

(1) Fixing agent clears all silver halide crystals from the emulsion
(2) Water keeps the fixer solution neutral
(3) Rapid oxidation of the solution is prevented by the use of a preservative
(4) The hardener shrinks and hardens the emulsion
(5) Hypo removes all unexposed silver halide crystals

a. 3, 4, 5
b. All of the above statements are true
c. 1, 2, 5
d. 3, 4
e. 1, 2

83. Which of the following statements are true concerning automatic processing chemistry?

(1) Developer is kept at 90° to 95° C
(2) Fixer is an acidic solution
(3) The preservative helps prevent rapid oxidation by room air
(4) Developer is an alkaline solution
(5) The restrainer prevents the reducing agents from developing the unexposed silver halide crystals
(6) Water is the solvent in which chemicals are mixed
(7) The activator softens and swells the film's emulsion so chemistry can come in contact with the silver halide crystals
(8) The hardener in the developer controls the swelling of the emulsion so that silver halide crystals do not escape out into solution

a. All of the statements are true
b. 1, 2, 3, 4, 5, 6, 7
c. 2, 3, 4, 5, 6, 7
d. 1, 2, 3, 4, 5, 6
e. 3, 5, 6, 7

84. The function of the wash tank is to:

a. Neutralize all chemistry
b. Stop development
c. Rinse away unexposed silver halide crystals
d. Remove chemistry from film
e. Shrink emulsion with hot water

85. Which of the following statements best describes the transport system of an automatic processor?

a. Moves film through processor with a series of rollers and racks and agitates chemistry
b. Moves film through the processor and maintains solution strength
c. Moves film through the developer and fixer and agitates chemistry
d. Moves film through the processor, maintains solution strength, and activates replenishment system
e. Moves film through the processor

86. Which of the following statements best describes the replenishment system of an automatic processor?

    a. Adds fresh developer, fixer, and water each time a film is fed into the processor
    b. Adds fresh developer and fixer each time a film is fed into the processor
    c. Adds fresh developer as film is being fed into the processor
    d. Maintains solution strength and temperature as film is fed into the processor
    e. Adds fresh chemistry to processor each time it is mixed

87. Which of the following statements best describes the recirculation system of an automatic processor?

    a. Adds fresh chemistry and maintains temperature
    b. Maintains developer temperature at 90-95° F
    c. Agitates developer solution, maintains temperature, removes by-products of chemical reactions
    d. Maintains chemistry temperature and concentration
    e. All of the above

88. Which of the following statements best describes the dryer system of an automatic processor?

    a. Helps to seal emulsion with heat, dries film, works at approximately 120° C
    b. Dries film as it passes between tubes blowing hot air
    c. Dries film after it leaves fixer and seals emulsion with hot air
    d. Removes water from film and humidity from air inside processor
    e. Helps to seal emulsion with heat, dries film, works at approximately 120° F

89. Which of the following statements describe the maintenance schedule for an automatic processor?

    (1) Wash tank should be drained at the end of each work day
    (2) Entire processor should be cleaned weekly
    (3) Fresh developer should be added daily after cleaning developer tank
    (4) Lid on processor should be left ajar at shutdown to allow for escape of chemical evaporation
    (5) Several 14- x17-inch films should be run through the processor at start up
    (6) Crossover racks should be cleaned at start up and shutdown
    (7) All tanks, racks, and rollers should be thoroughly cleaned monthly
    (8) Starter solution should be added to developer and fixer when refilling after cleaning

    a. 1, 4, 5, 6, 7, 8
    b. 1, 2, 4, 5, 6, 7
    c. 1, 3, 4, 6, 7
    d. 1, 4, 5, 6, 7
    e. 1, 3, 4, 5, 6, 7

90. When performing sensitometric testing on an automatic processor, the acceptable range of variation for speed and contrast is:

    a. ± .05
    b. ± .10
    c. ± .01
    d. ± .25
    e. ± 2.5

91. When performing sensitometric testing on an automatic processor, the acceptable range of variation for base plus fog is:

    a. ± .05
    b. ± .10
    c. ± .01
    d. ± .25
    e. ± 2.5

92. Sensitometric testing of automatic processors should be performed:

    a. Weekly
    b. Monthly
    c. Daily
    d. Several times each day
    e. Only when there appears to be a malfunction

93. Emulsion scratches that run the length of the film in the direction of film travel are usually caused by:

    a. Pi lines
    b. Improper cleaning of rollers
    c. Inadequate replenishment
    d. Guide shoes out of adjustment
    e. Film jam

94. Contamination of developer by fixer will cause:

    a. Developer contamination
    b. A chemical reaction that will release the odor of ammonia
    c. Increased fog on the radiograph
    d. Decreased contrast
    e. All of the above

95. Jamming of films in the processor may be caused by:

    a. All of the below
    b. Rollers out of alignment
    c. Racks improperly seated in place
    d. Inadequate replenishment
    e. Chemical buildup on rollers

The following graph (Fig. 4-2) provides H & D curves for the same film processed under varying conditions. Use it to answer questions 96–100:

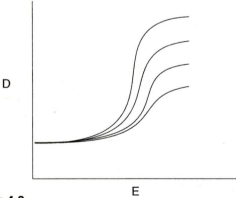

Figure 4-2

96. Which curve represents the film's response to inadequate drying?

    a. A
    b. B
    c. C
    d. D
    e. None of the curves indicates this condition

97. Which curve represents the film's response to extended development time?

    a. A
    b. B
    c. C
    d. D
    e. None of the curves indicates this condition

98. Which curve represents the film's response to developer under replenishment?

    a. A
    b. B
    c. C
    d. D
    e. None of the curves indicates this condition

99. Which curve represents the film's response to chemical contamination?

    a. A
    b. B
    c. C
    d. D
    e. None of the curves indicates this condition

100. Which curve represents the film's response to decreased developer temperature?

    a. A
    b. B
    c. C
    d. D
    e. None of the curves indicates this condition

Chapter 5

Review of Radiographic Procedures (Anatomy, Positioning, Procedures, Pathology)

> *Some people dream of worthy accomplishments, while others stay awake and do them.*

▼

▲ Basic Principles of Positioning and Procedures

A. Part placement
  1. Part should be placed on the cassette in such a way as to image all anatomy required for the procedure
  2. Allow for tight collimation
B. Alignment
  1. The long axis of the body part should correspond to the long axis of the film
  2. Exception being when cassette must be rotated in order to fit the entire part on the film
C. Two or more projections on the same film
  1. Lead strip should always be used to mask unexposed portion of the cassette
  2. Using only collimation may cause overlap of images; radiograph not as pleasing to view
  3. Long axis of the bone should be oriented in the same direction for both projections
D. Precise visualization
  1. Positioning must be absolutely accurate
  2. No rotation of image present
E. Patient identification
  1. I.D. marker on cassette should always be placed where it will not superimpose over required anatomy
  2. Patient information should include name and date of exam
F. Anatomic markers
  1. Right or left markers must always appear on the radiograph by using a radiopaque marker placed on the cassette

  2. Stickers, grease pencils, or felt-tip writing placed on the radiograph after processing are not considered legal markings. These should only be used in rare circumstances
  3. Radiopaque markers must be placed just inside the collimation field but not superimposed over required anatomy
G. Other markers
  1. Time—time indicators should always be used when radiographs are taken at specifically timed intervals
  2. Direction—if the film was taken erect, the lead marker indicating erect or upright must appear on the radiograph
  3. Inspiration/expiration—must be used for comparison studies of the chest
  4. Internal/external—must be used when both forms of rotation constitute part of an examination
  5. Numerical markers—must be used when taking a series of films in sequence, e.g., during trauma or surgical cases when the same projection is taken several times in a short period of time
H. Routines
  1. Minimum of two views per exam
  2. Exception being for certain cases where a single survey radiograph suffices
  3. A minimum of two projections, 90 degrees from one another, must always be taken
    a. Superimposition of structures may prevent the visualization of some pathological conditions
    b. Lesions or foreign bodies require precise localization
    c. Fractures must be seen from two points precisely 90 degrees from each other
    d. Minimum of three projections (AP or PA, lateral, and oblique) required for proper visualization of joints

▲ Positioning Terminology

Anterior or ventral—refers to forward or front

Caudal, inferior—away from the head

Central—mid area

Cranial, cephalic, superior—toward the head

Distal—farthest from the origin or point of reference

Lateral—away from the median plane of the body or from the middle of a part

Medial—toward the median plane of the body or toward the middle of a part

Posterior, dorsal—back of a part (not used to describe foot)

Proximal—nearer origin or point of reference

Dorsal recumbent—supine, lying on back

Ventral recumbent—prone, lying face down

Right lateral recumbent—lying on right side

Left lateral recumbent—lying on left side

Projection—path of the central ray

Position—placement of the body

View—image as seen by the image receptor (opposite of projection)

Oblique—body rotated from AP, PA, or lateral

RAO—oblique angle that places right anterior portion of the body closest to the film

LAO—oblique angle that places left anterior portion of the body closest to the film

LPO—oblique angle that places left posterior part of the body closest to the film

RPO—oblique angle that places right posterior portion of the body closest to the film

Decubitus position—patient lying down; central ray parallel to the floor (horizontal)

Left or right lateral decubitus—patient lying on left or right side; central ray parallel to the floor (horizontal); AP or PA projection

Dorsal decubitus—patient lying down on back; central ray parallel to the floor (horizontal)

Ventral decubitus—patient lying on abdomen; central ray parallel to the floor (horizontal)

Tangential—central ray skims between body parts or skims body surface; shows profile of body part, projects it free of superimposition

Axial—longitudinal angulation of the central ray with the long axis of the body part; projection which refers to images obtained with central ray angled 10 degrees or more along long axis of part

▲ Topography

A. Cervical region
   1. C1—mastoid tip
   2. C2, C3—gonion
   3. C5—thyroid cartilage
   4. C7—vertebra prominens

B. Thoracic region
   1. T1—2 inches above sternal notch
   2. T2, T3—level of manubrial notch and superior margin of scapula
   3. T4, T5—level of sternal angle
   4. T7—level of inferior angle of scapula
   5. T10—level of xiphoid tip

C. Lumbar region
   1. L3—costal margin
   2. L3, L4—level of umbilicus
   3. L4—level of most superior aspect of iliac crest

D. Sacrum and pelvic region
   1. S1—level of anterior superior iliac spine (ASIS)
   2. Coccyx—level of pubic symphysis and greater trochanters

E. Lines
   1. Orbitomeatal line (OML)
      a. Line from outer canthus of the eye to the auricular point
      b. Seven-degree angle with infraorbitomeatal line (IOML)
      c. Eight-degree angle with the glabellomeatal line
      d. Also called the *radiographic baseline*
   2. Infraorbitomeatal line (also called *Reid's baseline*)
      a. Line from just below the eye to the auricular point
      b. Seven-degree angle with the orbitomeatal line
   3. Glabellomeatal line
      a. Line from the glabella to the auricular point
      b. Eight-degree angle with the orbitomeatal line
   4. Acanthomeatal line (AML)
      a. Line from acanthion to the auricular point

▲ Motion Control

A. Involuntary motion (controlled with short exposure time and high speed film-screen combination)
   1. Cardiac motion
   2. Peristalsis
   3. Muscular spasm
   4. Chills
   5. Pain

B. Voluntary motion
   1. Belligerence
   2. Excitement
   3. Fear
   4. Nervousness
   5. Painful discomfort
   6. Age (children, elderly)
   7. Controlled by the use of the following:
      a. Clear communications
      b. Sandbags
      c. Sponges
      d. Tape
      e. Short exposure time
      f. Patient comfort

g. Compression bands
h. Use of Pigg-o-stat (for infants)
i. Use of sheets for mummification techniques (for children)
j. Instructions—clearly explain the examination to the patient
k. Obtain signature on consent form if required
l. Ask patient if there are any questions to be answered, ensuring informed consent
m. Describe examination in terminology the patient will understand
n. Describe exactly what will be done to the patient including the approximate number of radiographs to be taken and the duration of the exam
o. Explain the reasons for removal of clothing and the extent of gowning
p. Explain the reason for removal of all radiopaque objects in the area of interest
q. Describe the required respiration and the reasons for its use

▲ Exposure Modification

A. Use of optimum radiographic technique will ensure proper visualization of body parts
B. Exposure technique may need to be modified because of:
   1. Pathological conditions
   2. Age of the patient
   3. Conditions under which the radiographs are being taken (e.g., mobile radiography, crosstable projections)

▲ Gonadal Shielding

A. Used when gonads are within the primary beam or within 5 cm of the primary beam
B. Used if the shielding does not interfere with the purpose of the exam
C. Used on patients of reproductive age and younger

▲ Body Habitus

A. Hypersthenic
   1. Massive build
   2. Represents 5% of the population
   3. Thorax is broad and deep
   4. Ribs almost horizontal
   5. Thoracic cavity shallow
   6. Lungs short, narrow above and broad at the base
   7. Heart short and wide
   8. Diaphragm is high
   9. Upper abdominal cavity broad, lower part small
   10. Stomach and gallbladder high, horizontal
   11. Colon is high

B. Sthenic
   1. Slight modification of hypersthenic
   2. Most common body habitus
   3. Present in 50% of the population
C. Hyposthenic
   1. Between asthenic and sthenic
   2. Present in 35% of the population
D. Asthenic
   1. Slender build
   2. Present in 10% of the population
   3. Thorax narrow and shallow
   4. Ribs slope sharply downward
   5. Thoracic cavity is long
   6. Lungs are long, broader above than at the base
   7. Heart long and narrow
   8. Diaphragm low and abdominal cavity short
   9. Stomach and gallbladder are low, vertical, near the midline
   10. Colon low, median position

▲ Pediatric Radiography: General Principles

A. Appropriate introduction of radiographer to child and parent
B. Radiographer demonstrates positive attitude towards the child
C. Maintain clear communication with child and parent
D. Determine extent of parental involvement
E. Report suspected child abuse (nonaccidental trauma) to the appropriate radiologist, attending physician, radiology supervisor, or nurse
F. Determine type of immobilization to be used for the examination
   1. Immobilization board
   2. Pigg-o-stat
   3. Sandbags
   4. Tape
   5. Compression bands
   6. Sheets and towels
G. Practice ALARA principle
   1. Gonadal shielding of children
   2. Tight collimation
   3. Pieces of lead used as contact shields
   4. Low mAs techniques
   5. No repeat films
   6. High speed film-screen combinations
H. Determine if patient preparation was adequately carried out
I. Interview the parent and write down the appropriate history
J. Briefly discuss case with radiologist to determine specifically which projections are needed and the extent of gonadal shielding that should be used in cases where this may be in doubt

▲ *Trauma: General Principles*

A. Do no additional harm to the patient

B. Work quickly and confidently, observing universal precautions

C. Be prepared to modify conventional positions in response to patient condition

D. If patient is immobilized, transfer to the x-ray table with as much help as possible

E. In the case of skull and cervical spine injuries:
 1. A crosstable lateral cervical spine must be obtained before moving the patient in any way
 2. The radiograph must be approved by a physician before moving the patient or removing a cervical collar or sandbags

F. Each body part requires at least two radiographs taken at 90-degree angles to one another

G. Projections should, to the degree the patient's condition permits, approach routine positioning, with the cassette placed as close to the body part as possible

H. Central ray entrance and exit points should be as close to routine as possible

I. For long bone radiography
 1. Always include the joint nearest the trauma
 2. The joint farthest from the trauma should also be included, if possible; otherwise, separate radiographs should be taken of that joint

J. Splints or bandages
 1. Should not be removed unless permission has been obtained from the physician
 2. Exposure technique may need to be modified to compensate for splints and bandages

K. Allow the patient as much control over movement as possible

L. Whether patient is conscious or unconscious, explain your movements clearly in order to gain whatever cooperation is possible

M. Be prepared to perform several examinations at once
 1. For example, all AP projections should be taken in an uninterrupted sequence, then all lateral positions, etc.
 2. Reduces the number of times the x-ray tube must be moved
 3. Allows the overall procedure to be completed more quickly

N. Provide lead aprons for anyone who may need to be in the room caring for a critically injured patient

O. Move extremities carefully so as not to further displace fractures or cause internal hemorrhage

P. Maintain a cooperative spirit
 1. With other health care professionals who are attempting to care for the patient at the same time
 a. Medical technologists
 b. Respiratory therapists
 c. Physicians
 d. Nurses
 e. May all need to be caring for the patient simultaneously during the performance of radiographic examinations in cases of severe trauma
 f. Radiographer is a vital part of a trauma team and needs to work in harmony with the other health care professionals present for the proper care of the patient

Q. Inability of the patient to move and difficulty obtaining routine projections must never be used as an excuse to submit radiographs of poor quality
 1. Severely traumatized patient needs fully diagnostic radiographs in order to receive optimum care
 2. Radiographer must be proficient in radiographic exposure and positioning so that high quality radiographs may be obtained under difficult conditions

▲ *Review of Anatomy Relevant to Radiography*

Planes of the Body

A. Median sagittal plane (MSP or midsagittal plane)
 1. Passes vertically through the midline of the body from front to back
 2. Divides body into equal right and left portions
 3. Any plane parallel to the MSP is called a *sagittal plane*

B. Midcoronal plane
 1. Passes vertically through the midaxillary region of the body and through the coronal suture of the cranium at right angles to the MSP
 2. Divides body into anterior and posterior portions
 3. Any plane passing vertically through the body from side to side is called a *coronal plane*

C. Transverse plane (*axial plane*)
 1. Passes crosswise through the body at right angles to its longitudinal axis and to the MSP and coronal planes
 2. Divides body into superior and inferior portions

Clinical Divisions of the Abdomen

A. Divided into four quadrants by a transverse plane and the MSP intersecting at the umbilicus

B. Names of the quadrants:
 1. Right upper quadrant
 2. Right lower quadrant
 3. Left upper quadrant
 4. Left lower quadrant

Anatomic Divisions of the Abdomen

A. Abdomen is divided into nine regions using four planes
 1. Two transverse planes
 2. Two sagittal planes

B. Planes are called *Addison's planes*
C. Transverse planes are drawn
  1. At the levels of the tip of the ninth costal cartilage
  2. At the superior margin of the iliac crest
D. Two sagittal planes are drawn
  1. Each midway between the anterior superior iliac spines of the pelvis and the MSP of the body
E. Nine regions of the body
  1. Superior
    a. Right hypochondrium
    b. Epigastrium
    c. Left hypochondrium
  2. Middle
    a. Right lumbar
    b. Umbilical
    c. Left lumbar
  3. Inferior
    a. Right iliac
    b. Hypogastrium
    c. Left iliac

Skeletal System

Functions

A. Provides a rigid support system
B. Protects delicate structures
C. Bones supply calcium to the blood and are involved in the formation of blood cells
D. Bones serve to provide attachment of muscles and form levers in the joint spaces allowing movement

Ossification

A. Cartilage is covered with perichondrium that is converted to periosteum
B. Diaphysis—central shaft
C. Epiphysis—located at both ends of the diaphysis
D. Growth in the length of the bone is provided by the metaphyseal plate located between the epiphyseal cartilage and the diaphysis
E. An osseous matrix is formed in the cartilage
F. Bone appears at the site where there was cartilage
G. Ossification is completed as the proximal epiphysis joins with the diaphysis between the twentieth and twenty-fifth year of life

Marrow

A. Fills spaces of spongy bone
B. Contains blood vessels and blood cells in various stages of development
C. Red bone marrow
  1. Site of formation of red blood cells and some white blood cells

  2. Found in spongy bone of adults
    a. Sternum
    b. Ribs
    c. Vertebrae
    d. Proximal epiphysis of long bones
D. Yellow bone marrow
E. Fatty marrow—replaces red bone marrow in the adult, except in areas mentioned above

Types of Bones

A. Long bones—e.g., femur and humerus
B. Short bones—e.g., wrist and ankle bones
C. Flat bones—e.g., ribs, scapulae
D. Irregular bones—e.g., vertebrae and sesamoids (patella)

Descriptive Terminology for Bones

A. Projections
  1. Process—prominence
  2. Spine—sharp prominence
  3. Tubercle—rounded projection
  4. Tuberosity—larger rounded projection
  5. Trochanter—very large bony prominence
  6. Crest—ridge
  7. Condyle—round process of an articulating bone
  8. Head—enlargement at end of bone
B. Depressions
  1. Fossa—pit
  2. Groove—furrow
  3. Sulcus—synonymous with groove
  4. Sinus—cavity within a bone
  5. Foramen—opening
  6. Meatus—tubelike

Division of the Skeleton

A. Axial skeleton
  1. Seventy-four bones
  2. Upright axis of the skeleton
  3. Consists of:
    a. Skull
    b. Hyoid bone
    c. Vertebral column
    d. Sternum
    e. Ribs
B. Appendicular skeleton
  1. One hundred twenty-six bones
  2. Bones attached to the axial skeleton
    a. Upper and lower extremities
    b. Auditory ossicles—6 bones

Articulations

A. Classified according to:
 1. Structure
 2. Composition
 3. Mobility
B. Fibrous joints (*synarthroses*)
 1. Surfaces of bones almost in direct contact, with limited movement
 2. Generally immovable
 3. No joint cavity or capsule
 4. Examples: skull sutures
C. Cartilaginous joints (*amphiarthroses*)
 1. No joint cavity; contiguous bones united by cartilage and ligaments
 2. Slightly movable
 3. Examples: intervertebral disks, pubic symphysis
D. Synovial joints (*diarthroses*)
 1. Approximating bone surfaces covered with cartilage
 2. Freely movable
 3. Bones held together by a fibrous capsule lined with synovial membrane and ligaments
 4. Examples of movement:
   a. Hinge—permits motion in one plane only (elbow)
   b. Pivot—permits rotary movement in which a ring rotates round a central axis (proximal radioulnar articulation)
   c. Saddle—opposing surfaces are concavo-convex, allowing flexion, extension, adduction, and abduction (carpometacarpal joint of thumb)
   d. Ball and socket—capable of movement in an infinite number of axes; rounded head of one bone moves in a cuplike cavity of the approximating base (hip)
   e. Gliding—articulation of contiguous bones allows only gliding movements (wrist, ankle)
   f. Condyloid—permits movement in two directions at right angles to one another; circumduction occurs, rotation does not (radiocarpal joints)
E. Bursae
 1. Sacs filled with synovial fluid; located where tendons or muscles slide over underlying parts
 2. Some bursae communicate with a joint cavity
 3. Prominent bursae found at the elbow, shoulder, hip, and knee
F. Movements
 1. Gliding
   a. Simplest kind of motion in a joint
   b. Motion of a joint that does not involve any angular or rotary movements
 2. Flexion—decreases the angle formed by the union of two bones
 3. Extension—increases the angle formed by the union of two bones
 4. Abduction—occurs by moving part of the appendicular skeleton away from the median plane of the body
 5. Adduction—occurs by moving part of the appendicular skeleton towards the median plane of the body
 6. Circumduction
   a. Occurs in ball and socket joints
   b. Circumscribes the conic space of one bone by the other bone
 7. Rotation—turning on an axis without being displaced from that axis

Skull Morphology

A. Mesocephalic skull
 1. Considered the "typical" skull
 2. Petrous ridge forms 47-degree angle with MSP
B. Brachycephalic skull
 1. Petrous ridge forms 54-degree angle with MSP
 2. Short from front to back
 3. Broad side to side
 4. Shallow from vertex to base
C. Dolichocephalic
 1. Petrous ridge forms 40-degree angle with MSP
 2. Long from front to back
 3. Narrow side to side
 4. Deep from vertex to base

Axial Skeleton

Skull

A. Cranium (Figs. 5-1 and 5-2)
  1. Superior portion formed by the frontal parietal and occipital bones
  2. Lateral portions formed by the temporal and sphenoid bones
  3. Cranial base formed by the temporal, sphenoid, and ethmoid bones
  4. Fontanelles—soft spots in which ossification is incomplete at birth

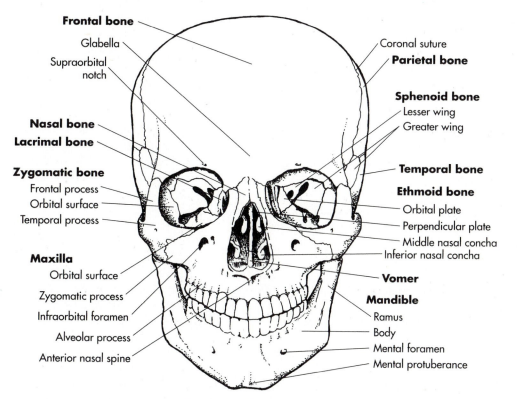

Figure 5-1 Skull: anterior view.

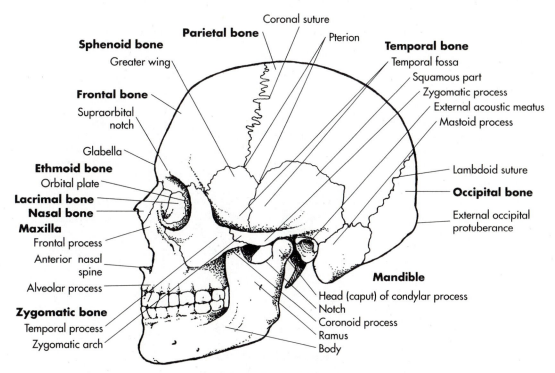

Figure 5-2 Skull: lateral view.

B. Frontal bone
  1. Forms the forehead
  2. Contains the frontal sinuses
  3. Forms the roof of the orbits
  4. Union with the parietal bones forms the coronal suture
C. Parietal bones
  1. Union with the occipital bone forms the lambdoidal suture
  2. Union with the temporal bone forms the squamous suture
  3. Union with the sphenoid bone forms the coronal suture
D. Temporal bones
  1. Contains the external auditory meatus and middle and inner ear structures
  2. Squamous portion—above the meatus; zygomatic process—articulates with the zygoma to form the zygomatic arch
  3. Petrous portion
    a. Contains organs of hearing and equilibrium
    b. Prominent elevation on the floor of the cranium
  4. Mastoid portion
    a. Protuberance behind the ear
    b. Mastoid process
  5. Mandibular fossa—articulates with the condyle on the mandible
  6. Styloid process—anterior to the mastoid process; several neck muscles attach here
  7. Jugular foramen—located between the petrous portion and the occipital bones; opening from which cranial nerves IX, X, and XI exit
E. Sphenoid Bone
  1. Bounded by the ethmoid and frontal bones anteriorly and the temporal and occipital bones posteriorly
  2. Greater wings—lateral projections (Fig. 5-3)

a. Form outer wall and floor of the orbits
b. Foramen rotundum—round, located horizontally in the anteromedial portion of the greater wing adjacent to the lateral wall of the sphenoid sinus; maxillary division of cranial nerve V exits
c. Foramen ovale—oval, located laterally and posteriorly to foramen rotundum; mandibular division of cranial nerve V exits
d. Foramen spinosum—located near posterior angle of the greater wing, lateral and posterior to foramen ovale; transmits an artery to the meninges
e. Foramen lacerum—contains the internal carotid artery
f. Superior orbital fissure—transmits cranial nerves III and IV and part of the cranial nerve V
  3. Lesser wings
    a. Posterior part of the roof of the orbits
    b. Optic foramen—cranial nerve II exits
  4. Body
    a. Sella turcica—holds the pituitary gland (*hypophysis*)
    b. Contains the sphenoid sinuses
    c. Medial and lateral pterygoid processes located here
F. Ethmoid Bone
  1. Contributes to the formation of the base of the cranium, the orbits, and the roof of the nose
  2. Perpendicular plate—forms the superior part of the nasal septum
  3. Horizontal plate (*cribriform plate*)
    a. Located at right angles to the perpendicular plate
    b. Olfactory nerves pass through
    c. Contains the crista galli—meninges of the brain attached to this process
  4. Lateral masses
    a. Form the orbital plates

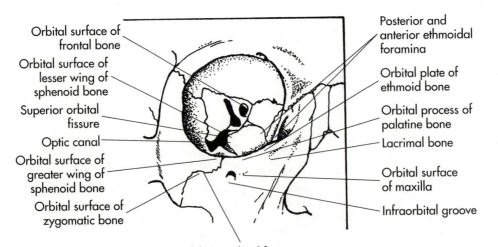

Figure 5-3 Right orbit.

b. Contain the superior and middle conchae (lateral walls of the nose)

c. Contain the ethmoid sinuses

G. Occipital bone
1. Forms the posterior part of the cranium
2. Foramen magnum—spinal cord enters to attach to the brain stem
3. Condyles (2)
   a. On both sides of the foramen magnum
   b. Articulate with depressions on the C1 vertebrae
4. External occipital protuberance—located on the posterior surface

Facial Bones

A. Appear suspended from the middle and anterior parts of the cranium

B. Ethmoid and frontal bones also contribute to the framework of the face

C. All the facial bones, except the mandible, touch the maxilla
1. Alveolar process—forms the upper jaw containing the maxillary teeth
2. Forms the floor of the orbits; infraorbital foramen is inferior from the orbit
3. Forms the walls of the nasal cavities and the hard palate (palatine process)
4. Maxillary sinus—large air space

D. Mandible (Fig. 5-4)
1. Body—central horizontal portion
   a. Chin—symphysis in midline
   b. Alveolar process—contains the mandibular teeth

c. Mental foramen
   (1) Below the first bicuspid on the outer surface
   (2) Transmits nerves and blood vessels
2. Ramus—upward process on both sides of the posterior body of the mandible
   a. Condyle—articulates with the mandibular fossa
   b. Coronoid process—attachment site for the temporalis muscle
   c. Mandibular foramen—located on the inner surface

E. Zygomatic bone
1. Prominence of cheek—attaches to the zygomatic process of the temporal bone to form the zygomatic arch
2. Other margin of the orbit

F. Lacrimal—medial part of the wall of the orbit

G. Nasal bones—upper bridge of the nose

H. Inferior nasal concha
1. Horizontally placed along the lateral wall of the nasal fossa
2. Inferior to the middle and superior conchae of the ethmoid

I. Palatine bones
1. Horizontal plates—form the posterior part of the hard palate
2. Perpendicular plates—form the sphenoid palatine foramen

J. Vomer
1. Plowshare-shaped
2. Forms the lower part of the nasal septum

K. Hyoid
1. U-shaped bone
2. Body

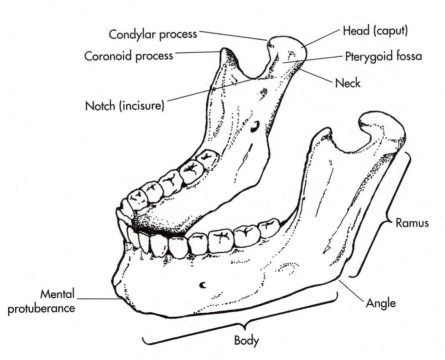

Condylar process

Coronoid process

Notch (incisure)

Head (caput)

Pterygoid fossa

Neck

Ramus

Mental protuberance

Angle

Body

Mandible: anterolateral superior view

Figure 5-4 Mandible.

3. Greater horn
4. Lesser horn
5. Suspended by ligaments from the styloid process

Vertebral Column

A. Part of the axial skeleton
   1. Supports the head
   2. Gives base to the ribs
   3. Encloses the spinal cord
B. Vertebrae
   1. Consists of 34 bones composing the spinal column
     a. Cervical—7 bones
     b. Thoracic—12 bones
     c. Lumbar—5 bones
     d. Sacral—5 bones
     e. Coccygeal—4 to 5 bones
   2. In the adult, the vertebrae of the sacral and coccygeal regions are united into two bones, the sacrum and the coccyx
C. Curvatures—from a lateral view, there are four curves, alternately convex and concave ventrally
   1. Two convex curves are the cervical and lumbar
   2. Two concave curves are the thoracic and sacral
D. Vertebra morphology
   1. Each vertebra differs in size and shape but has similar components
   2. Body—central mass of bone
     a. Weight-bearing
     b. Forms anterior part of vertebrae
   3. Pedicles of the arch—two thick columns that extend backward from the body to meet the laminae of the neural arch
   4. Processes-7 (one spinous [except C1], two transverse, two superior articular, and two inferior articular)
     a. Spinous process extends backward from the point of the union of the two laminae
     b. Transverse processes project laterally on both sides from the junction of the laminae and the pedicle
     c. Articular processes arise near the junction of the pedicle and the laminae—superior processes project upward; inferior processes project downward
     d. Surfaces of the processes are smooth
     e. Inferior articular processes of the vertebrae fit into the superior articular processes below
     f. Form true joints but the contacts established serve to restrict movement

E. Distinguishing features
  1. Cervical region—triangular shape
    a. All have foramina in the transverse processes (upper six transmit the vertebral artery)
    b. Spinous processes are short
      (1) C3 to C5 are bifurcated
      (2) C7 is long prominence felt at the back of the neck
    c. Have small bodies (except for C1 vertebra)
    d. C1 vertebra (atlas) (Fig. 5-5)
      (1) No body
      (2) Anterior and posterior arches and two lateral masses
      (3) Superior articular processes join with the condyles of the occipital bone
    e. C2 vertebra (axis)—process on the upper surface of the body (dens or odontoid) forms a pivot about which the axis rotates

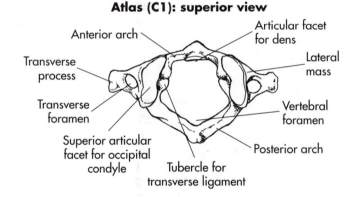

Atlas (C1): superior view

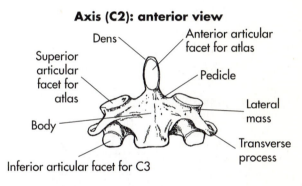

Axis (C2): anterior view

Atlas (C1): inferior view

Axis (C2): posterosuperior view

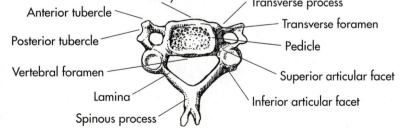

Cervical vertebra: superior view

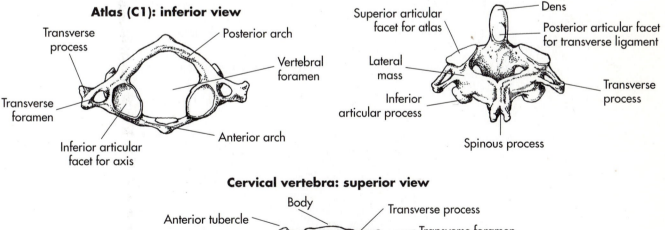

Figure 5-5 Atlas (C1): superior view, atlas (C1): inferior view; axis (C2): anterior view, axis (C2): posterior view; cervical vertebra: superior view.

2. Thoracic region (Fig. 5-6)
   a. Presence of facets for articulation with the ribs
   b. Processes are larger and heavier than those of the cervical region
   c. Spinous process is projected downward at a sharp angle
   d. Circular vertebral foramen
3. Lumbar region (Fig. 5-7)
   a. Large and heavy bodies
   b. Four transverse lines separate the bodies of the vertebrae on the pelvic surface
   c. Triangular shape—fitted between the halves of the pelvis
   d. Four pairs of dorsal sacral foramina communicate with four pairs of pelvic sacral foramina
4. Sacral vertebrae
   a. Formed by fusion of five sacral segments in curved, triangular bone

   b. Base directed obliquely, superiorly, anteriorly
   c. Apex directed posteriorly, inferiorly
   d. Longer, narrower, more vertical in males than females
   e. Body of sacrum has sacral promontory—prominent ridge at upper anterior margin
5. Coccygeal vertebrae
   a. Four to five modular pieces fused together
   b. Triangular shape with the base above and the apex below
6. Defects
   a. Lordosis—exaggerated lumbar concavity
   b. Scoliosis—lateral curvature of any region
   c. Kyphosis—exaggerated convexity in the thoracic region

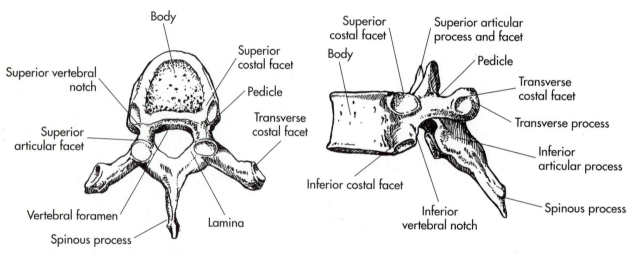

Superior view **Lateral view**

Figure 5-6 Thoracic vertebra: superior view; thoracic vertebra: lateral view.

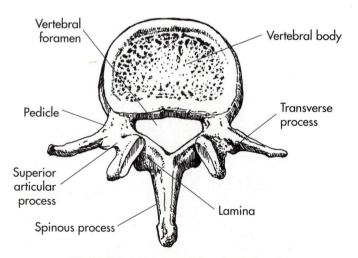

Figure 5-7 Lumbar vertebra: superior view.

Bones of the Thorax

A. Sternum
1. Forms the medial part of the anterior chest wall
2. Manubrium (upper part)—clavicle and first rib articulate with the manubrium; contains notch on superior border called *jugular (manubrial) notch*
3. Body (middle blade)—Ribs articulate with the body via the costal cartilages
4. Xiphoid (blunt cartilaginous tip)

B. Ribs—12 pairs (Fig. 5-8)
1. Each rib articulates with both the body and the transverse process of its corresponding thoracic vertebra
2. The second to ninth ribs articulate with the body of the vertebra above
3. Ribs curve outward, forward, and then downward
4. Anteriorly, each of the first seven ribs joins a costal cartilage that attaches to the sternum (Fig. 5-8)
5. Next three ribs (eighth to tenth) join the cartilage of the rib above
6. Eleventh and twelfth ribs do not attach to the sternum and are called floating ribs

Appendicular Skeleton

Upper Extremity

A. Shoulder—clavicle and scapula (Fig. 5-9A)
1. Clavicle
   a. Articulates with the manubrium at the sternal end
   b. Articulates with the scapula at the lateral end
   c. Slender S-shaped bone that extends horizontally across the upper part of the thorax
2. Scapula (Fig. 5-9B)
   a. Triangular bone with the base upward and the apex downward
   b. Lateral aspect contains the glenoid cavity (fossa) that articulates with the head of the humerus
   c. Spine extends across the upper part of the posterior surface; expands laterally and forms the acromion (point of shoulder)
   d. Coracoid process projects anteriorly from the upper part of the neck of the scapula

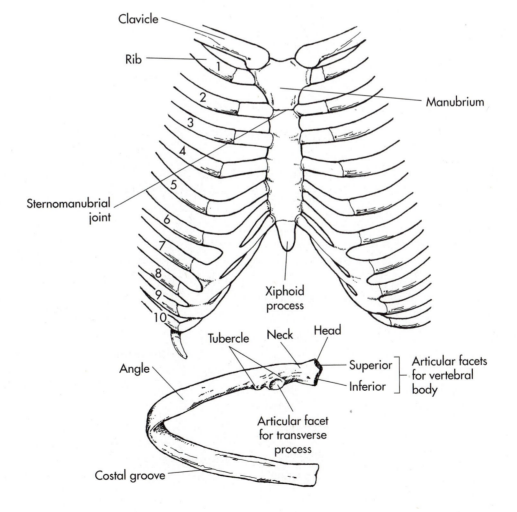

Figure 5-8 Sternocostal articulations: anterior view; middle rib: posterior view.

Humerus and scapula

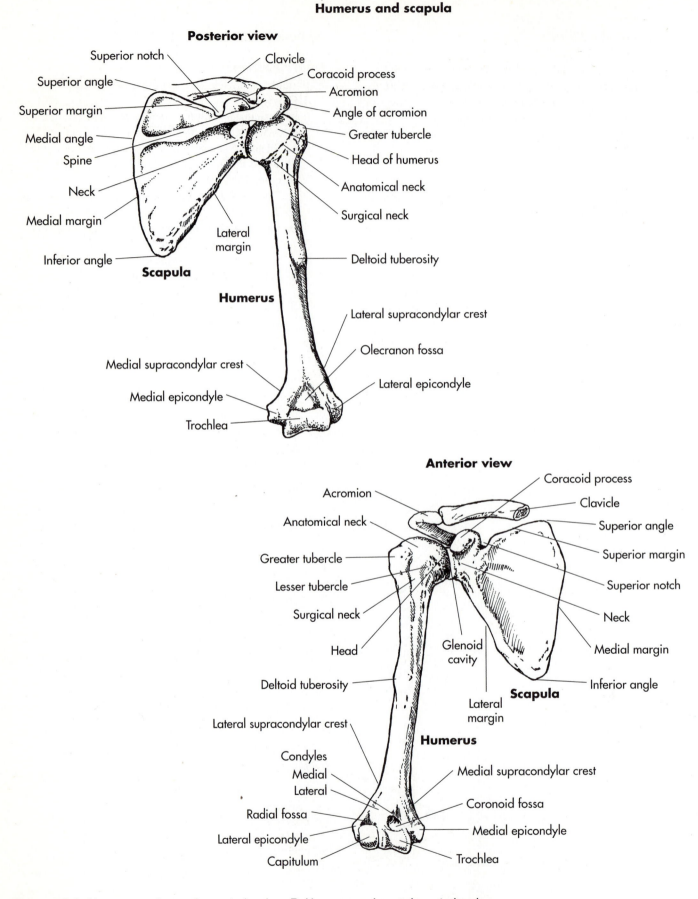

Posterior view

Superior notch
Superior angle
Superior margin
Medial angle
Spine
Neck
Medial margin
Inferior angle
Clavicle
Coracoid process
Acromion
Angle of acromion
Greater tubercle
Head of humerus
Anatomical neck
Surgical neck
Lateral margin
Scapula
Deltoid tuberosity
Humerus
Lateral supracondylar crest
Olecranon fossa
Lateral epicondyle
Medial supracondylar crest
Medial epicondyle
Trochlea

Anterior view

Acromion
Anatomical neck
Greater tubercle
Lesser tubercle
Surgical neck
Head
Deltoid tuberosity
Lateral supracondylar crest
Condyles
Medial
Lateral
Radial fossa
Lateral epicondyle
Capitulum
Coracoid process
Clavicle
Superior angle
Superior margin
Superior notch
Neck
Medial margin
Inferior angle
Scapula
Glenoid cavity
Lateral margin
Humerus
Medial supracondylar crest
Coronoid fossa
Medial epicondyle
Trochlea

Figure 5-9 A. Humerus and scapula: posterior view, **B.** Humerus and scapula: anterior view.

B. Humerus
1. Consists of a shaft (*diaphysis*) and two ends (*epiphyses*)
2. Proximal end has a head that articulates with the glenoid cavity (*fossa*) of the scapula
3. Greater and lesser tubercles lie below the head
   a. Intertubercular groove (*bicipital groove*) is located between them; long tendon of the biceps attaches here
   b. Surgical neck is located below the tubercles
4. Radial groove runs obliquely on the posterior surface; radial nerve is located here
5. Deltoid muscles attach in a V-shaped area in the middle of the shaft called the deltoid tuberosity

6. Distal end has two projections, the medial and lateral epicondyles
   a. Capitulum—articulates with the radius
   b. Trochlea—articulates with the ulna
C. Forearm (Fig. 5-10)
1. Radius
   a. Lateral bone of the forearm
   b. Radial tubercle (*tuberosity*) is located below the head on the medial side
   c. Proximal end has disklike head
   d. Neck located just inferior to head
   e. Distal end is broad for articulation with the wrist
   f. Has styloid process on its lateral side

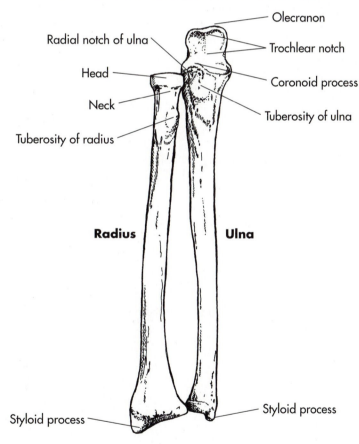

Radius and ulna in supination: anterior view

Olecranon

Radial notch of ulna

Trochlear notch

Head

Coronoid process

Neck

Tuberosity of ulna

Tuberosity of radius

Radius

Ulna

Styloid process

Styloid process

Figure 5-10 Forearm.

2. Ulna
   a. Medial bone of the forearm
   b. Conspicuous part of the elbow joint (*olecranon*)
   c. Curved surface that articulates with the trochlea of the humerus is the trochlear notch
   d. Lateral side is concave (*radial notch*); articulates with the head of the radius
   e. Distal end contains the styloid process
D. Hand and wrist (Fig. 5-11)
   1. Carpal bones—8
      a. Arranged in two rows of four

   b. (From lateral to medial, proximal row) scaphoid, lunate, triquetrum, pisiform
   c. (From lateral to medial, distal row) trapezium, trapezoid, capitate, and hamate
2. Metacarpal bones—5
   a. Framework of the hand
   b. Numbered 1 through 5, beginning on the lateral side
   c. Phalanges—14
      (1) Form the fingers
      (2) Three phalanges in each finger; two phalanges in the thumb

Right hand: palmar view　　　　**Right hand: dorsal view**

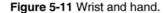

Figure 5-11 Wrist and hand.

Lower Extremity

A. Hip (os coxae or innominate) (Fig. 5-12)
  1. Constitutes the pelvic girdle
  2. United with the vertebral column
  3. Union of three parts that is marked by a cup-shaped cavity (*acetabulum*)
  4. Ilium
    a. Prominence of the hip
    b. Superior border is the crest
    c. Anterior superior iliac spine (ASIS)—projection at the anterior tip of the crest (just inferior to the ASIS is the anterior inferior iliac spine)
    d. Corresponding projections on the posterior part are the posterior superior and posterior inferior iliac spines
    e. Greater sciatic notch—located beneath the articular surface
    f. Most is a smooth concavity (*iliac fossa*)
    g. Posteriorly it is rough and articulates with the sacrum in the formation of the sacroiliac joint
  5. Pubic bone
    a. Anterior part of the innominate bone
    b. Symphysis pubis—joining of the right and left pubic bones at the midline
    c. Body and two rami
      (1) Body forms one fifth of the acetabulum
      (2) Superior ramus extends from the body to the median plane; superior border forms the pubic crest

  (3) Inferior ramus extends downward and meets with the ischium
  (4) Pubic arch is formed by the inferior rami of both pubic bones
  6. Ischium
    a. Forms the lower and back part of the innominate bone
    b. Body
      (1) Forms two fifths of the acetabulum
      (2) Ischial tuberosity supports the body in a sitting position
    c. Ramus—passes upward to join the inferior ramus of the pubis
    d. Opening created by this ring is known as the obturator foramen

B. Pelvis
  1. Formed by the right and left hip bones, sacrum, and coccyx
  2. Greater pelvis
    a. Bounded by the ilia and lower lumbar vertebrae
    b. Gives support to the abdominal viscera
  3. Lesser pelvis
    a. Brim of the pelvis corresponds to the sacral promontory
    b. Inferior outlet is bounded by the tip of the coccyx, ischial tuberosities, and inferior rami of the pubic bones
  4. Female pelvis
    a. Shows adaptations related to functions as a birth canal
    b. Wide outlet
    c. Angle of the pubic arch is obtuse

Coxal bone: lateral view

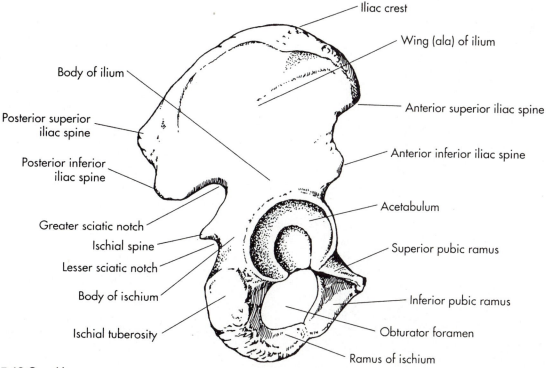

Figure 5-12 Coxal bone.

5. Male pelvis
   a. Shows adaptations that contribute to power and speed
   b. Heart-shaped outlet
   c. Angle of the pubic arch is acute
C. Femur (Fig. 5-13)
   1. Longest and strongest bone of the body

2. Proximal end has a rounded head that articulates with the acetabulum
3. Constricted portion—neck
4. Greater and lesser trochanters connected by intertrochanteric crest
5. Slightly arched shaft; is concave posteriorly
6. Distal end has two condyles separated on the posterior side by the intercondyloid fossa

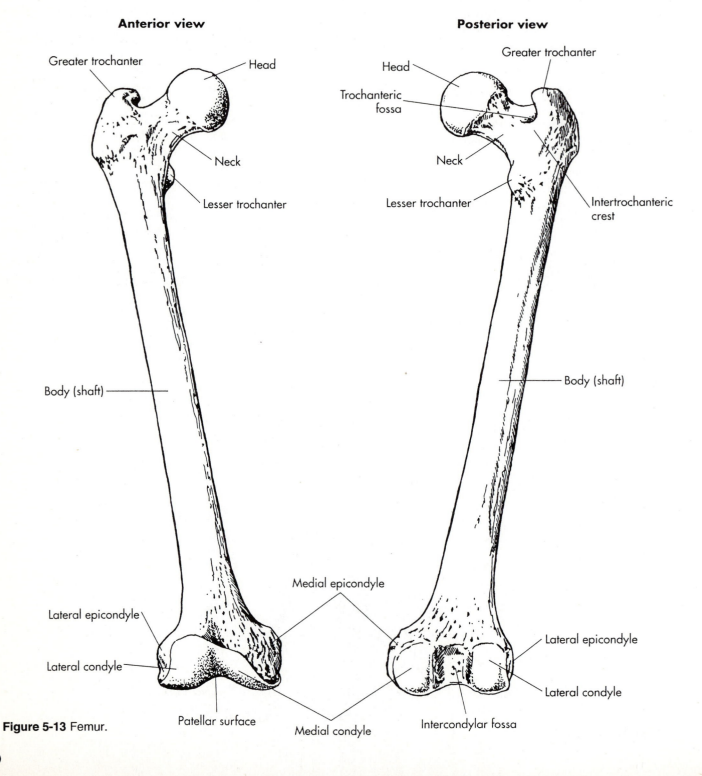

Anterior view

Greater trochanter

Head

Neck

Lesser trochanter

Body (shaft)

Lateral epicondyle

Lateral condyle

Patellar surface

Medial epicondyle

Medial condyle

Posterior view

Head

Greater trochanter

Trochanteric fossa

Neck

Lesser trochanter

Intertrochanteric crest

Body (shaft)

Lateral epicondyle

Lateral condyle

Intercondylar fossa

Figure 5-13 Femur.

D. Patella
　1. Sesamoid bone
　2. Embedded in the tendon of the quadriceps muscle
　3. Articulates with the femur
E. Leg (Fig. 5-14)
　1. Tibia—medial bone
　　a. Proximal end has two condyles that articulate with the femur

b. Triangular shaft
　(1) Anterior—shin
　(2) Posterior—soleal line
　(3) Distal—medial malleolus that articulates with the lattice that forms the ankle joint
2. Fibula—lateral bone
　a. Articulates with the lateral condyle of the tibia but does not enter the knee joint
　b. Distal end projects as the lateral malleolus

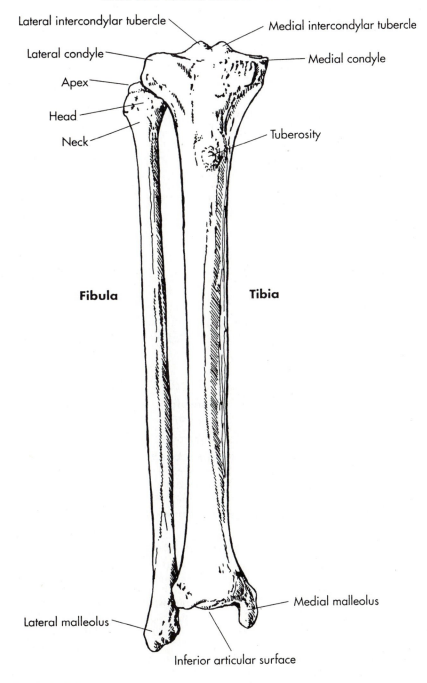

Tibia and fibula: anterior view

Lateral intercondylar tubercle
Medial intercondylar tubercle
Lateral condyle
Medial condyle
Apex
Head
Neck
Tuberosity
Fibula
Tibia
Lateral malleolus
Medial malleolus
Inferior articular surface

Figure 5-14 Tibia and fibula.

F. Ankle, foot, and toes (Fig. 5-15 A and B)
1. Adapted for supporting weight but similar in structure to the hand
2. Talus
   a. Occupies the uppermost and central portion of the tarsus

b. Distributes the body weight from the tibia above to the other tarsal bones
3. Calcaneus (os calcis, heel)—located beneath the talus
4. Navicular—located in front of the talus on the medial side; articulates with three cuneiform bones distally

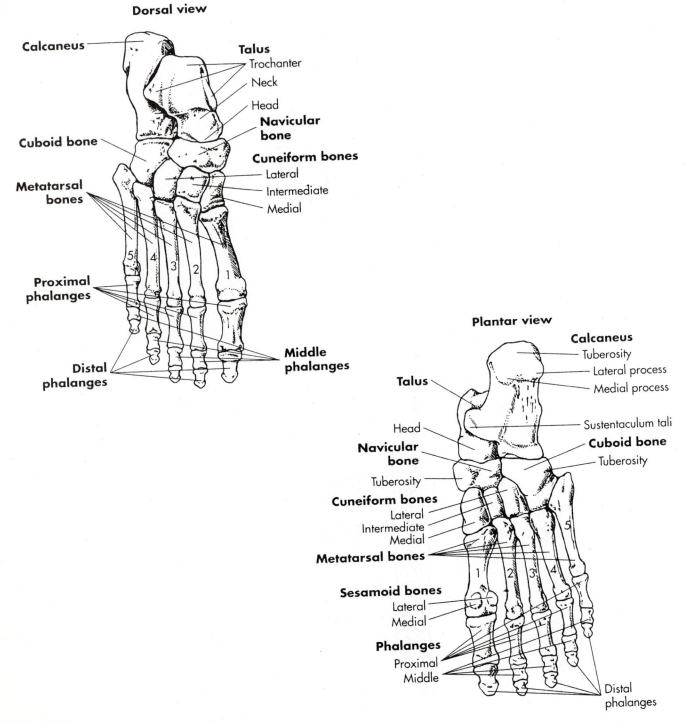

Figure 5-15A Foot. Dorsal view, plantar view.

5. Cuboid—lies along the lateral border of the navicular bone

6. Metatarsals
   a. First, second, and third metatarsals lie in front of the three cuneiform bones
   b. Fourth and fifth metatarsals lie in front of the cuboid bone

7. Phalanges
   a. Distal to the metatarsals
   b. Two in the great toe; three in each of the other four toes

8. Longitudinal arches of the foot—2
   a. Lateral—formed by the calcaneus, talus, cuboid, and fourth and fifth metatarsal bones
   b. Medial—formed by the calcaneus, talus, navicular, cuneiform and first, second, and third metatarsal bones

9. Transverse arches—formed by the tarsal and metatarsal bones

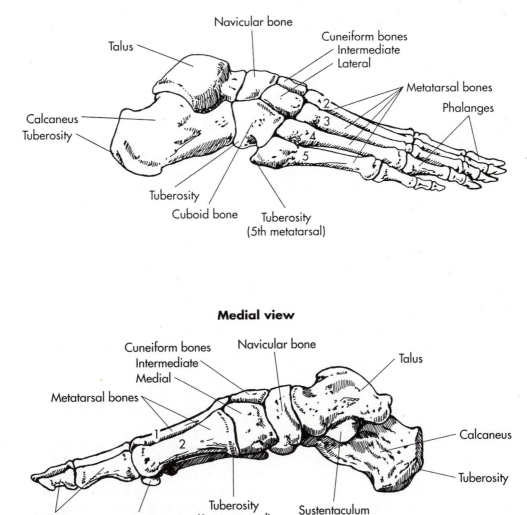

Lateral view

Medial view

Figure 5-15B Foot. Lateral view, medial view.

Nervous System

A. Adapts to environmental influences
   1. By stimulating skeletal, cardiac, and smooth muscles
   2. Adaptation by the muscular system is almost immediate
B. Organized into various systems
   1. Central nervous system (CNS)
      a. Consists of the brain and spinal cord
   2. Peripheral nervous system (PNS)
      a. Contains the nerves to and from the body wall that connect to the CNS
      b. Also known as the somatic division because it is under voluntary control
   3. Autonomic nervous system (ANS)
      a. Not under conscious control (involuntary)
      b. Provides stimulus for the viscera and smooth and cardiac muscles
      c. Sympathetic division includes motor (afferent) nerves from the ANS
      d. Parasympathetic division involves motor (efferent) nerves from the ANS
C. Nerve cell—neuron
   1. Dendrite carries impulse toward the cell body under normal conditions
   2. Axon carries impulse away from the cell body and makes contact with the next cell; release of chemicals starts impulse in the next neuron
   3. Myelin sheath—fatty substance around some cell axons provides insulation
   4. Neurons can carry impulses in different directions
      a. Afferent neurons carry the sensory information to the CNS
      b. Efferent neurons carry the motor information away from the CNS
   5. Central neurons are found entirely within the CNS; relay information within the system
      a. Spinal cord is approximately 45.8 cm long; occupies the upper two thirds of the vertebral canal
      b. There are 31 pairs of spinal nerves; each has a dorsal (afferent) route and a ventral (efferent) route
D. Brain—consists of four regions
   1. Cerebrum
      a. Seat of conscious activities
      b. Largest portion of the brain
      c. Located most superiorly
      d. Cerebral cortex—thin outside layer; gray color; consists of several layers of cells; convoluted surface
      e. Longitudinal fissure—divides into two hemispheres
      f. Corpus callosum—heavy band of white fibers; forms the floor of the longitudinal fissure
      g. Central fissure—posterior to the midline
      h. Frontal lobe—anterior to the central fissure
      i. Parietal lobe—posterior to the central fissure
      j. Temporal lobe—below the lateral fissure
      k. Occipital lobe—posterior part of the brain
      l. Broca's area—controls the muscular part of speech
      m. Somatesthetic area—interprets body sensations
      n. Visual area—fibers from the medial part of the retina cross to opposite sides in the brain; fibers from the lateral portion do not cross
      o. Auditory area—superior central portion of the temporal lobe
      p. Prefrontal area—personality characteristics
   2. Cerebellum—coordinates balance and equilibrium
   3. Medulla oblongata
      a. Bulb of the spinal cord located inside the foramen magnum
      b. White on the outside, gray on the inside
      c. Controls three vital functions—cardiac, respiratory, and basal motor
      d. Also controls chewing, salivation, swallowing, emesis, lacrimation, blinking, coughing, and sneezing
      e. Pons—ropelike mass of white fibers; connects the halves of the cerebellum
   4. Mesencephalon
      a. Short part of the brain stem
      b. Above the pons
      c. Mostly white matter
E. Meninges—membranous coverings of the brain and spinal cord
   1. Dura mater
      a. Double layer around the brain
      b. Single layer around the spinal cord including the cauda equina
   2. Arachnoid
      a. Membrane just inside the dura mater
      b. Relatively thin
   3. Pia mater
      a. Soft covering that fits against the brain and spinal cord
      b. Contains an enormous amount of blood
   4. Subarachnoid space
      a. Threadlike structure where cerebrospinal fluid circulates
      b. Located between the pia mater and arachnoid
F. Cranial nerves
   1. Part of the PNS
   2. Originate at the base of the brain
   3. Twelve pairs of cranial nerves
   4. Referred to by name or by Roman numerals
   5. Provide motor impulses, sensory impulses, or mixed impulses

Heart

A. Composed of cardiac muscle and serves to pump the blood through the circulatory system
B. Located behind the sternum
C. The size of a human fist
D. The apex of the heart points down and to the left
E. Located in a space between the lungs and the thoracic cavity known as the mediastinum
F. Consists of four chambers—two atria and two ventricles
  1. Blood from the superior and inferior vena cava fills the right atrium and passes into the right ventricle through the tricuspid valve
  2. From the right ventricle the unoxygenated blood is sent to the lungs by passing through the semilunar valve and the pulmonary artery
  3. Oxygenated blood is sent from the lungs to the left atrium through the pulmonary veins; the left semilunar valve separates the left atrium from the pulmonary veins
  4. From the left atrium blood flows through the mitral valve into the left ventricle
  5. Blood enters circulation by passing through the left semilunar valve into the aorta
G. Heart wall consists of three layers
  1. Visceral pericardium or epicardium
  2. Myocardium—heaviest covering
  3. Endocardium—smooth continuous covering
  4. All valves and chambers are lined by endothelium
H. Heart beat
  1. Averages 70 to 72 beats per minute
  2. Cannot contract without nerve impulses
  3. Nerves regulate the rate of the beat
I. Cardiac cycle
  1. Consists of a relaxation-contraction cycle
  2. Lasts for approximately .8 second
J. Electrocardiogram is a record of the action current as it travels across the heart

Circulatory System

A. Overview
  1. The connection of the heart to the arteries, arterioles, capillaries, venules, and veins
  2. The lymphatic system, which also interacts with the circulatory system
B. Arteries
  1. Thick-walled elastic vessels
  2. End in arterioles
C. Arterioles
  1. The smallest branch of an artery
  2. Connected to venules by capillaries
D. Capillaries
  1. Connect arterioles to venules
  2. Are lined by a thin layer of endothelium
  3. Capillaries can dilate or constrict depending on the tissue's needs
  4. Red blood cells go through capillaries one cell at a time
E. Venules
  1. Connected to veins that carry blood toward the heart and carry unoxygenated blood (except in the pulmonary vein)
F. Veins
  1. Have the same layers as arteries, except they are thinner
  2. Veins will collapse without blood
  3. Valves in the veins help to resist the forces of gravity
G. Arteriovenous shunt (*anastomosis*)
  1. A large blood vessel that connects an artery and vein directly
  2. Skin color is caused by blood in the capillaries and anastomosis; important for heat distribution
  3. Found only in the hands, face, and toes where the body is exposed to weather

Arterial Systemic Circulation

A. Aorta
  1. Arises from the left ventricle of the heart
  2. First 5 cm is called the ascending aorta
  3. Two left and right coronary arteries branch off directly above the left semilunar valve and supply blood to the cardiac muscle
B. Aortic arch
  1. Loops back over the top of the heart and left of the trachea
  2. Continues down in back of the heart
  3. Three arteries come off the arch
    a. Brachiocephalic
      (1) Only a few centimeters in length
      (2) Right subclavian artery arises from brachiocephalic artery and supplies blood to the right shoulder
      (3) Right common carotid artery arises from brachiocephalic artery and supplies blood to the right side of the head
    b. Left common carotid artery supplies blood to the left side of the head
    c. Left subclavian artery supplies branches to the upper chest and scapula
C. Carotid arteries
  1. Supply the head
  2. Right carotid artery originates from the brachiocephalic artery
  3. Left carotid artery originates from the aortic arch
D. Subclavian arteries
  1. Provide blood to the shoulder and arm
  2. Left one comes from the aortic arch
  3. Right one comes from the brachiocephalic artery
  4. Pass over the first rib and under the clavicle
  5. Become the axillary arteries as they pass through the shoulder region

6. First branch off the subclavian artery is the vertebral artery

E. Vertebral artery
1. Passes up the neck through the transverse foramen of the cervical vertebrae
2. Enters the skull through the foramen magnum
3. The two paired arteries join on the ventral side of the medulla and become the basilar artery (this artery joins branches from the internal carotid artery to form the Circle of Willis, also called the cerebral arterial circle)

F. Axillary artery
1. Becomes the brachial artery at the humerus
2. Moves along the medial surface across the elbow region and then divides into radial and ulnar arteries

G. Radial artery
1. Moves along the radius and crosses it at the distal end
2. A pulse can be felt at the distal end
3. Moves across the metacarpals and deep into the palm
4. Forms a loop that connects with the ulnar artery

H. Ulnar artery
1. Travels down the medial surface of the forearm
2. Becomes the superficial palmar artery that joins with the radial artery
3. Digital arteries supply the fingers and branch off from the palmar loop

I. Descending aorta—consists of the thoracic and abdominal sections of the aorta
1. Thoracic aorta
   a. Starts after the left subclavian artery branches off the aortic arch
   b. Extends from T4-T5 to T12-L1
   c. Passes down and in front of the vertebral column and through the diaphragm
   d. Gives off several branches supplying the ribs, lungs, and diaphragm
   e. After it passes through the diaphragm it is called the abdominal aorta
2. Abdominal aorta
   a. Extends to the L4 vertebra
   b. Gives rise to the visceral and parietal arteries
   c. Celiac artery—visceral artery that is 1.5 cm long; it divides into:
      (1) Left gastric artery—smallest branch to the stomach
      (2) Hepatic artery—supplies most of the blood to the liver, divides at the liver
         (a) Cystic artery—serves the gallbladder
         (b) Gastric duodenal artery—divides to serve the stomach, pancreas, and duodenum
      (3) Splenic artery—largest branch to the spleen
   d. Superior mesenteric artery—supplies all of the small intestine except the duodenum and superior ascending and transverse portion of the colon; comes off the front of the aorta below the celiac artery

e. Inferior mesenteric artery—supplies blood for part of the transverse colon and all of the descending and sigmoid colon, rectum, and bladder
f. Renal artery—supplies the kidneys; located below the superior mesenteric artery
   (1) Right renal artery slightly longer and lower because the aorta is slightly left of the midline
   (2) Enters the kidney at the hilus
g. Suprarenal artery—branches off the aorta above the renal artery (may be branches of the renal arteries)
h. Aorta then bifurcates and becomes the right and left common iliac arteries

J. Common iliac arteries—bifurcate
1. Internal iliac artery supplies the pelvic wall and viscera
2. External iliac artery goes into the thigh
   a. Passes over the pelvic brim and under the inguinal ligament
   b. Becomes the femoral artery

K. Femoral artery—supplies thigh
1. Becomes the popliteal artery just above the knee and goes behind the knee to bifurcate
   a. Anterior tibial artery
   b. Posterior tibial artery
   c. Anterior and posterior tibial arteries spread out at the ankle and become the dorsal artery of the foot

Venous Systemic Circulation

A. Consists of one set of superficial veins and one set of deep veins
B. Veins have a higher blood capacity than the arteries but have lower blood pressure and velocity than the arteries
C. Three sets of veins that connect to the heart
1. Vena cavae-superior and inferior
   a. Serve the body
   b. Return unoxygenated blood
2. Coronary sinus
   a. Serves the heart
   b. Returns unoxygenated blood
3. Pulmonary veins
   a. Serve the lungs (two per lung)
   b. Return oxygenated blood to the left atrium
D. Superior vena cava
1. Begins at the level of the first rib
2. Is formed by two veins
   a. Left and right brachiocephalic veins (return blood from the head, shoulders, and arms)
   b. Each brachiocephalic vein is a union of the internal jugular vein with the subclavian vein
E. Jugular veins drain blood from the head
1. External jugular vein
   a. Drains the face and the scalp
   b. Is the union of three main veins that unite just below the ear and empty into the subclavian vein

2. Internal jugular vein
   a. Returns from the internal carotid vein
   b. Originates in the skull

F. Vertebral veins
   1. Arise outside of the skull at the level of the atlas
   2. Pass through the transverse foramen to the subclavian artery

G. Arms and shoulders are drained by the deep veins that run alongside the arteries

H. Inferior vena cava
   1. Formed by two common iliac veins at the L5 vertebra in front of the vertebral column

I. Azygos vein
   1. Branches off the inferior vena cava at the level of the renal veins
   2. Goes through the aortic hiatus of the diaphragm just below the heart
   3. Empties into the superior vena cava
   4. Picks up veins from the esophagus and bronchi

J. Other veins serving the abdomen and thorax are named for the region or organs that they serve

K. Veins of the lower extremities
   1. Deep veins have the same names as the arteries
   2. Superficial veins
      a. Great saphenous vein—drains the dorsalis pedis of the foot
      b. Small saphenous vein—drains the lateral side of the foot
      c. Popliteal vein—drains the lateral side of the leg

Lymphatic System

A. Carries lymph

B. Involved in the maintenance of fluid pressure

C. Contains lymph glands that filter foreign particles
   1. Tissue fluid is located in the intracellular spaces and is derived from the blood
   2. Is constantly moving
   3. Similar to plasma without large proteins

D. Lymph is tissue fluid that has been reabsorbed into lymphatic vessels

E. Valves are necessary in the lymphatic system
   1. To keep fluid flowing in the right direction
   2. Most valves are located in the arms and legs where gravity is a problem

F. Lymph nodes
   1. Spongy masses of tissue through which lymph filters
   2. Have more afferent vessels coming to the node than efferent vessels leaving the node

G. Lymphocytes are small white blood cells that originate from stem cells

H. Right lymphatic duct
   1. Drains the upper right quadrant of the thorax, right arm, and right side of the head
   2. Empties into the right subclavian vein

I. Thoracic duct
   1. Drains the rest of the body
   2. Begins at the cisterna chyli
   3. Passes up the left side of the vertebral column, through the aortic hiatus of the diaphragm, into the left subclavian vein

J. Lymphoidal tissue is found in various anatomic structures
   1. Spleen—the graveyard of red blood cells
   2. Thymus—atrophies after puberty but is involved in the cell-mediated immune system
   3. Tonsils—located in the oral cavity

Respiratory System

A. Respiratory tract—begins at the nostril opening and extends to the alveoli of the lungs

B. Air is drawn in through the nose where it is warmed, humidified, and cleansed

C. Nasal cavity is lined with olfactory epithelium in the sphenoethmoid recess and by respiratory epithelium in the lower part

D. Superior, middle, and inferior turbinates are located on the lateral surface of the nasal cavity

E. Frontal, ethmoidal, maxillary, and sphenoidal sinuses empty into the nasal cavity

F. Pharynx
   1. Second part of the respiratory tract
   2. Starts at the base of the skull and extends to the esophagus
   3. Divided into three parts
      a. Nasopharynx—located behind the nasal cavity
         (1) Eustachian tube (auditory tube)—connects the middle ear with the pharynx; open only during swallowing; functions to equalize pressure
         (2) Pharyngeal tonsils (adenoids)—located on the upper back wall of the nasopharynx; it is a mass of lymphoid tissue
      b. Oropharynx—extends from the soft palate to the base of the tongue; separated from the oral cavity by the palatine arches
      c. Laryngopharynx—extends from the hyoid bone to larynx

G. Larynx
   1. Located at the base of the tongue
   2. Made up of nine cartilages

H. Vocal chords
   1. Folds of mucous membranes
   2. Elastic connective tissue at the edges

I. Trachea
   1. Approximately 12 cm long
   2. Located in front of the esophagus
   3. Composed of 16 to 20 C-shaped rings that prevent its collapse
   4. At the end of the T4 vertebra, the trachea divides into left and right branches known as the primary bronchi

J. Primary bronchi
　1. Left primary bronchus is longer than the right and forms a sharp angle
　2. Right primary bronchus has a larger diameter than the left and comes off almost forming a straight line
K. Secondary bronchi branch off the primary bronchi
　1. Three secondary bronchi for the right lung, one per lobe
　2. Two secondary bronchi for the left lung, one per lobe
L. Tertiary bronchi
　1. Branch off the secondary bronchi
　2. Ten tertiary bronchi per lung because there are 10 segments per lung
M. Bronchioles—smaller branches of the tertiary bronchi
　1. Terminal bronchiole—not involved in gaseous exchange
　2. Respiratory bronchiole—branch off the terminal bronchiole; first site of diffusion of oxygen into the blood
N. Alveolar ducts
　1. Branch off the respiratory bronchiole
　2. Alveolar sacs attach to the alveolar ducts
O. Two cone-shaped lungs in the thoracic cavity
　1. Base rests on the diaphragm
　2. Apex is located at the level of the clavicle
　3. Right lung
　　a. Has three lobes—superior, middle, and inferior
　　b. Larger than the left lung
　4. Left lung
　　a. Smaller than the right lung because two thirds of the heart is located on the left side
　　b. Contains only two lobes
　5. Ten bronchiopulmonary segments per lung
　　a. Each has a branch from the tertiary bronchi
　　b. Used as points of reference for surgery
P. Cardiac notch—depression on the medial surface of the left lung
　1. Hilus
　　a. Point of attachment to a lung
　　b. Blood vessels, bronchial tree, and nerves enter at the hilus
Q. Pleura—serous membrane surrounding the visceral and parietal layers of each lung
　1. Space between the two layers is the pleural cavity
　2. Lungs are not located in the pleural cavity
R. Mechanics of respiration
　1. Involve changing the pressure in the lungs to cause inspiration or expiration
　2. Inspiration
　　a. Occurs when the air pressure in the lungs is decreased
　　b. Causes the volume of the lungs to increase
　　c. External intercostal muscles cause the ribs to elevate and increase the size of the chest cavity
　　d. Dome-shaped diaphragm between the thoracic and abdominal cavities pulls downward when contracted
　　e. Also increases the size of the chest cavity
　3. Expiration
　　a. Basically a passive movement
　　b. Ribs fall down
　　c. Diaphragm is pushed up by the abdominal viscera
　　d. Abdominal muscles force the abdominal contents upward
　　e. Internal intercostal muscles pull the ribs downward

Digestive System

A. Digestive or alimentary tract
　1. Consists of a tube 6 meters long from the mouth to the anus
　2. Selectively absorbs nutrients and water for the body
B. Mouth
　1. Site at which food processing and digestion begins
　2. Secondary teeth tear and grind the food
C. Tongue
　　a. Fibromuscular organ
　　b. Contains the taste buds
　　c. Transmits the sensation of taste to the brain
　　d. Rolls the food into a bolus for swallowing
D. Saliva
　1. Added to help food become a bolus for easier passage down the esophagus
　2. Produced by three major paired glands and many minor glands
E. Salivary glands
　1. Parotid glands
　　a. Located in the preauricular region
　　b. Saliva travels down Stensen's duct (*parotid duct*) which opens opposite the second maxillary molar
　2. Sublingual glands
　　a. Lie under the tongue and rest against the mandible
　　b. Saliva travels down Bartholin's duct and enters the oral cavity through Rivinus's ducts (*lesser sublingual ducts*) on the sublingual fold
　3. Submandibular glands
　　a. Lie on the medial surface of the mandible
　　b. Saliva travels down Wharton's duct (*submandibular duct*) and is released into the mouth at the sublingual caruncles
F. Swallowing
　1. Bolus of food is conducted from the mouth and pharynx to the esophagus
　2. During swallowing, the soft palate is pushed back against the posterior pharyngeal wall, closing the passage to the nasopharynx
　3. Larynx is elevated, superior opening is protected by the epiglottis
　4. Bolus moves into esophagus
　5. Esophagus—a muscular tube located posterior to the trachea and connected to the stomach

6. Bolus moved through esophagus by peristalsis and gravity
G. Stomach—dilated portion of the alimentary canal lying in the upper abdomen just under the diaphragm (Figs. 5-16 and 5-17)
　1. Functions
　　a. Stores food
　　b. Digests—secretes pepsin, renin, and gastric lipase
　　c. Produces hydrochloric acid

2. Shaped like the letter *J*—internal surface is wrinkled (*rugae*)
　a. Cardiac portion—where esophagus enters
　b. Body—main part
　c. Fundus—bulge at the upper end, left of the esophageal area
　d. Pyloric portion—narrow distal end which connects with the small intestine

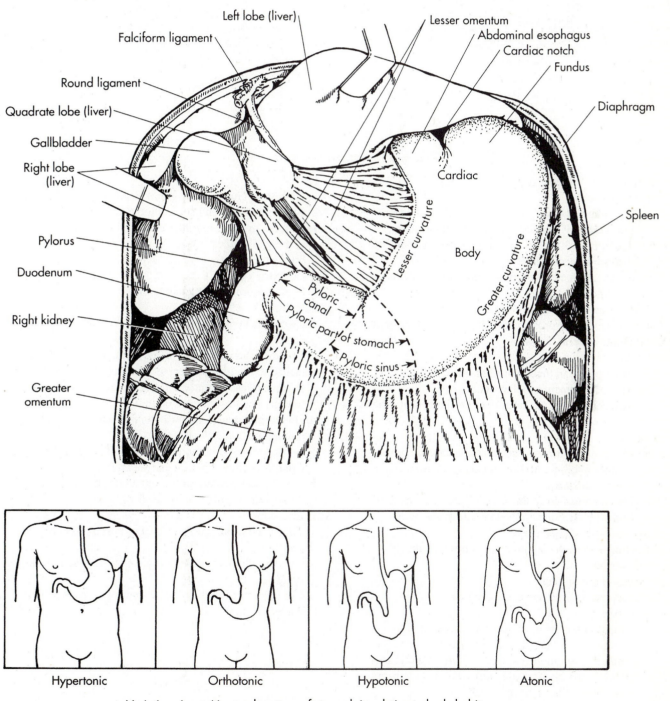

Variations in position and contour of stomach in relation to body habitus

Hypertonic　Orthotonic　Hypotonic　Atonic

Figure 5-16 Stomach.

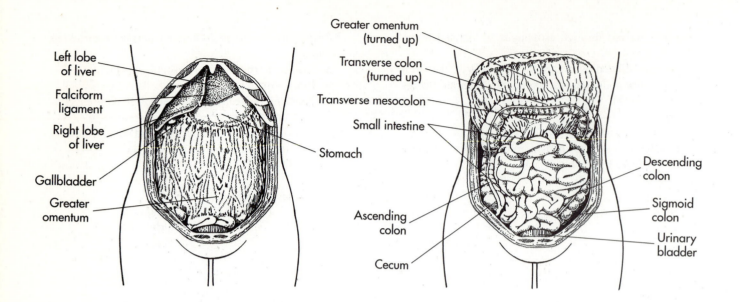

Figure 5-17 Abdominal viscera.

H. Small intestine—thin-walled muscular tube
   1. Three portions
      a. Duodenum (horseshoe-shaped)—bile and pancreatic secretions are added to the small intestine
      b. Jejunum (1.5 meters long)—greatest amount of absorption occurs here
      c. Ileum (2.5 meters long)—connects with the large intestine
   2. Secretes several enzymes and substances
I. Large intestine—approximately 1.5 meters long and divided into several divisions
   1. Cecum
      a. Blind pouch in the lower right quadrant
      b. Appendix attaches to the cecum
      c. Ileocecal sphincter separates the ileum from the cecum
   2. Colon
      a. Ascending—from the cecum to the hepatic flexure
      b. Transverse—from the hepatic flexure to the splenic flexure
      c. Descending—from the splenic flexure to the level of the pelvic bone on the left side of the body
   3. Sigmoid—S-shaped curve
   4. Rectum—from the sigmoid colon down to the pelvic diaphragm
   5. Anus—3 cm in length
J. Pancreas—endocrine and exocrine gland
   1. Exocrine
      a. Produces pancreatic juice that is collected by the pancreatic duct (Wirsung's duct) and carried away
      b. Joins the common bile duct to form Vater's ampulla (hepatopancreatic ampulla), which penetrates the walls of the abdomen
   2. Endocrine—releases insulin that controls blood glucose levels; also releases glucagon and somatostatin

K. Liver
   1. Largest and most active gland in the body
   2. Two main lobes and several lobules
   3. Lobules produce bile that is carried away and stored in the gallbladder
   4. Stores glycogen
   5. Detoxifies waste
   6. Plays major role in metabolism
L. Bile ducts
   1. Two main hepatic ducts join to form common hepatic duct
   2. Common hepatic duct unites with cystic duct (attached to the gallbladder) to form common bile duct
   3. In some cases, common bile duct joins pancreatic duct to enter hepatopancreatic ampulla
   4. Hepatopancreatic ampulla opens into descending duodenum
   5. In other cases, common bile duct and pancreatic duct enter duodenum directly and separately
   6. Distal end of common bile duct controlled by hepatopancreatic sphincter (*sphincter of Oddi*)
M. Gallbladder
   1. Thin-walled sac with capacity of approximately two ounces
   2. Concentrates and stores bile and evacuates bile during digestion
   3. Contraction of gallbladder is controlled by hormone cholecystokinin

Urinary System

A. Kidneys (Fig. 5-18)
   1. Paired bean-shaped organs on both sides of the vertebral column
   2. Renal artery and vein and the ureter (which leads to the bladder) are attached to the center of the kidney at the hilus

3. Outer part of the kidney is designated the cortex and the inner part, the medulla
   a. Medulla consists of several pyramids
   b. Apices of the pyramids project into the calices
   c. Nephron is the functional unit of the kidney
4. Kidney connected to the bladder by the ureters

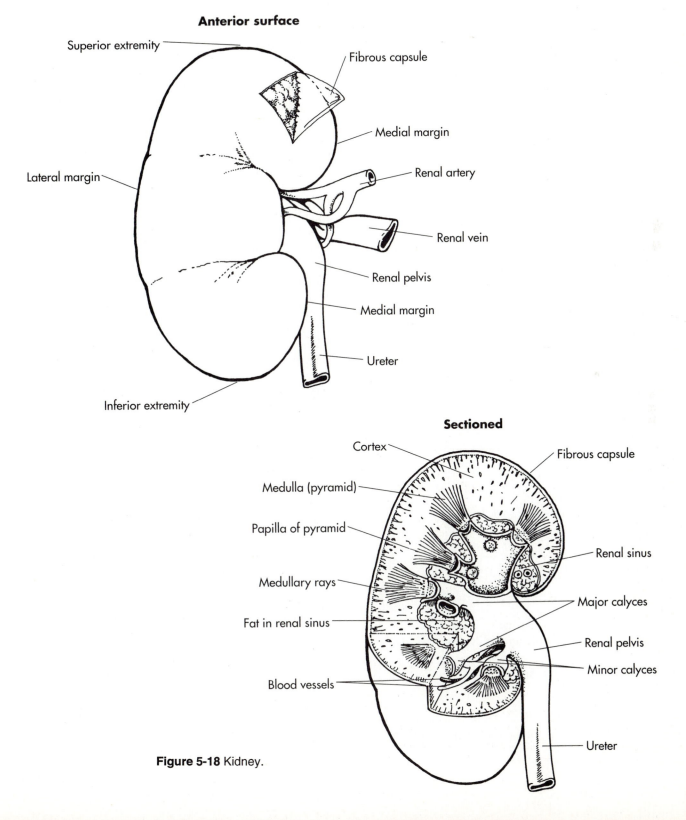

Figure 5-18 Kidney.

B. Ureters
   1. Approximately 27 cm long
   2. Urine flows down the ureters via peristalsis
C. Bladder
   1. Lies behind the symphysis pubis
   2. Serves as a reservoir for the urine
D. Urethra
   1. Connects the bladder to the exterior
   2. Female urethra is approximately 4 cm long
   3. Male urethra is approximately 20 cm long
E. Blood is filtered first in the glomeruli
   1. Passed through the glomerular membrane into Bowman's capsule and then into the proximal tubules
   2. Filtration rate is determined by the filtration pressure
   3. Modified as it passes through the tubules by means of reabsorption and secretion
      a. Proximal convoluted tubule
      b. Loop of Henle
      c. Distal collecting tubule
   4. Waste products are not reabsorbed

▲ Review of Radiographic Positioning, Procedures, and Pathology*

Skeletal System

Pathologies Imaged

(Note: Designation of harder or easier to penetrate does not necessarily signify that alteration of exposure technique is required.)

A. Acromegaly
   1. Endocrine disorder causing bones to become thick and coarse
   2. Harder to penetrate
B. Ankylosing spondylitis
   1. Inflammatory disease of the spine and adjacent structures causing severe pain and fusion of the joints involved
C. Bony cyst
   1. Fluid-filled sacs in fibrous tissue
   2. Easier to penetrate
D. Bursitis
   1. Inflammation of bursa, causing severe pain
   2. Harder to penetrate if calcium has deposited
E. Callus
   1. New bony deposit surrounding fractures in the process of healing
   2. Harder to penetrate

F. Club foot (talipes)
   1. Congenital malformation of the foot causing foot to be turned inward at the ankle
G. Congenital hip anomaly
   1. Caused by a malformation of the acetabulum in which the femoral head displaces superiorly and posteriorly
H. Disk herniation
   1. Protrusion of an intervertebral disk
I. Ewing's sarcoma
   1. Malignant destructive tumor of bone marrow
   2. Easier to penetrate
J. Fractures—disruption of bone tissue
   1. Complete fracture—discontinuity between two or more fragments
   2. Incomplete fracture—partial discontinuity; portion of the cortex is intact
   3. Closed fracture—overlying skin is intact
   4. Compound fracture—overlying skin is broken; bony fragments
   5. Transverse fracture—runs at right angle to the long axis of the bone
   6. Oblique fracture—runs approximately 45 degrees to the long axis of the bone
   7. Spiral fracture—encircles the shaft of the bone
   8. Avulsion fracture—small fragments of bone torn off bony prominences
   9. Comminuted fracture—fracture producing more than two fragments
   10. Compression fracture—causes compaction of the bone resulting in decreased length or width
   11. Stress fracture—fracture resulting from repeated stresses placed upon the bone
   12. Pathologic fracture—occurs as a result of bone disease
   13. Greenstick fracture—incomplete fracture with cortex intact on opposite side of the bone from the fracture
   14. Bowing fracture—occurs when stress, applied to the bone, causes it to bow but stops short of an actual fracture
   15. Undisplaced fracture—lack of angulation or separation of fractured bone
   16. Displacement—separation of bone fragments
   17. Angulation—deformity between the axis of major fragments of bone
   18. Dislocation—displacement of a bone from its normal site of articulation
   19. Subluxation—partial loss of continuity in a joint
   20. Fracture healing—characterized radiographically by calcium deposits across the fracture line that unite the fracture fragments
   21. Battered child syndrome—multiple fractures at various stages of healing located in long bones and the skull; also characterized by fractures at unusual sites (ribs, scapula, sternum, spine, clavicles)
   22. Colles' fracture—transverse fracture through the distal radius with posterior angulation and overriding of the distal fracture fragment

---

* Note: Student is reminded that positioning routines vary from text to text and department to department. What follows is a general review of common routines.

23. Boxer's fracture—transverse fracture of the neck of the fifth metacarpal, with palmar angulation of the distal fragment
24. Elbow fractures—in addition to bony involvement, radiograph will show dislocation of elbow fat pads; this necessitates the use of appropriate radiographic exposure
25. Pott's fracture—fracture of medial and lateral malleoli of the ankle with ankle joint dislocation
26. Bimalleolar fracture—fracture of both medial and lateral malleoli
27. Trimalleolar fracture—involves the posterior portion of the tibia and the medial and lateral malleoli
28. Jefferson fracture—comminuted fracture of the ring of the atlas involving both anterior and posterior arches and causing displacement of the fragments
29. Hangman's fracture—caused by acute hyperextension of the head on the neck; characterized by a fracture of the arch of C2 and anterior subluxation of C2 onto C3; primarily caused by motor vehicle accidents
30. Seat belt fracture—transverse fracture of lumbar vertebrae including substantial abdominal injuries

K. Hydrocephalus
   1. Abnormal accumulation of cerebrospinal fluid in the brain
   2. Harder to penetrate
L. Giant cell myeloma
   1. Benign or malignant tumor arising on bone with large bubble appearance
   2. Easier to penetrate
M. Gout
   1. Metabolic disorder in which urate crystals are deposited in the joints, most commonly the great toe, causing extreme swelling
   2. Harder to penetrate
N. Multiple myeloma
   1. Malignancy of plasma cells resulting in destruction of bone, failure of bone marrow, and impairment of renal function
   2. Easier to penetrate
O. Osteoarthritis
   1. Form of arthritis characterized by degeneration of one or several joints
   2. Easier to penetrate
P. Osteoblastic metastases
   1. Dense, sclerotic tumors in bone
   2. Harder to penetrate
Q. Osteochondroma
   1. Benign projection of bone in the young
   2. Harder to penetrate
R. Osteogenic sarcoma
   1. Destructive cancer at the end of long bones
   2. Easier to penetrate, except for sclerotic area
S. Osteoma
   1. Benign, small, round tumor

   2. Harder to penetrate
T. Osteogenesis imperfecta
   1. Inherited condition causing poor development of connective tissue and brittle and easily fractured bones
   2. Easier to penetrate
U. Osteomyelitis
   1. Bacterial infection of bone and bone marrow
   2. Easier to penetrate
V. Osteolytic metastases
   1. Arise in medullary canal to destroy bone
   2. Easier to penetrate
W. Osteomalacia
   1. Abnormal softening of bone
   2. Easier to penetrate
X. Osteopetrosis
   1. Inherited condition causing increased bone density
   2. Harder to penetrate
Y. Osteoporosis
   1. Abnormal demineralization of bone
   2. Easier to penetrate
Z. Paget's Disease (osteitis deformans)
   1. Nonmetabolic bone disease causing bone destruction and unorganized bone repair
   2. Difficult to image properly because some areas that are easier to penetrate are adjacent to structures that are harder to penetrate
AA. Rheumatoid arthritis
   1. Destructive collagen disease with inflammation and joint swelling
   2. Harder to penetrate
BB. Rickets
   1. Soft pliable bones resulting from deficiency of vitamin D and sunlight
   2. Easier to penetrate
CC. Scoliosis
   1. Abnormal lateral curvature of the spine
DD. Spina bifida
   1. Defect of posterior aspect of spinal canal caused by failure of vertebral arch to form properly
EE. Spondylolisthesis
   1. Spondylolysis with displacement
FF. Spondylolysis
   1. Defect in pars articularis, which is between the superior and inferior articular processes of a vertebra
   2. No displacement present

Digits (Fingers)

A. PA
   1. Patient position: seated
   2. Part position:
      a. Separate and center extended digit of interest with palmar surface of hand firmly against cassette
   3. Central ray: perpendicular, entering proximal interphalangeal joint

B. Lateral
1. Patient position: seated
2. Part position:
   a. Digit of interest is extended
   b. Close rest of digits into a fist
   c. Adjust digit of interest parallel to film plane
   d. Immobilize extended digit
3. Central ray: perpendicular, entering proximal interphalangeal joint
C. Oblique
1. Patient position: seated
2. Part position:
   a. Place patient's hand in lateral position, ulnar side down
   b. Centered to cassette
   c. Rotate palm 45 degrees toward cassette until digits are resting on support
   d. Immobilize separated digits
3. Central ray: perpendicular, entering proximal interphalangeal joint

Thumb

A. AP, lateral, oblique
1. Patient position: seated
2. Part position:
   a. AP—patient's hand is turned in extreme internal rotation, thumb resting on cassette, other fingers held out of the way
   b. Lateral—hand in natural arched position, palm down, adjust hand to put thumb in true lateral
   c. Oblique—abduct thumb, palm down
3. Central ray (all projections): perpendicular to the metacarpophalangeal joint

Hand

A. PA
1. Patient position: seated
2. Part position:
   a. Patient rests forearm on table, with palmar surface firmly against cassette
   b. Spread digits slightly
3. Central ray: perpendicular to third metacarpophalangeal joint
B. Oblique
1. Patient position: seated, rests forearm on table with hand on cassette in lateral position, ulnar side down
2. Part Position:
   a. Rotate hand medially
   b. Place digits on a 45-degree radiolucent support to demonstrate interphalangeal joints
   c. Adjust digits parallel to cassette
3. Central ray: perpendicular to third metacarpophalangeal joint

C. Lateral
1. Patient position: seated, rests ulnar surface of forearm on table with hand in true lateral position
2. Part position:
   a. Extend digits with first digit (thumb) placed at a right angle to palm of hand
   b. As an option, patient may "fan" fingers and place on positioning sponge to reduce superimposition of phalanges
   c. Center metacarpophalangeal joints to cassette
   d. Adjust palmar surface of hand perpendicular to cassette
3. Central ray: perpendicular to second metacarpophalangeal joint

Wrist

A. PA
1. Patient position: seated, forearm resting on table
2. Part position:
   a. Center carpus to cassette area
   b. Patient's digits are flexed slightly to place wrist in contact with cassette
3. Central ray: perpendicular to midcarpal area (Fig. 5-19)

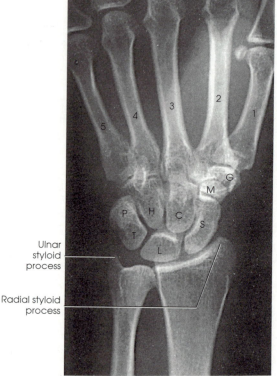

Figure 5-19 PA wrist. *S*, scaphoid; *L*, lunate; *T*, triquetrum; *P*, pisiform; *G*, trapezium; *M*, trapezoid; *C*, capitate; and *H*, hamate. From Ballinger, P: Merrill's atlas of radiographic positions and radiologic procedures, ed 8, St. Louis, 1995, Mosby.

B. Lateral
1. Patient position: elbow is flexed 90 degrees, with forearm and arm in contact with table
2. Part Position: center carpals and adjust hand so wrist is lateral
3. Central ray: perpendicular to wrist joint (Fig. 5-20)

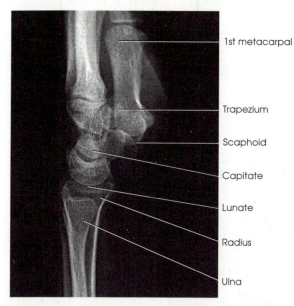

Figure 5-20 Lateral wrist. From Ballinger, P: Merrill's atlas of radiographic positions and radiologic procedures, ed 8, St. Louis, 1995, Mosby.

C. Oblique
1. Patient position: seated, ulnar surface of wrist on cassette
2. Part position:
   a. Center carpus to cassette area
   b. From true lateral, rotate part approximately 45 degrees medially and support on sponge
3. Central ray: perpendicular to cassette, entering mid-carpal area just distal to radius (Fig. 5-21)
D. Scaphoid (navicular)
1. Patient position: elbow is flexed 90 degrees, with forearm and arm in contact with table
2. Part position:
   a. Center carpals to cassette area
   b. Place patient's wrist in extreme ulnar flexion
3. Central ray: perpendicular to scaphoid; option to delineate fracture may require angulation of 10 to 15 degrees proximally (toward elbow) or distally; another approach is to elevate distal end of cassette approximately 20 degrees

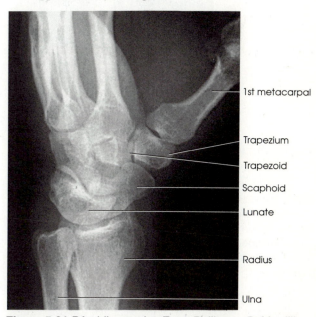

Figure 5-21 PA oblique wrist. From Ballinger, P: Merrill's atlas of radiographic positions and radiologic procedures, ed 8, St. Louis, 1995, Mosby.

Forearm

A. AP

1. Patient position: seated
2. Part position: supinate hand and center forearm to cassette to include joint(s) of interest
3. Central ray: perpendicular to midpoint of forearm (Fig. 5-22)

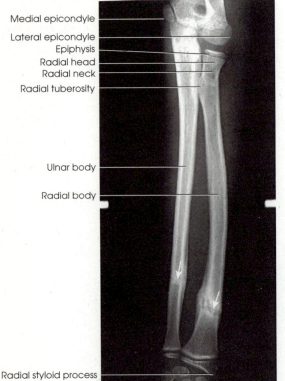

Medial epicondyle
Lateral epicondyle
Epiphysis
Radial head
Radial neck
Radial tuberosity

Ulnar body

Radial body

Radial styloid process

Figure 5-22 AP forearm with fractured radius and ulna. From Ballinger, P: Merrill's atlas of radiographic positions and radiologic procedures, ed 8, St. Louis, 1995, Mosby.

B. Lateral

1. Patient position: seated, with humerus and forearm in contact with table; elbow flexed
2. Part position:
   a. Elbow is flexed 90 degrees
   b. Adjust hand to lateral position (thumb up)
   c. Center forearm to cassette to include joint(s) of interest
3. Central ray: perpendicular to midpoint of forearm (Fig. 5-23)

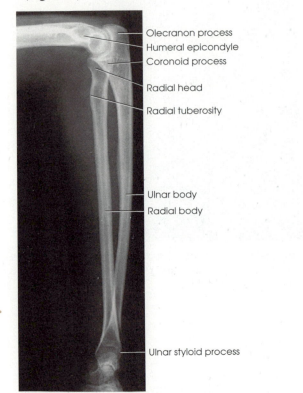

Olecranon process
Humeral epicondyle
Coronoid process

Radial head

Radial tuberosity

Ulnar body
Radial body

Ulnar styloid process

Figure 5-23 Lateral forearm. From Ballinger, P: Merrill's atlas of radiographic positions and radiologic procedures, ed 8, St. Louis, 1995, Mosby.

Elbow

A. AP
1. Patient position: seated, with arm extended
2. Part position:
    a. Extend patient's elbow
    b. Supinate hand
    c. Center elbow joint to cassette
    d. Patient may have to lean slightly laterally to ensure AP alignment
3. Central ray: perpendicular to elbow joint (Fig. 5-24)

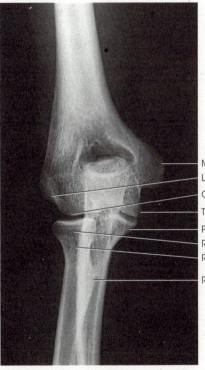

Medial epicondyle
Lateral epicondyle
Capitulum (capitellum)
Trochlea
Proximal ulna
Radial head
Radial neck
Radial tuberosity

Figure 5-24 AP elbow. From Ballinger, P: Merrill's atlas of radiographic positions and radiologic procedures, ed 8, St. Louis, 1995, Mosby.

B. Lateral
1. Patient position: seated, with elbow flexed 90 degrees; humerus and forearm resting on table
2. Part position:
    a. Center 90-degree flexed elbow joint to cassette
    b. Adjust wrist and hand in lateral position
3. Central ray: perpendicular to elbow joint (Fig. 5-25)

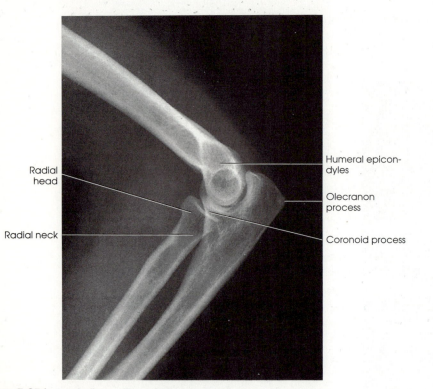

Radial head

Radial neck

Humeral epicondyles

Olecranon process

Coronoid process

Figure 5-25 Lateral elbow. From Ballinger, P: Merrill's atlas of radiographic positions and radiologic procedures, ed 8, St. Louis, 1995, Mosby.

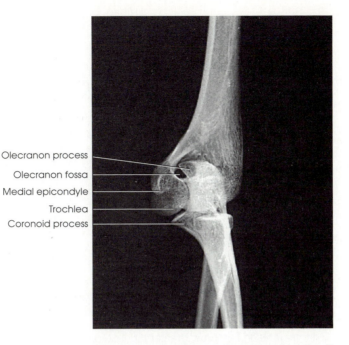

Olecranon process
Olecranon fossa
Medial epicondyle
Trochlea
Coronoid process

Figure 5-26 AP oblique elbow. From Ballinger, P: Merrill's atlas of radiographic positions and radiologic procedures, ed 8, St. Louis, 1995, Mosby.

C. Medial oblique
  1. Patient position: seated, with arm extended
  2. Part position:
    a. Pronate patient's hand
    b. Medially rotate arm
    c. Adjust anterior surface of elbow (epicondyles) at an angle of 40 to 45 degrees
  3. Central ray: perpendicular to elbow joint (Fig. 5-26)
D. Lateral oblique
  1. Patient position: seated, with arm extended
  2. Part position:
    a. Rotate patient's hand laterally
    b. Adjust posterior surface of elbow at a 40-degree angle to cassette
  3. Central ray: perpendicular to elbow joint

Humerus

A. AP
  1. Patient position: erect or supine
  2. Part position:
    a. Unless it is contraindicated, supinate patient's hand and adjust humerus with epicondyles parallel to cassette (keep humerus in neutral position if fracture is suspected or if reexamining healing fracture with a hanging cast)
    b. If patient is recumbent, elevate and support opposite shoulder
    c. Center humerus to cassette
  3. Central ray: perpendicular to midpoint of humerus
B. Lateral
  1. Patient position: erect or supine
  2. Part position:
    a. Unless it is contraindicated, slightly abduct the arm and center arm to cassette
    b. Medially rotate forearm until epicondyles are perpendicular to cassette
  3. Central ray: perpendicular to midpoint of humerus

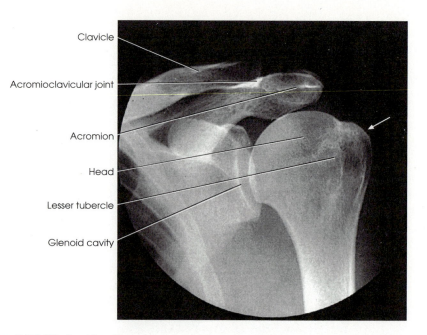

Clavicle

Acromioclavicular joint

Acromion

Head

Lesser tubercle

Glenoid cavity

Figure 5-27 AP shoulder. External rotation humerus; greater tubercle (arrow). From Ballinger, P: Merrill's atlas of radiographic positions and radiologic procedures, ed 8, St. Louis, 1995, Mosby.

Shoulder

A. AP
  1. Patient position: erect or supine
  2. Part position:
    a. Center area of coracoid process to cassette
    b. Rotate patient slightly to place affected scapula parallel to cassette
    c. Adjust hand in: (1) external rotation to obtain AP projection of humerus, or (2) internal rotation for lateral position of humerus
    d. Respiration: suspended
  3. Central ray: perpendicular to coracoid process (Fig. 5-27)
B. Transthoracic lateral
  1. Patient position: erect or supine
  2. Part position:
    a. Raise patient's uninjured arm and rest on head
    b. Elevate uninjured shoulder as much as possible
    c. Respiration: full inspiration or slow breathing
  3. Central ray: adjust patient to project humerus between vertebral column and sternum; unless it is contraindicated, adjust humeral epicondyles perpendicular to cassette; CR perpendicular to median coronal plane, exiting surgical neck of affected humerus; if patient cannot elevate unaffected shoulder, the central ray may be angled 10 to 15 degrees cephalad

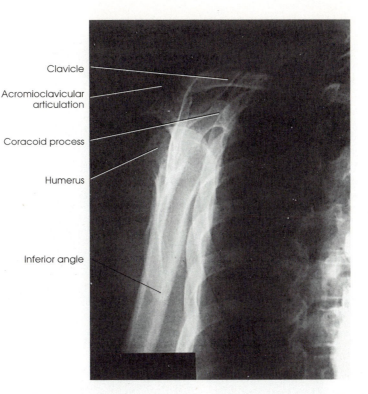

Clavicle

Acromioclavicular articulation

Coracoid process

Humerus

Inferior angle

Figure 5-28 PA oblique shoulder (scapular Y). From Ballinger, P: Merrill's atlas of radiographic positions and radiologic procedures, ed 8, St. Louis, 1995, Mosby.

C. PA oblique (scapular Y)
   1. Patient position: erect or prone oblique
   2. Part position:
     a. Center anterior surface of affected shoulder to cassette
     b. Rotate patient so midcoronal plane forms 60-degree angle from cassette
     c. Respiration: suspended
   3. Central ray: perpendicular to shoulder joint at level of scapulohumeral joint (Fig. 5-28)

Acromioclavicular Articulations

A. AP
   1. Patient position: upright, if condition permits
   2. Part position:
     a. Adjust midpoint of cassette to level of acromioclavicular (A-C) joints
     b. Center MSP of patient's body to midline of cassette, if both A-C joints can be demonstrated on one radiograph
     c. Otherwise, center to each individual A-C joint for two separate exposures
     d. To demonstrate A-C separation, sandbags of equal weight should be attached to each wrist and a second radiograph obtained without weights
     e. Respiration: suspended
   3. Central ray: perpendicular to cassette, midway between A-C joints or perpendicular to each A-C joint

Clavicle

A. PA
   1. Patient position: erect or prone; may take AP for patient comfort
   2. Part position:
     a. Center clavicle to center of cassette midway between midline of body and coracoid process
     b. Head may be turned away from affected side
     c. Respiration: suspended
   3. Central ray: perpendicular to midshaft of clavicle
B. PA axial
   1. Patient position: erect or prone; may take AP for patient comfort
   2. Part position:
     a. Center clavicle to midline of table with cassette midway between MSP and coracoid process
     b. Head may be turned away from affected side
     c. Respiration: suspended
   3. Central ray: angle 25 to 30 degrees caudad, centered to the midshaft of the clavicle (25 to 30 degrees cephalad, if performed AP)

Scapula

A. AP
   1. Patient position: supine or upright (upright preferred when shoulder is tender)
   2. Part position:

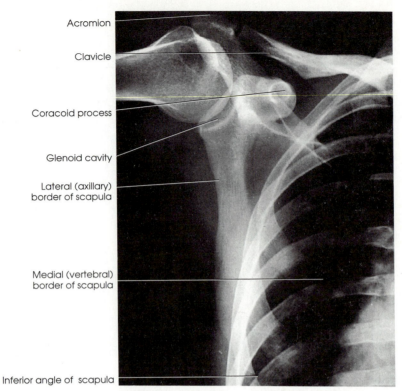

Acromion

Clavicle

Coracoid process

Glenoid cavity

Lateral (axillary)
border of scapula

Medial (vertebral)
border of scapula

Inferior angle of scapula

Figure 5-29 AP scapula. From Ballinger, P: Merrill's atlas of radiographic positions and radiologic procedures, ed 8, St. Louis, 1995, Mosby.

a. Abduct patient's arm
b. Flex elbow
c. Support hand near head
d. Center palpated scapular area to cassette approximately 2 inches inferior to coracoid process
e. Respiration: quiet breathing
3. Central ray: perpendicular to cassette at midscapular area approximately 2 inches inferior to coracoid process (Fig. 5-29)
B. Lateral
1. Patient position: prone oblique or upright (upright preferred when shoulder is tender)
2. Part position:
a. Place patient in an oblique position with affected scapula centered to cassette
b. Extend affected arm across anterior thorax
c. Palpate axillary and vertebral borders of scapula and adjust body rotation so scapula is lateral and will be projected free of rib cage
d. Respiration: suspended
3. Central ray: perpendicular to medial border of protruding scapula

Toes

A. AP
1. Patient position: supine or seated on table, knees flexed with feet separated

2. Part position: center toes with plantar surface flat against cassette
3. Central ray: 15 degrees cephalad, if positioning wedge is not used; enters the second metatarsophalangeal joint
B. Oblique
1. Patient position: supine or seated on table, knees flexed with feet separated
2. Part position: Center patient's toes over cassette area and medially rotate leg and foot until a 30- to 45-degree angle is formed from cassette to plantar surface of foot
3. Central ray: perpendicular entering third metatarsophalangeal joint

Foot

A. AP
1. Patient position: supine or seated on table, knees flexed with feet separated
2. Part position:
a. Plantar surface firmly resting on cassette
b. Center foot to cassette
c. Adjust midline of foot parallel to long axis of cassette
3. Central ray: 10 degrees toward the heel, entering base of third metatarsal

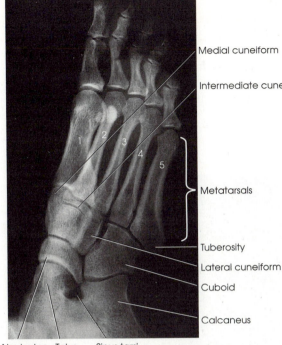

Figure 5-30 AP oblique projection foot, medial rotation. From Ballinger, P: Merrill's atlas of radiographic positions and radiologic procedures, ed 8, St. Louis, 1995, Mosby.

B. Medial oblique
   1. Patient position: supine or seated on table, knees flexed with feet separated
   2. Part position:
      a. Center patient's foot to cassette
      b. Rotate leg medially until foot plantar surface forms angle of 30 degrees to cassette
   3. Central ray: perpendicular to base of third metatarsal (Fig. 5-30)
C. Lateral (mediolateral)
   1. Patient position:
      a. With the patient lying upon the affected side, adjust leg and foot in lateral position
      b. Patella perpendicular to table
   2. Part position: center foot and adjust plantar surface perpendicular to cassette
   3. Central ray: perpendicular to midpoint of cassette, entering base of third metatarsal

Calcaneus

A. Axial (plantodorsal)
   1. Patient position: supine or seated with leg fully extended
   2. Part position:
      a. Center cassette to ankle
      b. Draw the plantar surface of foot perpendicular to cassette

3. Central ray: 40 degrees cephalad to long axis of foot, entering midline at level of base of fifth metatarsal
B. Lateral
   1. Patient position:
      a. With the patient lying on the affected side, adjust leg and foot in lateral position
      b. Patella perpendicular to table
   2. Part position: center calcaneus to cassette, about 1 to 1.5 inches distal to medial malleolus
   3. Central ray: perpendicular to midportion of calcaneus

Ankle

A. AP

1. Patient position: supine or seated on table with small support under knee
2. Part position:
   a. Center ankle to cassette
   b. Dorsiflex foot
   c. Adjust ankle with toes pointing vertically
3. Central ray: perpendicular to ankle joint midway between malleoli (Fig. 5-31)

B. Lateral

1. Patient position: supine, roll onto affected side
2. Part position:
   a. Rotate patient's ankle to lateral position
   b. Adjust foot in lateral position
   c. Center ankle to cassette
3. Central ray: vertically through medial malleolus (Fig. 5-32)

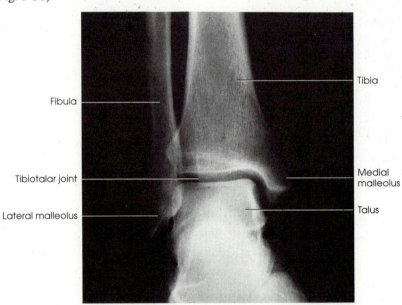

Figure 5-31 AP ankle. From Ballinger, P: Merrill's atlas of radiographic positions and radiologic procedures, ed 8, St. Louis, 1995, Mosby.

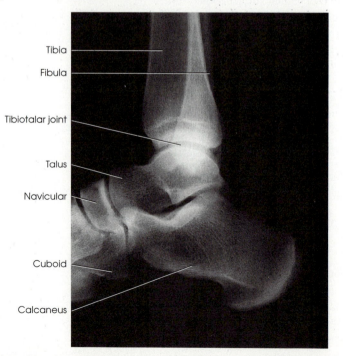

Figure 5-32 Lateral ankle. From Ballinger, P: Merrill's atlas of radiographic positions and radiologic procedures, ed 8, St. Louis, 1995, Mosby.

C. Medial oblique
　　1. Patient position: supine or seated on table
　　2. Part position:
　　　　a. Rotate patient's leg and foot medially
　　　　b. Adjust degree of medial rotation for: (1) mortise joint: until malleoli are parallel with film (15 to 20 degrees), or (2) bony structure: to 45 degrees rotation
　　3. Central ray: vertically midway between malleoli

Leg

A. AP
　　1. Patient position: supine with leg extended
　　2. Part position:
　　　　a. Center leg to cassette
　　　　b. Adjust leg to AP position
　　　　c. Both joints should be included
　　3. Central ray: vertically to midpoint of leg
B. Lateral
　　1. Patient position: supine and roll onto affected side
　　2. Part position:
　　　　a. Center leg to cassette
　　　　b. Adjust leg to lateral position
　　　　c. Patella perpendicular
　　　　d. Both joints should be included
　　3. Central ray: perpendicular to midpoint of leg (Fig. 5-33)

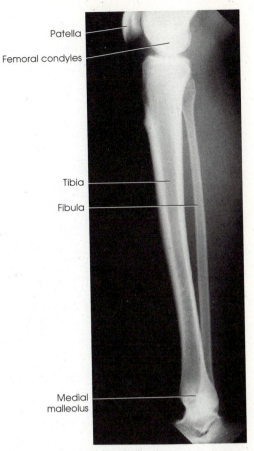

Figure 5-33 Lateral tibia and fibula. From Ballinger, P: Merrill's atlas of radiographic positions and radiologic procedures, ed 8, St. Louis, 1995, Mosby.

115

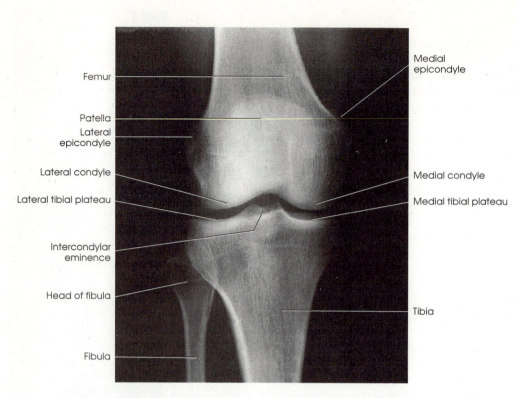

Femur

Patella

Lateral
epicondyle

Lateral condyle

Lateral tibial plateau

Intercondylar
eminence

Head of fibula

Fibula

Medial
epicondyle

Medial condyle

Medial tibial plateau

Tibia

Figure 5-34 AP knee. From Ballinger, P: Merrill's atlas of radiographic positions and radiologic procedures, ed 8, St. Louis, 1995, Mosby.

Knee

A. AP
1. Patient position: supine and with leg extended, adjust patient's body so pelvis is not rotated
2. Part position:
   a. Center knee to cassette
   b. Adjust leg to AP position
3. Central ray: 5 to 7 degrees cephalad to a point $\frac{1}{2}$ inch inferior to patellar apex (Fig. 5-34)

B. Lateral
1. Patient position: turn patient onto affected side with knee flexed (usually 20 to 30 degrees)
2. Part position:
   a. Flex and center knee
   b. Center cassette approximately 1 inch distal to medial epicondyle
   c. Patella perpendicular to film
3. Central ray: 5 degrees cephalad, entering knee joint inferior to medial condyle

C. Intercondylar fossa (Tunnel)
1. Patient position: kneeling on radiographic table with affected knee flexed 70 degrees from full extension
2. Part position:
   a. Center patient's knee to cassette
   b. Place at level of patellar apex
   c. Knee flexed 70 degrees from full extension
3. Central ray: perpendicular to long axis of lower leg, entering midpopliteal area

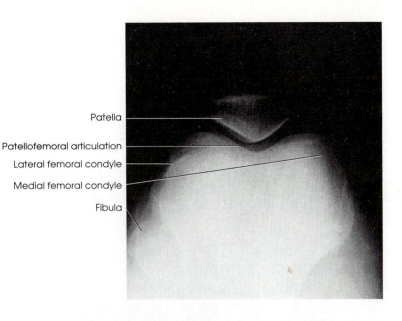

Patella

Patellofemoral articulation

Lateral femoral condyle

Medial femoral condyle

Fibula

Figure 5-35 Tangential patella: Settegast method. From Ballinger, P: Merrill's atlas of radiographic positions and radiologic procedures, ed 8, St. Louis, 1995, Mosby.

Patella

A. PA
 1. Patient position: prone with knee extended
 2. Part position:
    a. Center patella
    b. Adjust to be parallel with cassette plane
    c. Heel generally rotated 5 to 10 degrees laterally
 3. Central ray: perpendicular to midpopliteal area
B. Tangential
 1. Patient position: prone with foot resting on table
 2. Part position: Flex affected knee so tibia and fibula form a 50- to 60-degree angle from table
 3. Central ray: 45 degrees cephalad through patellofemoral joint (Fig. 5-35)
C. Lateral
 1. Patient position: lying on affected side
 2. Part position: flex knee 5 to 10 degrees, femoral epicondyles superimposed
 3. Central ray: perpendicular to patella

Femur

A. AP
 1. Patient position: supine with toes up
 2. Part position:
    a. Center affected thigh to midline of table
    b. Internally rotate lower limb approximately 15 degrees
    c. Both joints should be included
    d. Apply gonad shielding as appropriate
 3. Central ray: perpendicular to midfemur

B. Lateral
 1. Patient position: lying on affected side with knee slightly flexed
 2. Part position:
    a. To include hip joint, rotate patient's unaffected hip posteriorly to prevent superimposition of unaffected hip
    b. Center femur to midline of table
    c. Both joints should be included
    d. Apply gonad shielding as appropriate
 3. Central ray: perpendicular to midfemur

Pelvis

A. AP
 1. Patient position: supine
 2. Part position:
    a. Center MSP to table
    b. Adjust to AP position
    c. Internally rotate feet and lower limb 15 degrees
    d. Center cassette approximately 2 inches superior to level of greater trochanter
    e. Use gonad shielding as appropriate
    f. Respiration: suspended
 3. Central ray: perpendicular to midpoint of film 2 inches superior to symphysis pubis

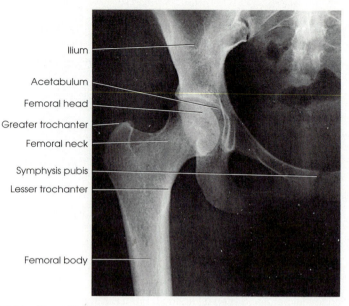

Ilium
Acetabulum
Femoral head
Greater trochanter
Femoral neck
Symphysis pubis
Lesser trochanter
Femoral body

Figure 5-36 AP hip. From Ballinger, P: Merrill's atlas of radiographic positions and radiologic procedures, ed 8, St. Louis, 1995, Mosby.

Hip

A. AP
  1. Patient position: supine
  2. Part position:
      a. Rotate lower limb 15 degrees medially
      b. Center hip to cassette
      c. Respiration: suspended
  3. Central ray: perpendicular to a point 2 inches medial to ASIS and at level of superior margin of greater trochanter (Fig. 5-36)
B. Lateral
  1. Patient position: from supine position, turn patient toward affected side to posterior oblique body position
  2. Part position:
      a. Flex affected knee
      b. Center affected hip to midline of table
      c. Extend unaffected knee
      d. Respiration: suspended
  3. Central ray: perpendicular to a point midway between ASIS and symphysis pubis
C. Axiolateral
  1. Patient position: supine with level of greater trochanter elevated to center of cassette
  2. Part position:
      a. Flex knee and hip of unaffected side
      b. Elevate and rest on suitable support
      c. Adjust pelvis to supine position
      d. Unless it is contraindicated, rotate affected leg 15 to 20 degrees internally
      e. Respiration: suspended
  3. Central ray: perpendicular to long axis of femoral neck and cassette

Cervical Vertebrae

A. Atlas and axis
1. Patient position: erect or supine
2. Part position:
   a. MSP centered to cassette at level of C2
   b. Arms by sides
   c. Shoulders in same plane
   d. Have patient open mouth wide
   e. Adjust head so line from lower edge of upper incisors to mastoid process is perpendicular to cassette
   f. Respiration: phonate "ah" during exposure
3. Central ray: perpendicular to cassette, centered to open mouth (Fig. 5-37)

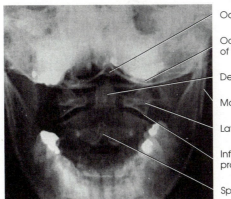

Occipital base

Occlusal surface of teeth

Dens (odontoid process)

Mandibular ramus

Lateral mass of atlas

Inferior articular process of atlas

Spinous process of axis

Figure 5-37 Open-mouth atlas and axis. From Ballinger, P: Merrill's atlas of radiographic positions and radiologic procedures, ed 8, St. Louis, 1995, Mosby.

B. AP
   1. Patient position: erect or supine
   2. Part position:
      a. MSP centered to cassette
      b. Arms by sides
      c. Center cassette at level of C4
      d. Adjust a line between upper occlusal plane and mastoid tip, perpendicular to cassette
      e. Respiration: suspended
   3. Central ray: 15 to 20 degrees cephalad, entering slightly inferior to thyroid cartilage (Fig. 5-38)

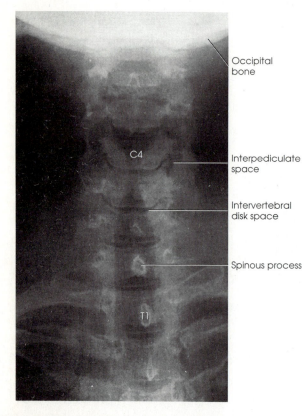

Occipital bone

Interpediculate space

Intervertebral disk space

Spinous process

Figure 5-38 AP axial cervical vertebrae. From Ballinger, P: Merrill's atlas of radiographic positions and radiologic procedures, ed 8, St. Louis, 1995, Mosby.

C. Lateral
  1. Patient position: seated or standing in lateral position
  2. Part position:
      a. Center coronal plane through mastoid tips to cassette
      b. Adjust patient's shoulders to same horizontal level and body to true lateral position
      c. Elevate chin slightly
      d. Relax shoulders
      e. Weights may be attached to wrists to help lower shoulders
      f. Seventy-two inches SID recommended
      g. Respiration: expiration
  3. Central ray: perpendicular to cassette entering C4 (Fig. 5-39)

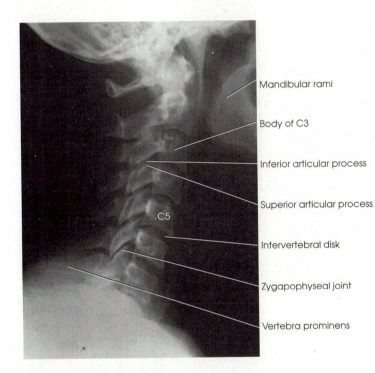

Figure 5-39 Lateral cervical vertebrae. From Ballinger, P: Merrill's atlas of radiographic positions and radiologic procedures, ed 8, St. Louis, 1995, Mosby.

D. LPO and RPO (AP oblique)
   1. Patient position: seated or standing
   2. Part position:
      a. Rotate body to 45 degrees
      b. Side of interest farthest from cassette
      c. Have patient slightly extend chin while looking forward
      d. Center spine to cassette
      e. Take both obliques
      f. Respiration: suspended
   3. Central ray: 15 to 20 degrees cephalad, entering C4 (Fig. 5-40)

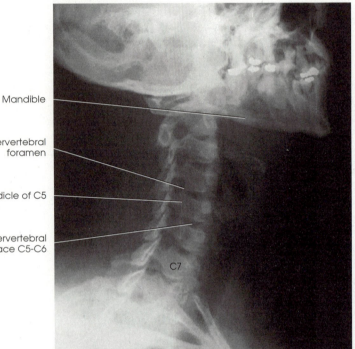

Mandible

Intervertebral foramen

Pedicle of C5

Intervertebral disk space C5-C6

C7

Figure 5-40 RAO position demonstrating right side. From Ballinger, P: Merrill's atlas of radiographic positions and radiologic procedures, ed 8, St. Louis, 1995, Mosby.

Thoracic Vertebrae

A. AP
1. Patient position: supine or upright
2. Part position:
   a. MSP centered to cassette
   b. Top of film $1\frac{1}{2}$ to 2 inches above shoulders
   c. Arms by sides
   d. Shoulders in same plane
   e. Respiration: shallow or suspended expiration
3. Central ray: perpendicular to T7, 3 to 4 inches distal to jugular (manubrial) notch
B. Lateral
1. Patient position: lateral recumbent or erect
2. Part position:
   a. Elevate patient's head to spine level
   b. Extend arms forward
   c. Place radiolucent support under lower thoracic region until spine is horizontal to table top
   d. Respiration: shallow or suspended expiration
3. Central ray: perpendicular to cassette entering level of T7, approximately 3 to 4 inches below sternal angle (Fig. 5-41)

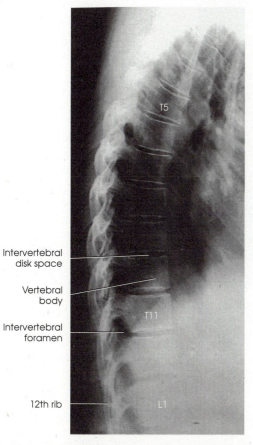

Figure 5-41 Lateral thoracic spine. From Ballinger, P: Merrill's atlas of radiographic positions and radiologic procedures, ed 8, St. Louis, 1995, Mosby.

C. Cervicothoracic (Twining)
 1. Patient position: lateral, seated or standing
 2. Part position:
    a. Midcoronal plane centered to grid
    b. Arm adjacent to Bucky is elevated
    c. Center film to the level of T2
    d. Body in true lateral position
    e. Respiration: suspended
 3. Central ray: perpendicular to cassette, entering at level of T2 (Fig. 5-42)

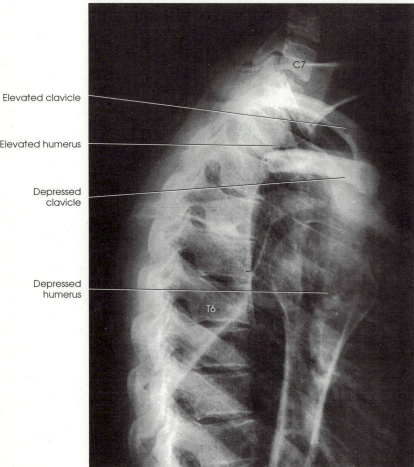

Figure 5-42 Lateral cervicothoracic region: Twining method. From Ballinger, P: Merrill's atlas of radiographic positions and radiologic procedures, ed 8, St. Louis, 1995, Mosby.

Lumbar Vertebrae

A. AP
  1. Patient position: supine
  2. Part position:
       a. MSP centered to table
       b. Flex patient's knees and hips enough to place back in firm contact with table
       c. Center cassette at level of iliac crest (L4)
       d. Respiration: suspended
  3. Central ray: perpendicular to midline, entering level of iliac crests (Fig. 5-43)

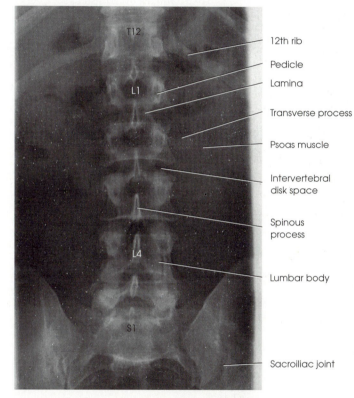

Figure 5-43 AP lumbar spine. From Ballinger, P: Merrill's atlas of radiographic positions and radiologic procedures, ed 8, St. Louis, 1995, Mosby.

3. Central ray: perpendicular to L5 at a point 1½ inches anterior to palpated spinous process of L5 and 1½ inches inferior to iliac crest

D. LPO and RPO (AP obliques)
1. Patient position: posterior oblique; side closest to cassette is side of interest
2. Part position:
   a. Adjust and support body obliquity to 45 degrees
   b. Adjust arms to a comfortable position
   c. Center spine to midline of table
   d. Center cassette at level of L3
   e. Take obliques of both sides
   f. Respiration: suspended
3. Central ray: perpendicular to L3, 1 to 2 inches above level of iliac crest entering elevated side 2 inches laterally from patient's midline

Sacroiliac Joints

A. LPO and RPO (AP oblique)
1. Patient position: supine
2. Part position:
   a. Elevate and support side of interest 25 to 30 degrees from table
   b. Align sagittal plane passing 1 inch medial to ASIS of elevated side centered to film
   c. Center to table
   d. Take both obliques
   e. Respiration: suspended
3. Central ray: perpendicular to cassette, 1 inch medial to elevated ASIS

Sacrum

A. AP
1. Patient position: supine
2. Part position:
   a. Center MSP to center of table
   b. Respiration: suspended
3. Central ray: 15 degrees cephalad, entering 2 inches superior to symphysis pubis

B. Lateral
1. Patient position: lateral with hips and knees flexed
2. Part position:
   a. Support body to place long axis of spine horizontal
   b. Align coronal plane passing 3 inches posterior to median coronal plane
   c. Center to midline of table
   d. Respiration: suspended
3. Central ray: perpendicular to cassette, entering 3 inches posterior to median coronal plane at level of ASIS

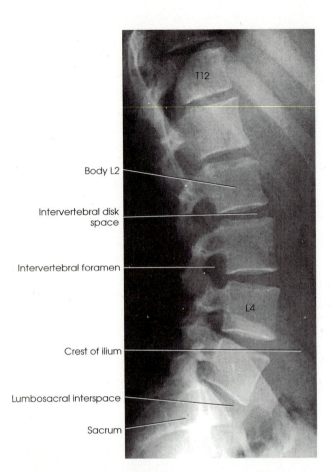

Figure 5-44 Lateral lumbar spine. From Ballinger, P: Merrill's atlas of radiographic positions and radiologic procedures, ed 8, St. Louis, 1995, Mosby.

B. Lateral
1. Patient position: lateral with hips and knees flexed
2. Part position:
   a. Center midaxillary line of body and L4 to table
   b. Extend patient's arms forward
   c. Place radiolucent support under lower thorax and adjust spine parallel to table
   d. Check for true lateral position
   e. Respiration: suspended
3. Central ray: perpendicular to cassette, entering midaxillary line at level of iliac crests (Fig. 5-44)

C. Lateral L5-S1
1. Patient position: lateral with hips and knees flexed
2. Part position:
   a. Center 1½ inches posterior to midaxillary line and 1½ inches below iliac crest
   b. Extend arms forward
   c. Place radiolucent support under lower thorax and adjust spine parallel to table
   d. Check for true lateral position
   e. Collimate tightly
   f. Respiration: suspended

Coccyx

A. AP
1. Patient position: supine
2. Part position:
   a. Center MSP to center of table
   b. Respiration: suspended
3. Central ray: 10 degrees caudad, entering 2 inches superior to symphysis pubis

B. Lateral
1. Patient position: lateral with hips and knees flexed
2. Part position:
   a. Support body to place long axis of spine horizontal
   b. Align coronal plane passing approximately 5 inches posterior to median coronal plane
   c. Center to midline of table
   d. Respiration: suspended
3. Central ray: perpendicular to cassette, entering palpated coccyx located approximately 5 inches posterior to median coronal plane

Scoliosis Series

A. PA (to minimize exposure to breast tissue; AP may be performed using compensating filters)
1. Patient position: seated or standing
2. Part position:
   a. First radiograph: MSP centered to film; film adjusted to include 1 inch of the iliac crests; arms at sides
   b. Second radiograph: MSP centered to film; elevate hip or foot of convex side of curve 3 or 4 inches on a block
3. Central ray: perpendicular to the midpoint of the film

Thorax

Pathologies Imaged

A. Adult respiratory distress syndrome
1. Acute life-threatening respiratory distress
2. Large amount of fluid in interstitial and alveolar spaces
3. Harder to penetrate

B. Asthma
1. Pulmonary disorder with increased mucus production in bronchi, causing hyperventilation of the lungs
2. Bronchi harder to penetrate
3. Lungs easier to penetrate

C. Atelectasis
1. Collapse of lung tissue
2. Harder to penetrate

D. Bronchial adenoma
1. Neoplasm occurring in a bronchus causing atelectasis and pneumonitis
2. Harder to penetrate

E. Bronchiectasis
1. Dilatation and destruction of bronchial walls
2. Consolidation present
3. Harder to penetrate

F. Bronchogenic carcinoma
1. Lung cancer arising from the bronchial mucosa
2. Harder to penetrate

G. Chronic bronchitis
1. Debilitating pulmonary disease with substantial increase of mucus production in the trachea and bronchi
2. Harder to penetrate unless evolved into emphysema, which is easier to penetrate

H. Chronic obstructive pulmonary disease
1. Progressive condition marked by diminished capabilities of inspiration and expiration
2. Harder to penetrate

I. Croup
1. Acute viral infection of infant's respiratory system
2. Lateral soft tissue neck radiograph taken to show subepiglottic narrowing

J. Cystic fibrosis
1. Inherited pathology of exocrine glands
2. Marked by increased mucus secretion in lungs and bronchi
3. Harder to penetrate

K. Emphysema
1. Overinflation of alveolar walls
2. Easier to penetrate
3. Should not be imaged using automatic exposure controls because minimum reaction time of equipment usually results in overexposure and subsequent repeat films

L. Empyema
1. Pus in the pleural space
2. Harder to penetrate

M. Histoplasmosis
1. Infection caused by inhaling fungal spores
2. Harder to penetrate

N. Hyaline membrane disease
1. Respiratory distress syndrome of the newborn (RDS)
2. Acute lung disease in newborn; characteristics include airless alveoli and rapid respirations
3. Harder to penetrate

O. Legionnaires' disease
1. Form of acute bacterial pneumonia
2. Harder to penetrate

P. Pleural effusion
1. Accumulation of fluid in intrapleural spaces
2. Harder to penetrate

Q. Pneumoconiosis
1. Lung disease caused by inhaling dust (usually mineral dust from the environment or workplace)
2. Silicosis—caused by prolonged inhalation of silicon dioxide (sand)

3. Anthracosis—caused by prolonged inhalation of anthracite (coal dust)
4. Asbestosis—caused by prolonged inhalation of asbestos
5. Siderosis—caused by prolonged inhalation of iron dust
6. All are harder to penetrate

R. Pneumonia
   1. Acute inflammation of the lungs
   2. Harder to penetrate

S. Pneumothorax
   1. Air in the pleural space which causes the lung to collapse
   2. Easier to penetrate

T. Pulmonary metastases
   1. Spread of cancer into the lungs from a primary site
   2. Harder to penetrate

U. Tuberculosis
   1. Chronic infection of the lungs caused by acid-fast bacillus
   2. More difficult to penetrate

Chest

A. PA
   1. Patient position:
      a. Standing or seated erect
      b. Back of hands on hips
      c. Top of cassette 1 to 2 inches above shoulders
   2. Part position:
      a. MSP centered
      b. Chin extended and looking straight ahead
      c. Roll shoulders forward
      d. SID of 72 inches recommended
      e. Respiration: full inspiration (expose at end of second inspiration)
   3. Central ray: perpendicular to MSP at level of T7 (Fig. 5-45)

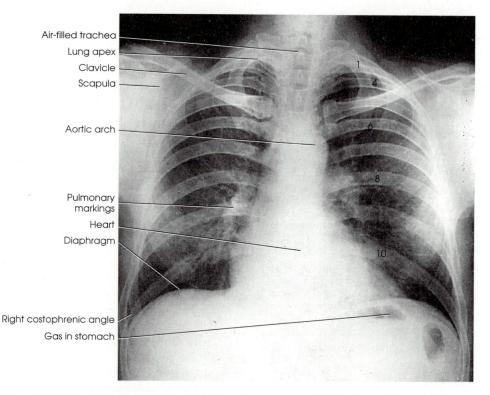

Figure 5-45 PA chest. From Ballinger, P: Merrill's atlas of radiographic positions and radiologic procedures, ed 8, St. Louis, 1995, Mosby.

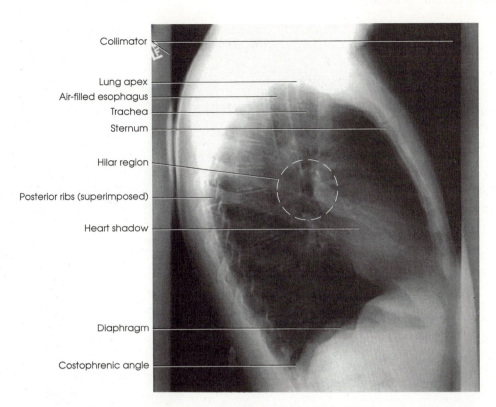

Collimator

Lung apex
Air-filled esophagus
Trachea
Sternum

Hilar region

Posterior ribs (superimposed)

Heart shadow

Diaphragm

Costophrenic angle

Figure 5-46 Left lateral chest. From Ballinger, P: Merrill's atlas of radiographic positions and radiologic procedures, ed 8, St. Louis, 1995, Mosby.

B. Lateral
  1. Patient position:
    a. Standing or seated erect
    b. Left side against cassette unless otherwise specified
    c. Top of cassette 1 to 2 inches above shoulder
  2. Part position:
    a. MSP parallel to cassette
    b. Adjacent shoulder resting against cassette holder
    c. Arms raised and crossed over head
    d. Center thorax to cassette
    e. SID of 72 inches recommended
    f. Respiration: full inspiration (expose at end of second inspiration)
  3. Central ray: perpendicular to cassette, entering patient approximately 2 inches anterior to midaxillary plane at level of T7 (Fig. 5-46)
C. LAO and RAO (PA obliques)
  1. Patient position:
    a. Standing or seated
    b. Adjust coronal plane 45 degrees (or 60 degrees) from plane of cassette
    c. Top of cassette 2 inches above shoulders
    d. Side farthest from cassette is usually side of primary interest

  2. Part position:
    a. Shoulder nearest cassette rolled posteriorly
    b. Hand placed on hip
    c. Arm farthest from cassette placed on top of cassette holder
    d. Center thorax to cassette
    e. SID of 72 inches recommended
    f. Both 45-degree obliques (or 60-degree obliques) may be taken
    g. Respiration: full inspiration
  3. Central ray: perpendicular at level of T7
D. AP lordotic
  1. Patient position:
    a. Standing approximately 1 foot in front of cassette
    b. When patient is properly positioned, top of cassette should be approximately 3 inches above shoulders

  2. Part position:
    a. MSP centered with no rotation
    b. Flex patient's elbows
    c. Hands, with palms out, on hips
    d. Patient leans backward in extreme lordotic position
    e. SID of 72 inches recommended
    f. Respiration: full inspiration

3. Central ray: perpendicular to cassette, entering midsternum

E. Lateral decubitus
1. Patient position: lateral recumbent
2. Part position:
   a. Lying on affected or unaffected side, depending upon existing condition
   b. Elevate dependent side on firm pad
   c. Extend patient's arms above head
   d. Adjust thorax in true lateral position
   e. Place top of cassette approximately 2 inches above shoulders
   f. Respiration: full inspiration
3. Central ray: horizontal and perpendicular to cassette, entering T7

Ribs

A. AP
1. Patient position: erect or recumbent
2. Part position:
   a. Center midsaggital plane to midline of grid
   b. Above diaphragm: center to T7; top of cassette should be 1 to 2 inches above shoulders; shoulders rotated anteriorly; respiration: full inspiration
   c. Below diaphragm: center thorax with bottom of cassette at level of iliac crests; respiration: full expiration
3. Central ray: perpendicular to T7 for upper ribs; perpendicular to T12 for lower ribs

B. LPO and RPO (AP obliques)
1. Patient position: erect or recumbent
2. Part position:
   a. Rotate body 45 degrees with the affected side toward cassette
   b. Center midway between MSP and lateral surface of body to center of grid
   c. Abduct arm nearest cassette
   d. Place hand on head
   e. Abduct opposite limb
   f. Place hand on hip
   g. Respiration: above diaphragm, full inspiration; below diaphragm, full expiration
3. Central ray: perpendicular to cassette; above diaphragm: center at level of T7; below diaphragm: center at level of T10

Sternum

A. RAO (PA oblique)
1. Patient position: prone position for RAO (right PA oblique)
2. Part position:
   a. Center sternum to cassette

Figure 5-47 Sternum RAO (right PA oblique). From Ballinger, P: Merrill's atlas of radiographic positions and radiologic procedures, ed 8, St. Louis, 1995, Mosby.

(Labels on image: Left clavicle; Jugular notch; Sternoclavicular joint; 1st Rib; Manubrium; Sternal angle; Body; Xiphoid process)

   b. Rotate body 15 to 20 degrees to prevent superimposition of vertebral and sternal images
   c. Respiration: shallow breathing or suspended expiration
3. Central ray: perpendicular, exiting midsternum (Fig. 5-47)

B. Lateral
1. Patient position: lateral, either seated or standing
2. Part position:
   a. Top of cassette 1 to 2 inches above jugular notch
   b. Shoulders and arms rotated posteriorly
   c. Center sternum to cassette
   d. Adjust to true lateral position
   e. Respiration: full inspiration
3. Central ray: perpendicular to center of midsternum

Sternoclavicular Joints

A. PA
   1. Patient position: prone or upright, MSP centered to table
   2. Part position:
      a. Cassette centered to T3
      b. Arms along side of body, palms up, shoulders in same plane
      c. Bilateral exam: patient's head rests on chin, MSP vertical to table
      d. Unilateral exam: Turn head toward affected side, rest cheek on table
   3. Central ray: perpendicular to T3
B. RAO
   1. Patient position: prone or upright
   2. Part position:
      a. Rotate patient to an oblique position to place vertebral shadow behind sternoclavicular joint nearest film (10 to 15 degrees)
      b. Center joint to midline of film
   3. Central ray: perpendicular to affected joint

Skull

Cranium

A. PA or Caldwell (Figs. 5-48 and 5-49)
  1. Patient position: prone or seated erect
  2. Part position:
     a. Head resting on forehead and nose
     b. MSP perpendicular to midline of grid device
     c. OML perpendicular to cassette
     d. Respiration: suspended
  3. Central ray:
     a. Caldwell method—direct central ray 15 degrees caudad to OML, exiting nasion, for survey examination
     b. PA—perpendicular to cassette, exiting nasion, to examine frontal bone

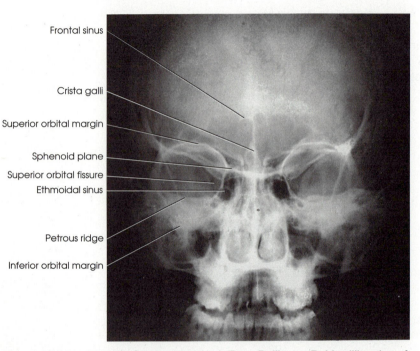

Figure 5-48 PA axial skull. Caldwell method. From Ballinger, P: Merrill's atlas of radiographic positions and radiologic procedures, ed 8, St. Louis, 1995, Mosby.

Frontal sinus
Crista galli
Superior orbital margin
Sphenoid plane
Superior orbital fissure
Ethmoidal sinus
Petrous ridge
Inferior orbital margin

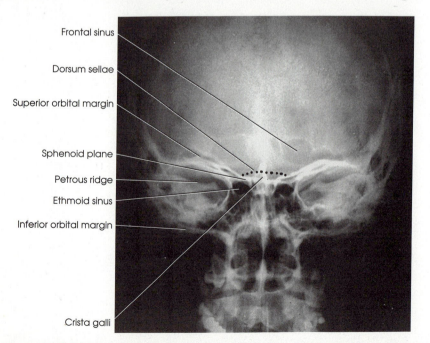

Frontal sinus
Dorsum sellae
Superior orbital margin
Sphenoid plane
Petrous ridge
Ethmoid sinus
Inferior orbital margin
Crista galli

Figure 5-49 PA skull. From Ballinger, P: Merrill's atlas of radiographic positions and radiologic procedures, ed 8, St. Louis, 1995, Mosby.

B. Lateral (Fig. 5-50)
1. Patient position: seated erect or semiprone
2. Part position:
   a. Center a point to the cassette that is 2 inches superior to the external auditory meatus (EAM)
   b. MSP parallel to cassette
   c. IOML parallel to transverse axis of cassette
   d. Interpupillary line (IPL) perpendicular to cassette
   e. Respiration: suspended
3. Central ray:
   a. Perpendicular, entering 2 inches superior to EAM for survey exam
   b. When sella turcica is of primary interest, cassette is centered and central ray enters ¾ inches superior and ¾ inches anterior to EAM

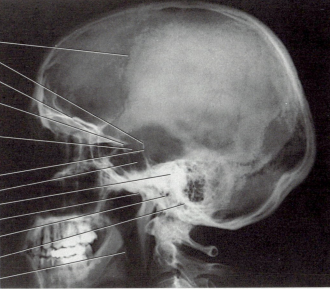

Coronal suture
Posterior clinoid process
Orbital roof (plate)
Anterior clinoid process

Hypophyseal fossa

Dorsum sellae
Sphenoidal sinus
Petrous portion of temporal bone
Temporomandibular joint
External acoustic meatus
Mastoid region
Mandibular rami

Figure 5-50 Lateral skull. Caldwell method. From Ballinger, P: Merrill's atlas of radiographic positions and radiologic procedures, ed 8, St. Louis, 1995, Mosby.

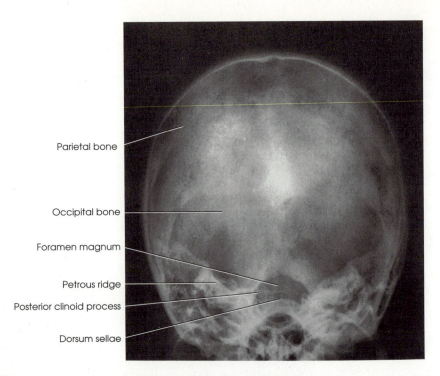

Parietal bone

Occipital bone

Foramen magnum

Petrous ridge

Posterior clinoid process

Dorsum sellae

Figure 5-51 AP axial skull. From Ballinger, P: Merrill's atlas of radiographic positions and radiologic procedures, ed 8, St. Louis, 1995, Mosby.

C. AP axial (Towne) (Fig. 5-51)
  1. Patient position: supine or seated erect
  2. Part position:
    a. Center MSP to midline of grid device
    b. Adjust to be perpendicular
    c. Flex patient's head and adjust OML perpendicular to cassette
    d. Place top of film at level of cranial vertex
    e. Respiration: suspended
  3. Central ray:
    a. Direct through foramen magnum with caudal angle of 30 degrees to OML or 37 degrees to IOML, entering 2 to $2\frac{1}{2}$ inches above glabella
D. Submentovertex (full basal)
  1. Patient position: seated erect at head unit or supine on elevated table support
  2. Part position:
    a. Extend patient's neck
    b. Rest head on vertex
    c. Center and adjust MSP perpendicular to cassette
    d. Adjust IOML parallel to plane of cassette
    e. Respiration: suspended
  3. Central ray: direct perpendicular to IOML, entering between angles of mandible

Optic Foramen (Fig. 5-52)

A. Parieto-orbital oblique (Rhese)
1. Patient position: prone or seated erect
2. Part position:
   a. Center affected orbit to cassette
   b. Rest head on zygoma, nose, and chin
   c. Adjust AML perpendicular to cassette
   d. Rotate MSP 53 degrees from cassette
   e. Respiration: suspended
3. Central ray: perpendicular, entering 1 inch superior and posterior to top of ear attachment, exiting affected orbit

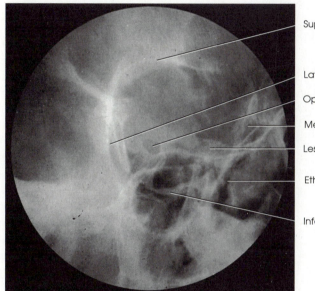

Superior orbital margin

Lateral orbital margin

Optic canal (foramen)

Medial orbital margin

Lesser wing of sphenoid

Ethmoidal sinus

Inferior orbital margin

Figure 5-52 Parieto-orbital oblique projection. Rhese method for optic canal. From Ballinger, P: Merrill's atlas of radiographic positions and radiologic procedures, ed 8, St. Louis, 1995, Mosby.

Facial Bones

A. Lateral (Fig. 5-53)
1. Patient position: semiprone or seated erect
2. Part position:
    a. Center zygoma
    b. Adjust MSP parallel to cassette
    c. IOML parallel to transverse axis of cassette
    d. IPL perpendicular to cassette
    e. Respiration: suspended
3. Central ray: perpendicular, entering lateral surface of
   zygomatic bone

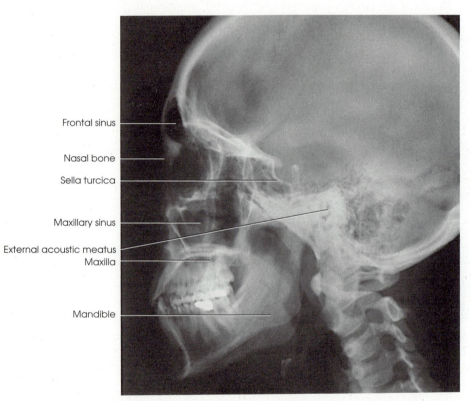

Figure 5-53 Lateral facial bones. From Ballinger, P: Merrill's atlas of radiographic positions and radiologic procedures, ed 8, St. Louis, 1995, Mosby.

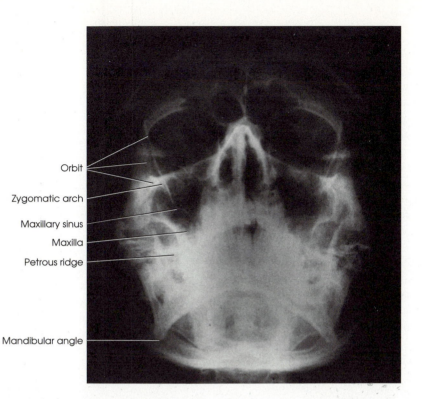

Figure 5-54 Parietocanthial facial bones. Waters method. From Ballinger, P: Merrill's atlas of radiographic positions and radiologic procedures, ed 8, St. Louis, 1995, Mosby.

B. Parietoacanthial (Waters) (Fig. 5-54)
1. Patient position: prone or seated erect
2. Part position:
   a. Center and adjust MSP perpendicular to cassette
   b. Rest patient's head on extended chin
   c. Adjust OML to form 37-degree angle to film plane
   d. Respiration: suspended
3. Central ray: perpendicular, exiting acanthion

Nasal Bones
A. Lateral (performed as a bilateral exam)
1. Patient position: semiprone or seated erect
2. Part position:
   a. Center nasion to cassette
   b. Adjust MSP parallel to cassette
   c. IOML parallel to transverse axis of cassette
   d. IPL perpendicular to cassette
   e. Respiration: Suspended
3. Central ray: perpendicular to the bridge of the nose, entering ¾ inch distal to nasion

Zygomatic Arches
A. Bilateral tangential (basal)
1. Patient position: seated erect or supine on elevated table support
2. Part position:
   a. Have patient extend head and rest on vertex
   b. Center and adjust MSP perpendicular to cassette
   c. Adjust IOML parallel to cassette

   d. Respiration: suspended
3. Central ray: perpendicular to IOML, entering midway between zygomatic arches approximately 1 inch posterior to outer canthi
B. Unilateral tangential (May)
1. Patient position: prone or seated erect at vertical grid device
2. Part position:
   a. Extend patient's neck and rest chin on grid device
   b. Rotate MSP 15 degrees away from side being examined
   c. Center cassette 3 inches distal to most prominent point of zygoma
   d. IOML parallel to plane of film
   e. Respiration: suspended
3. Central ray:
   a. Perpendicular to IOML
   b. Directed through zygomatic arch 1.5 inches posterior to outer canthus

Mandible
A. PA
1. Patient position: prone or seated erect
2. Part position:
   a. Have patient rest head on nose and chin
   b. For mandibular body, center cassette at level of lips
   c. For rami and TMJ, center to tip of nose
   d. MSP perpendicular to film
   e. Respiration: suspended

3. Central ray:
   a. For mandibular body, direct perpendicular to cassette at level of lips
   b. For rami and condylar processes, direct midway between TMJs at 30-degree cephalad angle

B. Axiolateral oblique (for mandibular body)
  1. Patient position: semiprone or seated erect
  2. Part position:
   a. Adjust cassette under affected cheek
   b. Extend patient's neck to place long axis of mandibular body parallel to cassette
   c. Center to first molar region
   d. Adjust broad surface of mandibular body parallel to cassette
   e. Respiration: suspended
  3. Central ray: Direct slightly posteriorly to mandibular angle farthest from film at a 25-degree cephalad angle

C. Axiolateral oblique (for mandibular ramus)
  1. Patient position: semiprone or seated erect
  2. Part position:
   a. Center cassette ½ inch anterior and 1 inch inferior to affected side EAM
   b. Extend patient's chin
   c. Adjust broad surface of ramus parallel to cassette
   d. Respiration: suspended
  3. Central ray: direct 25 degrees cephalad, entering 2 inches distal to the mandibular angle on side farthest from film

D. Submentovertex (basal)
  1. Patient position: seated erect or supine on elevated table support
  2. Part position:
   a. Extend neck and rest head on vertex
   b. Center and adjust MSP perpendicular to cassette
   c. Adjust IOML parallel to plane of film
   d. Respiration: suspended
  3. Central ray: perpendicular to IOML, entering midway between mandibular angles

Temporomandibular Articulations (Open and Closed Mouth Laterals)

A. Patient position: seated erect or semiprone
B. Part position:
  1. Center a point ½ inch anterior and 1 inch inferior to EAM to cassette
  2. MSP angled 15 degrees (nose toward film)
  3. AML adjusted parallel to transverse axis of cassette
  4. IPL perpendicular to cassette
  5. After first exposure with mouth closed and patient not permitted to move, cassette is changed and second exposure made with patient's mouth fully open
  6. Respirations: suspended
  7. Central ray: direct 15 degrees caudad, exiting TMJ against cassette

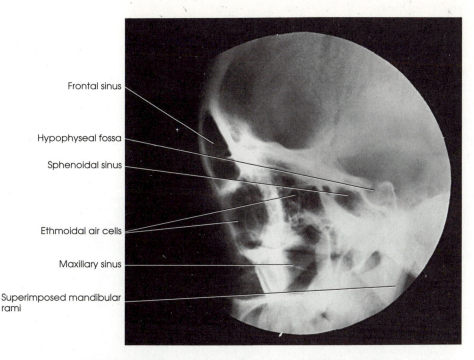

Frontal sinus

Hypophyseal fossa

Sphenoidal sinus

Ethmoidal air cells

Maxillary sinus

Superimposed mandibular rami

Figure 5-55 Lateral sinuses. Waters method. From Ballinger, P: Merrill's atlas of radiographic positions and radiologic procedures, ed 8, St. Louis, 1995, Mosby.

Paranasal Sinuses (Fig. 5-55)

A. Lateral
  1. Patient position: seated erect
  2. Part position:
    a. Center cassette ½ to 1 inch posterior to outer canthus
    b. Adjust patient's head to true lateral position
    c. MSP parallel and interpupillary line perpendicular to cassette
    d. IOML adjusted parallel to transverse axis of cassette
    e. Respiration: suspended
  3. Central ray: perpendicular, entering ½ to 1 inch posterior to outer canthus

B. PA axial (Caldwell)
  1. Patient position: seated erect at vertical grid device
  2. Part position:
    a. Rest patient's head on forehead and nose
    b. MSP perpendicular to midline of cassette
    c. OML perpendicular to cassette
    d. Respiration: suspended
  3. Central ray: direct to nasion at angle of 15 degrees caudal to the OML

C. Parietoacanthial (Waters)
  1. Patient position: seated erect; use horizontal central ray to demonstrate fluid level
  2. Part position:
    a. Center and adjust MSP perpendicular to cassette
    b. Rest patient's head on extended chin
    c. Adjust OML to form 37-degree angle to cassette
    d. Respiration: suspended
  3. Central ray: horizontal and perpendicular to cassette, exiting acanthion

D. Submentovertex (basal) (Fig. 5-56)
1. Patient position: seated erect at vertical grid device
2. Part position:
   a. Extend patient's head and rest on vertex
   b. Center and adjust MSP perpendicular to cassette
   c. Adjust IOML parallel to cassette
   d. Respiration: suspended
3. Central ray: perpendicular to IOML through sella turcica, approximately ¾ inch anterior to level of EAM

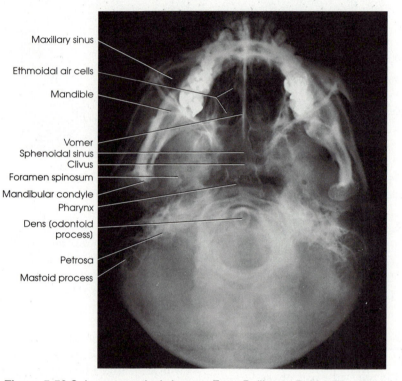

Maxillary sinus

Ethmoidal air cells

Mandible

Vomer
Sphenoidal sinus
Clivus
Foramen spinosum
Mandibular condyle
Pharynx
Dens (odontoid process)

Petrosa
Mastoid process

Figure 5-56 Submentovertical sinuses. From Ballinger, P: Merrill's atlas of radiographic positions and radiologic procedures, ed 8, St. Louis, 1995, Mosby.

Gastrointestinal System

Pathologies Imaged

A. Acute cholecystitis
1. Inflammation of gallbladder
B. Cancer of the colon and rectum
1. Leading cause of death from cancer in the United States
2. More typical form is annular carcinoma, with classic "apple-core" pattern when imaged using barium enema
C. Cancer of the esophagus
1. Malignant neoplasm
2. Imaged during barium study
D. Cancer of the stomach
1. May appear as gross changes in the stomach wall or as a large mass
2. Imaged during barium study
3. Harder to penetrate
E. Cholelithiasis
1. Gallstones
2. Harder to penetrate
F. Crohn's disease
1. Chronic inflammation of the bowel
2. Sometimes separated by normal segments of bowel
G. Diverticulitis
1. Inflammation of diverticula
H. Diverticulosis
1. Presence of diverticula, pouchlike herniations through the wall of the colon
I. Esophageal varices
1. Varicose veins at distal end of esophagus
J. Esophagitis
1. Inflammation of esophageal mucosal lining
K. Gastritis
1. Inflammation of the stomach
L. Hiatus hernia
1. Condition in which a portion of the stomach protrudes through the diaphragm
M. Ileus
1. Intestinal obstruction
2. Adynamic ileus—ileus caused by immobility of the bowel
3. Mechanical ileus—ileus caused by mechanical obstruction
N. Intussusception
1. Prolapse of one segment of bowel into another section of bowel
O. Irritable bowel syndrome
1. Abnormal increase in small and large bowel motility
P. Large bowel obstruction
1. Characterized by massive accumulation of gas proximal to obstruction
2. Absence of gas distal to obstruction
3. High risk of bowel perforation
4. Extent of obstruction determines ease or difficulty of penetration
Q. Peptic ulcer disease
1. Loss of mucous membrane in a portion of the gastrointestinal system
2. Imaged using barium study
3. Has craterlike appearance
R. Pyloric stenosis
1. Narrowing of pyloric sphincter
S. Small bowel obstruction
1. Seen as distended loops of bowel filled with gas
2. Bowel proximal to obstruction may be filled with fluid
3. Extent of obstruction determines ease or difficulty of penetration
T. Ulcerative colitis
1. Severe inflammation of the colon and rectum characterized by ulceration
U. Volvulus
1. Twisting of bowel on itself, causing an obstruction

General Survey Exams

Abdomen

A. AP (kidney, ureter, bladder [KUB])
  1. Patient position: supine
  2. Part position:
    a. Center MSP to table
    b. Shoulders in same transverse plane
    c. Support under knees
    d. Center cassette at level of iliac crests
    e. Apply gonad shielding as appropriate
    f. Respiration: expiration
  3. Central ray: perpendicular to midline at level of iliac crests

B. AP (upright)
  1. Patient position: erect
  2. Part position:
    a. Center MSP to table or upright grid device
    b. Shoulders in same transverse plane
    c. Center cassette 2 to 3 inches above iliac crests to include diaphragm
    d. Apply gonad shielding as appropriate
    e. Respiration: expiration
  3. Central ray: horizontal, entering MSP 2 to 3 inches superior to iliac crests

C. Lateral decubitus (Fig. 5-57)
  1. Patient position:
    a. Lateral recumbent (usually left side down), lying on pad
    b. Arms above level of diaphragm
    c. Knees slightly flexed
  2. Part position:
    a. MSP centered to grid device
    b. Center cassette at level of iliac crest
    c. Apply gonad shielding as appropriate
    d. Respiration: expiration
  3. Central ray: horizontal and parallel to the MSP at level of iliac crest

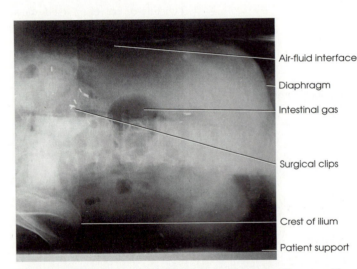

Air-fluid interface

Diaphragm

Intestinal gas

Surgical clips

Crest of ilium

Patient support

Figure 5-57 AP abdomen, left lateral decubitus position resulting in air marked by the air-fluid interface. From Ballinger, P: Merrill's atlas of radiographic positions and radiologic procedures, ed 8, St. Louis, 1995, Mosby.

Gallblabber

A. PA

1. Patient position: prone
2. Part position:
   a. Center right side of abdomen to midline of table
   b. Center cassette according to patient habitus over right upper quadrant
   c. Respiration: expiration
3. Central ray: perpendicular to center of cassette

B. LAO (PA oblique)

1. Patient position: recumbent with left arm posterior, right arm by head
2. Part position:
   a. Elevate right side 15 to 40 degrees to desired obliquity (thin patients require more rotation)
   b. Support patient on flexed knee and elbow
   c. Center localized gallbladder area to cassette
   d. Respiration: expiration
3. Central ray: perpendicular to center of cassette

Upper Gastrointestinal System

Esophagus

A. RAO (PA oblique)

1. Patient position: recumbent with right arm posterior, left arm by head
2. Part position:
   a. Elevate patient's left side to obliquity of 35 to 40 degrees
   b. Support patient on flexed knee and elbow
   c. Align esophagus and center at level of T5 or T6

   d. Feed barium to patient
   e. Respiration: suspended
3. Central ray: perpendicular to cassette, entering level of T5 or T6

Stomach

A. PA

1. Patient position: prone
2. Part position:
   a. Center at level of pylorus (approximately midway between xiphoid process and umbilicus)
   b. Center halfway between midline and lateral border of abdominal cavity for 10- x 12-inch cassette or MSP for 14- x 17-inch cassette
   c. Respiration: expiration
3. Central ray: perpendicular to cassette at level of pylorus (L2)

B. RAO (PA oblique) (Fig. 5-58)

1. Patient position: recumbent with right arm posterior, left arm by head
2. Part position:
   a. Elevate left side and support patient to obliquity of 40 to 70 degrees
   b. Longitudinal plane midway between vertebrae and anterior surface of elevated side is centered to cassette
   c. Center at level of duodenal bulb
   d. Respiration: expiration
3. Central ray: perpendicular to center of cassette midway between vertebral column and lateral border of abdominal cavity at level of L2

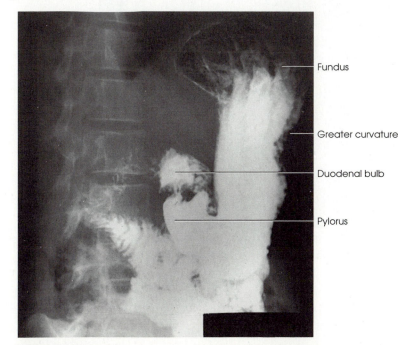

Fundus

Greater curvature

Duodenal bulb

Pylorus

Figure 5-58 Single contrast PA oblique stomach, RAO position. From Ballinger, P: Merrill's atlas of radiographic positions and radiologic procedures, ed 8, St. Louis, 1995, Mosby.

C. Lateral
1. Patient position: recumbent (right lateral) or erect (left lateral)
2. Part position:
   a. Center cassette between midaxillary plane and anterior abdominal surface
   b. Center at level of pylorus
   c. Adjust to true lateral
   d. Respiration: expiration
3. Central ray: perpendicular to center of cassette midway between midaxillary line and anterior surface of abdomen at the level of L1 for recumbent or L3 for upright position

Small Bowel
A. PA
1. Patient position: prone
2. Part position:
   a. MSP centered to table
   b. Center cassette at level of iliac crest (may be slightly higher for early time exposures)
   c. Respiration: suspended
3. Central ray: perpendicular to cassette entering midline at level of iliac crest (or slightly above)

Lower Gastrointestinal System

Colon
A. PA (Fig. 5-59)
1. Patient position: prone
2. Part position:
   a. MSP centered to table
   b. Center cassette at level of iliac crest
   c. Respiration: suspended
3. Central ray: perpendicular to cassette entering level of iliac crest
B. PA axial
1. Patient position: prone
2. Part position:
   a. MSP centered to table
   b. Center cassette at level of iliac crest
   c. Respiration: suspended
3. Central ray:
   a. 30 to 40 degrees caudad
   b. For demonstration of retrosigmoid area using smaller cassette, central ray enters midline at level of ASIS

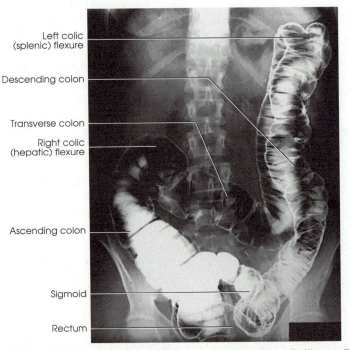

Left colic (splenic) flexure

Descending colon

Transverse colon

Right colic (hepatic) flexure

Ascending colon

Sigmoid

Rectum

Figure 5-59 Double-contrast PA large intestine. From Ballinger, P: Merrill's atlas of radiographic positions and radiologic procedures, ed 8, St. Louis, 1995, Mosby.

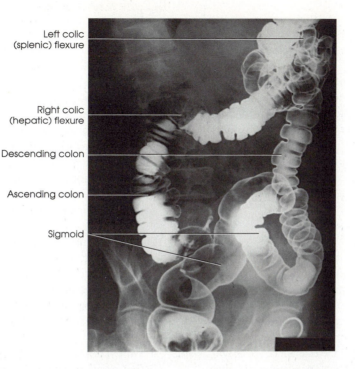

Left colic
(splenic) flexure

Right colic
(hepatic) flexure

Descending colon

Ascending colon

Sigmoid

Figure 5-60 Double-contrast PA oblique large intestine. From Ballinger, P: Merrill's atlas of radiographic positions and radiologic procedures, ed 8, St. Louis, 1995, Mosby.

C. LAO and RAO (PA oblique) (Fig. 5-60)
1. Patient position: PA oblique
2. Part position:
  a. Patient rotated 35 to 45 degrees
  b. Either right or left side up
  c. Center abdomen to table
  d. Cassette centered at level of iliac crest
  e. Respiration: suspended
3. Central ray: perpendicular to cassette entering level of iliac crest
D. Lateral rectum
1. Patient position: lying on side
2. Part position:
  a. Adjust patient's body to true lateral position (right or left side down)
  b. Center midaxillary plane of abdomen to center of table
  c. Respiration; suspended
3. Central ray: perpendicular to cassette, entering midaxillary plane at level of ASIS
E. AP
1. Patient position: supine
2. Part position:
  a. MSP centered to table
  b. Cassette centered at level of iliac crest
  c. Respiration: suspended
3. Central ray: perpendicular to cassette entering level of iliac crest
F. AP axial

1. Patient position: supine
2. Part position
  a. MSP centered to table
  b. Cassette centered 2 inches above iliac crest
  c. Respiration: suspended
3. Central ray:
  a. 30 to 40 degrees cephalad, entering approximately 2 inches below level of ASIS
  b. When retrosigmoid is of interest, central ray enters inferior margin of symphysis pubis
G. Lateral decubitus
1. Patient position: lying on either right or left side
2. Part position:
  a. Arms above head
  b. Knees slightly flexed
  c. Cassette centered to abdomen at level of iliac crest
  d. Respiration: suspended
3. Central ray: horizontal, entering midline at level of iliac crest
H. LPO and RPO (AP oblique)
1. Patient position: AP oblique
2. Part position:
  a. Patient rotated 35 to 45 degrees from AP position; either right or left side up
  b. Center abdomen to table
  c. Cassette centered at level of iliac crest
  d. Respiration: suspended
3. Central ray: perpendicular to cassette at level of iliac crest

Operative Cholangiogram

A. AP or AP oblique
　1. Patient position: supine on operating table
　2. Part position:
　　a. Right upper quadrant centered to the film
　　b. Left side of body may be elevated into a 15- to 20-degree oblique angle to prevent bile ducts from being superimposed over the spine
　3. Central ray: perpendicular to the exposed biliary tract
　4. Procedure notes:
　　a. Surgeon directs filming sequence
　　b. Equipment must be properly cleaned and ready to use
　　c. Radiographer must be in proper operating room attire
　　d. Appropriate radiation protection standards must be maintained for the radiographer, as well as for the operating room staff, using distance and lead shielding
　　e. Exposure times must be as short as possible, with patient respiration controlled by the anesthetist
　5. Exam evaluation: patency of the bile ducts; the operation of the sphincter of the hepatopancreatic ampulla; and the presence of calculi

T-Tube Cholangiogram

A. RPO (Fig. 5-61)
　1. Patient position: supine on fluoroscopic table
　2. Part position: right upper quadrant centered to midline of table
　3. Central ray: perpendicular to the biliary tract
　4. Procedure notes:
　　a. T-tube placed in common bile duct during surgery, providing for drainage and enabling postoperative evaluation of the biliary tree
　　b. Lower concentration, water-soluble contrast agent used to fill biliary tree
　　c. Spot films and radiographs may be taken during the stages of injection of the contrast medium
　　d. Exam continues until contrast agent is visualized entering the duodenum
　　e. T-tube remains clamped until end of procedure
　5. Exam evaluation: patency of the bile ducts; the operation of the sphincter of the hepatopancreatic ampulla; and the presence of calculi
B. Lateral
　1. Patient position: right lateral recumbent
　2. Part position: centered to midline of table
　3. Central ray: perpendicular to the biliary tract
　4. Exam evaluation: right lateral demonstrates branching of ducts and provides right-angle view to detect otherwise unseen abnormalities

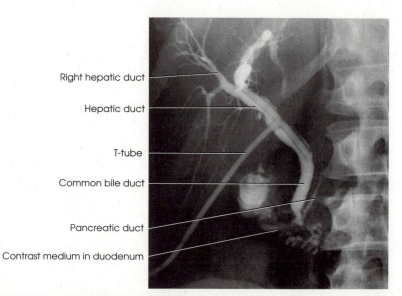

Right hepatic duct
Hepatic duct
T-tube
Common bile duct
Pancreatic duct
Contrast medium in duodenum

Figure 5-61 AP oblique postoperative cholangiogram, RPO position. From Ballinger, P: Merrill's atlas of radiographic positions and radiologic procedures, ed 8, St. Louis, 1995, Mosby.

Endoscopic Retrograde Cholangiopancreatography (ERCP)

A. Exam notes:
1. Used to evaluate biliary and pancreatic pathologies
2. Endoscope is passed into duodenum under fluoroscopic control
3. Contrast medium is injected into the common bile duct or pancreatic duct through a cannula passed through the endoscope
4. Patient is placed prone for spot films and radiographs
5. ERCP may be preceded by sonography, oral cholecystogram, or intravenous cholangiogram

Urinary System

Pathologies Imaged

A. Carcinoma of the bladder
1. Seen as solid mass arising from the bladder wall
2. Harder to penetrate
B. Cystitis
1. Inflammation of bladder and ureters
C. Glomerulonephritis
1. Inflammation of glomerulus of kidney
D. Polycystic kidney disease (PKD)
1. Enlarged kidneys containing numerous cysts
2. Harder to penetrate

E. Pyelonephritis
1. Inflammation of renal pelvis and parenchyma
F. Renal calculus
1. Kidney stone
2. Harder to penetrate stone, but overall technique is not increased to compensate
G. Renal carcinoma
1. Solid mass cancer that causes renal bulging or enlargement with impact on collecting system
2. Harder to penetrate
H. Renal cysts
1. Fluid-filled masses in kidney
2. Harder to penetrate
I. Wilm's tumor
1. Malignant cancer of kidney in children
2. Harder to penetrate

Urinary System Procedures

Intravenous Urography

A. KUB (AP) (Fig. 5-62)
1. Patient position: supine, centered to the table
2. Part position:
   a. Spine centered to the table
   b. Include entire renal outlines, bladder, and symphysis pubis, as well as the prostatic region on older male patients
3. Central ray: perpendicular to film, centered at level of iliac crest

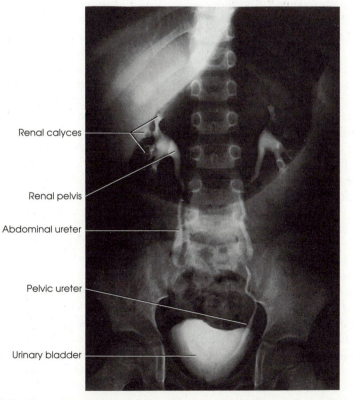

Renal calyces

Renal pelvis

Abdominal ureter

Pelvic ureter

Urinary bladder

Figure 5-62 Supine urogram at 15-minute interval with gas-filled stomach. From Ballinger, P: Merrill's atlas of radiographic positions and radiologic procedures, ed 8, St. Louis, 1995, Mosby.

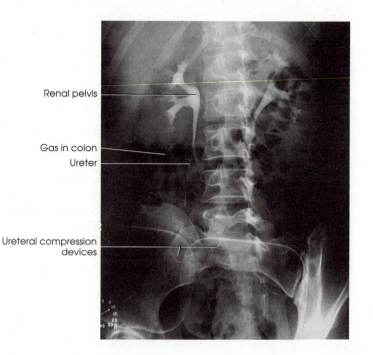

Renal pelvis

Gas in colon
Ureter

Ureteral compression
devices

Figure 5-63 Ten-minute postinjection urogram, AP oblique projection. From Ballinger, P: Merrill's atlas of radiographic positions and radiologic procedures, ed 8, St. Louis, 1995, Mosby.

B. Oblique (RPO, LPO) (Fig. 5-63)
  1. Patient position: supine
  2. Part position: patient's body rotated to a 30-degree oblique angle, kidney farthest from the film will be parallel to film and kidney nearest to the film will be perpendicular to film
  3. Central ray: perpendicular to film at iliac crest
C. AP bladder
  1. Patient position: supine
  2. Part position: supine, centered to film
  3. Central ray: perpendicular to film, centered at level of ASIS
D. Intravenous pyelogram (IVP) procedure notes
  1. Patient should be properly prepared with a low residue diet for 1 to 2 days before the exam and cleansing of the GI tract
  2. NPO after midnight the day of the exam, but not dehydrated
  3. A preliminary KUB is taken before injection to verify positioning, to visualize renal anatomy, or to detect the presence of lesions
  4. Thirty to one hundred milliliters (based on patient weight) of an iodinated contrast medium is injected; pelvicalyceal system will visualize in 2 to 8 minutes, with greatest visualization occurring in 15 to 20 minutes
  5. AP and oblique radiographs are made at specific intervals after injection of the contrast medium

6. All films must be carefully identified using right, left, upright, and "post-void" markers and numbers indicating postinjection time; stickers, felt-tip markers, and grease pencils should NOT be used to place identification on a radiograph
7. All film sizes needed for the exam should be made readily available before beginning procedure
8. AP upright positions may be used to demonstrate kidney mobility and the filled bladder
9. Oblique radiographs may be used to image kidney rotation or to localize tumor masses
10. Post-void radiographs may be taken to image tumor masses or prostatic enlargement
11. Tomography may be used during an IVP to blur gas patterns and to better image intrarenal lesions; this is termed *nephrotomography*

Cystography/Cystourethrography

A. Positioning
  1. AP
     a. Five-degree caudal angle on tube
     b. Film centered at level 2 to 3 inches above symphysis pubis
  2. Oblique (RPO, LPO)
     a. Patient rotated 40 to 60 degrees
     b. Pubic arch closest to table centered to midline of table

3. PA of bladder
    a. Patient centered
    b. Central ray enters 1 inch distal to tip of coccyx with a 10- to 15-degree cephalad angle
4. Lateral
    a. Bladder centered to film; cassette 2 to 3 inches above symphysis pubis
    b. Central ray centered and perpendicular to film

B. Procedure notes
1. Bladder is drained using catheter which has been put in place
2. Bladder is filled with contrast medium through urethral catheter
3. Once bladder is filled, clamp is closed to prevent contrast agent from draining
4. Filming follows filling of bladder
5. Cystourethrography may follow cystogram
    a. Patient is instructed to void contrast material from bladder while on fluoroscopic table
    b. Radiologist takes spot films during urination to evaluate urethra and to image reflux

Retrograde Pyelography

A. Positioning
1. AP
2. RPO
3. LPO

B. Procedure notes
1. Ureters are catheterized to allow filling of the pelvicalyceal system
2. Urologist performs procedure
3. Film is placed to include both kidneys and ureters
4. Following catheterization and introduction of contrast material, urologist directs filming sequence

Other Radiologic Examinations

A. Tomography
1. Uses motion of x-ray tube and film to blur unwanted structures from the image
2. X-ray tube and film are connected by a rigid rod that pivots around a fulcrum
3. Position of fulcrum corresponds to level in the body that will appear in focus on the radiograph (called the *objective plane*)
4. Structures above and below the objective plane are blurred beyond recognition
5. Angle of arc through which the x-ray tube travels is called *exposure angle*
    a. Exposure angle determines thickness of tomographic cut
    b. Wider angles provide thin cuts
    c. Narrower angles provide thick cuts
6. Thick-section tomography called *zonography*
7. Blurring pattern on radiograph determines detail visibility

8. Blurring pattern is determined by motion used
9. Types of motions
    a. Linear
    b. Circular
    c. Elliptical
    d. Hypocycloidal
    e. Spiral
10. Patient positioning must be extremely accurate
11. Equipment must be kept in proper working condition to prevent unwanted stray motion in linkages connecting x-ray tube, rod, and tray
12. Primary use of tomography is nephrotomography
13. Tomography largely displaced by computed tomography

B. Myelography
1. Pathologies imaged
    a. Herniated intervertebral disks
    b. Degenerative diseases of the CNS
    c. Space-occupying lesions
2. Pathologies imaged by displacing column of contrast material in the subarachnoid space
3. Lumbar puncture performed by physician at L3-L4 interspace allows injection of water soluble contrast agent into subarachnoid space
4. Small amount of spinal fluid is withdrawn for laboratory analysis
5. X-ray table is tilted up and down to distribute contrast medium
6. Contrast medium should not be allowed to enter cerebral ventricles; head must be kept hyperextended to compress cisterna magna when working with contrast medium in cervical region
7. Spot films are taken under fluoroscopic control in PA and oblique positions
8. Crosstable lateral radiographs are taken by radiographer to provide right-angle views
9. Contrast medium is absorbed by patient's body

C. Arthrography
1. Contrast exam of an encapsulated joint
    a. Knee
    b. Shoulder
    c. Hip
    d. Wrist
    e. TMJ
2. Pathologies imaged
    a. Joint trauma
    b. Meniscal tears
    c. Capsular damage
    d. Deformities secondary to arthritis
    e. Rupture of articular ligaments
3. Performed under local anesthetic using asepsis
4. Physician injects contrast material
5. Joint is manipulated to distribute contrast agent
6. Fluoroscopic spot films and radiographs may be taken
7. Arthrography gradually being replaced by MRI

D. Venography
   1. Pathologies imaged
      a. Embolism—lodging of an embolus in a blood vessel
      b. Thrombophlebitis—inflammation of a vein, accompanied by the formation of clots
      c. Thrombosis—formation of blood clot (*thrombus*) within a blood vessel
      d. Varicose veins—dilated veins with malfunctioning valves
      e. Vessel damage secondary to trauma
   2. Upper extremity venograms
      a. Performed to evaluate presence of thrombosis
      b. Contrast medium injected into superficial vein at elbow or wrist, by hand or with automatic injector
      c. Flow of contrast agent may be observed using fluoroscopy and spot filming; automatic film changer may be used
      d. Radiography performed using AP projection
      e. Radiograph should extend from site of injection to superior vena cava
      f. Contrast agent may be forced into deep veins by applying a tourniquet proximal to the injection site
   3. Lower extremity venograms
      a. Used to evaluate thrombosis in legs
      b. Contrast medium injected into superficial vein of foot, by hand or with automatic injector
      c. Flow of contrast agent may be observed using fluoroscopy and spot filming; automatic film changer may be used
      d. Radiography performed using AP projection of legs with 30-degree internal rotation
      e. Automatic long-leg film changer may be used for serial radiography 5 to 10 seconds apart
      f. Contrast agent may be forced into deep veins by applying a tourniquet proximal to the injection site
      g. Radiographs should extend from site of injection to inferior vena cava
E. Hysterosalpingography
   1. Pathologies imaged
      a. Abnormal uterine bleeding
      b. Amenorrhea
      c. Cervical stenosis
      d. Dysmenorrhea
      e. Fistulae
      f. Masses
      g. Neoplasms
      h. Patency of oviducts
      i. Polyps
      j. Uterine anomalies
   2. Therapeutic procedures
      a. Dilate oviducts
      b. Open oviducts
      c. Remove kinks

3. Preliminary radiograph centered 2 inches proximal to symphysis pubis
4. Physician introduces iodinated contrast agent through cervix and into uterus
5. Fluoroscopic spot films or radiographs (AP) are taken to image the uterus and contrast agent flow through the fallopian tubes
6. Images indicate shape of uterus, presence of pathologies, and patency of oviducts
7. Other radiographs may be taken in oblique or lateral positions
8. Contrast medium is absorbed by patient and excreted by urinary system

▲ *Review Questions*

Use the listing below to answer questions 1–8. Items may be used more than once.

    A. Hypersthenic habitus
    B. Sthenic habitus
    C. Hyposthenic habitus
    D. Asthenic habitus

1. Slender build   *D*

2. Massive build   *A*

3. Stomach and gallbladder are low, vertical, near the midline   *D*

4. Average build, present in about 35% of the population   *C*

5. Most common body habitus, present in about 50% of the population   *B*

6. Stomach and gallbladder high and horizontal   *A*

7. Thorax narrow and shallow   *D*

8. Thorax broad and deep   *A*

For the following questions, choose the single best answer.

9. Key points in performing pediatric radiography are:

    a. Work quickly, impersonally, use gonadal shielding, report suspected child abuse, keep parents in waiting room
    b. Work quickly, communicate clearly with child and parent(s), use gonadal shielding, report suspected child abuse
    c. Work quickly, impersonally, report suspected child abuse, keep parents in waiting room, always use Pigg-o-stat
    d. Work quickly, impersonally, use gonadal shielding only on abdominal exams, report suspected child abuse, keep parents in waiting room
    e. Work quickly, impersonally, report suspected child abuse

10. The most important point to remember when performing trauma radiography is:

    a. Use gonadal shielding because this patient will be having many follow-up exams
    b. Work quickly because the injuries may be life-threatening
    c. Do no additional harm to the patient
    d. Do only the projections ordered by the physician
    e. Acquire only two projections for each exam ordered

11. When performing trauma radiography:

    a. Splints, bandages, and cervical collars should be removed so they do not obstruct the anatomy that must be imaged
    b. Remove cervical collars only under the direction of a radiologist
    c. Remove cervical collars only under the direction of an ER physician or radiologist
    d. Splints, bandages, and cervical collars should be removed after preliminary films have been viewed by a physician so they do not obstruct the anatomy that must be imaged
    e. Speed is the single most important trait the radiographer must possess

Use the listing below to answer questions 12–16. Items may be used more than once.

    A. Transverse plane
    B. Midcoronal plane
    C. Median sagittal plane
    D. Sagittal plane
    E. Coronal plane

E 12. Any plane passing vertically through the body from side to side

C 13. Passes vertically through the midline of the body from front to back

A 14. Divides the body into superior and inferior portions

B 15. Passes vertically through the midaxillary region of the body and through the coronal suture of the cranium at right angles to the midsagittal plane

D 16. Any plane parallel to the MSP

Use the listing below to answer questions 17–21. Items may be used more than once.

A. Ball and socket joint
B. Pivot joint
C. Hinge joint
D. Saddle joint
E. Cartilaginous joint

17. No joint cavity, contiguous bones united by cartilage

18. Rounded head of one bone moves in a cup-like cavity

19. Permits motion in one plane only

20. Opposing surfaces are convex-concave, allowing great freedom of motion

21. Permits rotary movement in which a ring rotates around a central axis

For the following questions, choose the single best answer.

22. Which of the following pathologies would NOT be an indication for performing hysterosalpingography?

　a. Determine the patency of the oviducts
　b. Status of pregnancy
　c. Abnormal uterine bleeding
　d. Uterine polyps
　e. Neoplasms

23. Which of the following are true regarding venography?

(1) Performed to visualize thrombophlebitis, varicose veins, or vessel damage secondary to trauma
(2) Requires AP and lateral projections
(3) Use of exam is limited because deep veins cannot be imaged
(4) Injection is made into superficial veins
(5) Automatic film changers required for film imaging

　a. All are true
　b. 1, 4
　c. 2, 3, 5
　d. 1, 2, 4
　e. 1, 3, 4

24. Which of the following are true regarding contrast arthrography?

(1) Asepsis required
(2) May be performed on knee, shoulder, TMJ, hip, wrist
(3) Indications include trauma, capsular damage, meniscal tears, rupture of ligaments, arthritis
(4) Joint is manipulated by hand to distribute contrast medium

　a. 1, 2, 3, 4
　b. All except 4
　c. All except 1
　d. 2, 3
　e. 1, 2

25. Which of the following are true concerning myelography?

(1) Injection is always made at the L3-L4 interspace
(2) Oily, iodinated contrast agent is the medium of choice
(3) Indications include herniated intervertebral disks, space-occupying lesions, degenerative diseases of the CNS
(4) Contrast medium is distributed by manual manipulation of the subarachnoid space
(5) Head must be kept hyperflexed to prevent contrast medium from entering cerebral ventricles
(6) Spinal fluid may be withdrawn for laboratory analysis

　a. All are true
　b. None are true
　c. 1, 2, 3, 5
　d. 3, 6
　e. 1, 3, 4, 5

26. An exam that uses motion and blurring to view anatomy by setting the x-ray tube and film in motion is:

　a. Computed tomography
　b. Autotomography
　c. Conventional tomography
　d. Fluoroscopy
　e. All of the above

27. The proper centering point for a PA projection of the hand is the:

　a. Third metatarsophalangeal joint
　b. Third metacarpophalangeal joint
　c. Midshaft of the third metacarpal
　d. First metacarpophalangeal joint
　e. Third PIP joint

28. For the lateral projection of the wrist:

    a. The radius and ulna should be superimposed
    b. Radial surface must be in contact with the film
    c. Central ray is perpendicular to wrist
    d. All of the above
    e. More than one but not all of the above

29. For the lateral projection of the forearm:

    (1) The ulnar surface must be in contact with the film
    (2) Thumb should be in a relaxed position
    (3) Humerus and forearm should be in contact with the table
    (4) Elbow should be flexed 45 degrees
    (5) Central ray is directed to the injured joint

    a. 1, 2, 3, 4, 5
    b. 1, 2, 5
    c. 1, 3
    d. 2, 4, 5
    e. 3, 4

30. For the AP projection of the elbow:

    (1) Forearm and humerus should be at right angles
    (2) Central ray is directed perpendicular to the joint
    (3) Forearm and humerus should be parallel to the table
    (4) Hand must be pronated
    (5) Patient may have to lean laterally to ensure AP alignment

    a. 1, 2, 3, 4, 5
    b. 2, 3, 5
    c. 1, 4
    d. 2, 3, 4, 5
    e. 2, 5

31. For the lateral projection of the humerus:

    (1) The hand should be pronated
    (2) Patient may be upright or supine
    (3) Humeral epicondyles are placed perpendicular to cassette
    (4) Arm should be slightly adducted
    (5) Central ray is directed perpendicular to the midshaft

    a. 2, 3, 5
    b. 1, 4
    c. 1, 2, 3, 4, 5
    d. 1, 2, 3, 5
    e. 2, 3, 4, 5

32. For the PA oblique (scapular Y) projection of the shoulder:

    (1) Central ray is directed to the shoulder at a 10-degree cephalad angle
    (2) The anterior surface of the affected shoulder is centered to the cassette
    (3) Patient is rotated so midcoronal plane forms 60-degree angle with cassette
    (4) Patient continues shallow breathing during exposure

    a. 1, 2, 3, 4
    b. 2, 3, 4
    c. 2, 3
    d. 1, 2, 3
    e. 3, 4

33. For the AP projection of the acromioclavicular joints:

    a. To properly demonstrate A-C separation, both joints with and without weights should be demonstrated on one film if possible
    b. To properly demonstrate A-C separation, separate films must be acquired—with equal weights attached to both wrists and without weights
    c. The central ray is always directed midway between the A-C joints
    d. Patient should be seated upright and instructed to continue shallow breathing during the exposure

34. When radiographing the clavicle:

    (1) PA projection must always be used
    (2) Central ray angle of 25 to 30 degrees cephalad is used for the PA axial
    (3) Patient's head should be turned away from the affected side
    (4) AP projection may be used for patient comfort
    (5) Erect position may be used for patient comfort
    (6) Central ray angle of 25 to 30 degrees caudad is used for the PA axial

    a. 1, 2, 3, 4, 5
    b. 1, 3, 4, 5
    c. 2, 3, 4, 5
    d. 3, 4, 5, 6

35. For the lateral projection of the scapula:

    (1) Patient should be upright to reduce pain
    (2) Patient is positioned obliquely with unaffected scapula centered to the cassette
    (3) Body is adjusted by palpating axillary and vertebral borders of the scapula so the scapula is lateral
    (4) Scapula must be projected free of the rib cage

    a. 1, 3, 4
    b. 1, 2, 3, 4
    c. 3, 4
    d. 2, 3, 4

Use the listing below to answer questions 36–40. Items may be used more than once.

    A. Trimalleolar fracture
    B. Giant cell myeloma
    C. Osteoarthritis
    D. Pott's fracture
    E. Comminuted fracture

36. Fracture of medial and lateral malleoli of the ankle with ankle joint dislocation

37. Involves the posterior portion of the tibia and the medial and lateral malleoli

38. Fracture producing more than two fragments

39. Tumor arising on bone with large bubble appearance; may be benign or malignant

40. Characterized by the degeneration of one or several joints

For the following questions, choose the single best answer.

41. For AP radiography of the foot:

    (1) A trough compensating filter may be used
    (2) Dorsal surface rests on cassette
    (3) Central ray is directed 10 degrees anterior
    (4) Central ray is directed at the head of the third metatarsal

    a. 1, 2, 3, 4
    b. 1, 3, 4
    c. 2, 4
    d. 1, 2, 4
    e. None of these a through d are correct

42. When performing the AP axial projection for the os calcis:

    (1) Leg should be fully extended
    (2) The plantar surface of the foot should be parallel to the cassette
    (3) The central ray is directed 40 degrees cephalad to the long axis of the foot
    (4) The central ray enters the foot at the head of the fifth metatarsal
    (5) A cylinder cone may be used for this projection

    a. 1, 3, 5
    b. 2, 4
    c. 1, 2, 3, 4, 5
    d. 1, 3, 4, 5

43. For the medial oblique position of the ankle:

    (1) Leg and foot are rotated medially
    (2) Ankle is adjusted to a 90-degree angle
    (3) Medial rotation is adjusted to 45 degrees to demonstrate the mortise joint
    (4) Medial rotation is adjusted to 15 to 20 degrees to demonstrate the bony structure
    (5) Central ray is directed vertically midway between the malleoli

    a. 1, 2, 3, 4, 5
    b. 1, 5
    c. 1, 3, 4, 5
    d. 1, 2, 3, 4

44. For the lateral lower leg projection:

    (1) Leg is centered to cassette
    (2) May be performed table top or Bucky
    (3) Roll patient away from affected side
    (4) Patella should be perpendicular to cassette
    (5) Include both joints
    (6) Tibia and fibula should be superimposed
    (7) Central ray is directed to midpoint of leg

    a. 1, 2, 3, 4, 5, 6, 7
    b. 1, 2, 3, 4, 5, 7
    c. 1, 4, 5, 6, 7
    d. 1, 2, 4, 5, 7

45. When performing the lateral knee projection:

    (1) Patient turns onto affected side
    (2) Knee is flexed 20 to 30 degrees
    (3) Patella must be parallel to film
    (4) Central ray is directed 5 degrees caudad
    (5) Central ray enters knee joint inferior to the medial condyle

    a. 1, 2, 3, 4, 5
    b. 1, 2, 3, 5
    c. 1, 2, 5
    d. 1, 2, 4, 5

46. For the tangential projection of the patella:

    (1) Patient is prone
    (2) Affected knee is flexed so tibia and fibula form 50- to 60-degree angle with table
    (3) Central ray is directed 45 degrees cephalad through patellofemoral joint
    (4) Tangential patella may also be performed with the patient supine

    a. 1, 2, 3, 4
    b. 2, 3, 4
    c. 1, 2, 3
    d. 1, 2, 4

47. For the AP projection of the femur:

    a. The lower leg should be rotated laterally 15 degrees
    b. The central ray is directed toward the affected joint
    c. The patient is prone
    d. The lower leg is rotated medially 15 degrees

48. The central ray for an AP projection of the hip is:

    a. Directed parallel to a point 2 inches medial to the ASIS and at the level of the superior margin of the greater trochanter
    b. Directed parallel to a point 2 inches lateral to the ASIS and at the level of the superior margin of the greater trochanter
    c. Directed parallel to a point 2 inches medial to the ASIS and at the level of the inferior margin of the greater trochanter
    d. Directed perpendicular to a point 2 inches medial to the ASIS and at the level of the superior margin of the greater trochanter
    e. Directed perpendicular to a point 2 inches medial to the ASIS and at the level of the inferior margin of the greater trochanter

Use the listing below to answer questions 49–53. Items may be used more than once.

    A. Jefferson fracture
    B. Hangman's fracture
    C. Spondylolysis
    D. Spina bifida
    E. Osteoblastic metastases

49. Dense, sclerotic tumors in bone

50. Caused by acute hyperextension of the head on the neck; fracture of the arch of C2

51. Defect of the posterior aspect of the spinal canal caused by failure of the vertebral arch to properly form

52. Defect in pars articularis

53. Comminuted fracture of the ring of the atlas involving both anterior and posterior arches and causing displacement of the fragments

For the following questions, choose the single best answer.

54. For the lateral projection of the cervical spine:

    (1) Patient may be upright, seated, or supine, depending upon condition
    (2) SID of 72 inches should be used because of increased OID
    (3) Shoulders should lie in the same plane
    (4) Cervical collar should be removed so that it does not obstruct pertinent anatomy
    (5) Chin should be in contact with chest

    a. 1, 2, 3, 4, 5
    b. 1, 2, 3
    c. 1, 2, 3, 5
    d. 1, 2, 4, 5
    e. 1, 3, 5

55. For the lateral projection of the thoracic spine:

    (1) The head and spine should be in the same plane
    (2) The central ray is directed to T7, at a cephalad angle of 10 degrees
    (3) Patient should continue shallow breathing during exposure
    (4) Exam should not be performed in room with a falling load generator

    a. 1, 2, 3, 4
    b. 1, 3
    c. 1, 3, 4
    d. 1, 2, 3

56. For the lateral projection of L5-S1:

    (1) Patient is in lateral position
    (2) Hips and knees are extended
    (3) Cassette is centered at the level of the transverse plane that passes midway between the iliac crests and the ASIS
    (4) A cylinder cone may be used to greatly reduce the production of scatter radiation
    (5) Central ray is directed to a point 1½ inches anterior to palpated spinous process of L5

    a. 1, 2, 3, 4, 5
    b. 1, 2
    c. 1, 2, 3, 5
    d. 1, 3, 4, 5

57. The RPO and LPO positions for sacroiliac joints:

    a. Image the joint nearest the film
    b. Require the part to be angled at 10 to 15 degrees to coincide with the angle of the joints
    c. Image the joint farthest from the film
    d. Require the central ray to be angled 25 degrees cephalad
    e. Require both obliques to be taken upright for weight bearing studies

58. For the AP projection of the coccyx:

    a. The central ray should be directed 10 degrees caudad entering 2 inches superior to the symphysis pubis
    b. The central ray should be directed 10 degrees cephalad entering 2 inches superior to the symphysis pubis
    c. The central ray should be directed 25 degrees caudad entering 2 inches superior to the symphysis pubis
    d. The central ray should be directed 25 degrees caudad entering 4 inches superior to the symphysis pubis

Use the listing below to answer questions 59–64. Items may be used more than once.

    A. Atelectasis
    B. Bronchogenic carcinoma
    C. COPD
    D. Emphysema
    E. Pleural effusion

59. Pathology that is easy to penetrate *D*

60. Collapse of lung tissue; harder to penetrate *A*

61. Accumulation of fluid in intrapleural spaces; harder to penetrate *E*

62. AEC should not be used to image *D*

63. Lung cancer arising from bronchial mucosa *B*

64. Progressive condition marked by diminished capabilities of inspiration and expiration *C*

For the following questions, choose the single best answer.

65. For the AP projection of the ribs above the diaphragm:

    (1) Top of cassette placed 1 to 2 inches above shoulders
    (2) Shoulders relaxed, scapulae flat against table
    (3) Central ray to T7
    (4) Respiration on full expiration to depress diaphragm

    a. 1, 3
    b. 1, 2, 3, 4
    c. 1, 2, 3
    d. 1, 3, 4

66. For the RAO position of the sternum:

    a. Body should be rotated 45 to 60 degrees to prevent superimposition of sternum and spine
    b. Patient is supine
    c. Breathing should be shallow during exposure; falling load generator should not be used
    d. Best image is obtained with suspended breathing

67. When radiographing the sternoclavicular articulations:

    a. PA and lateral projections are required
    b. RAO or LAO positions are used to eliminate superimposition of joints onto vertebral shadow
    c. Patient should breathe during exposure; falling load generator should be used if possible
    d. AP projection is used to reduce magnification of joints

Use the listing below to answer questions 68–72. Items may be used more than once.

A. Hydrocephalus
B. Paget's disease
C. Osteoporosis
D. Rickets
E. Osteomalacia

68. Soft bones resulting from deficiency of vitamin D and sunlight

69. Bone disease causing bone destruction and unorganized bone repair; generally difficult to penetrate

70. Abnormal demineralization of bone, seen more often in females

71. Abnormal accumulation of CSF in the brain

72. Abnormal softening of bone; easier to penetrate

For the following questions, choose the single best answer.

73. For the direct PA projection of the skull the central ray is directed:

   a. 15 degrees caudad
   b. 25 degrees caudad
   c. Perpendicular to the film
   d. Perpendicular to the film, exiting the nasion
   e. Perpendicular to the film, exiting the nasion when the OML is perpendicular to the cassette

74. When radiographing the skull in the lateral position,

   a. The MSP must be perpendicular to the cassette, the IOML must be parallel to the cassette, the IPL must be parallel to the cassette
   b. The MSP and IOML are parallel to the cassette and the IPL is perpendicular to the cassette
   c. The MSP is perpendicular to the cassette and the IPL is parallel to the cassette
   d. The MSP and IOML are perpendicular to the cassette and the IPL is parallel to the cassette

75. For the parieto-orbital (Rhese) projection of the optic foramen:

   a. The head is resting on the forehead, nose, and zygoma
   b. The MSP forms an angle of 37 degrees from the perpendicular
   c. The central ray exits the unaffected orbit
   d. The head rests on the zygoma, nose, and chin while the MSP is rotated 53 degrees from the cassette

76. When performing the parietoacanthial (Waters) projection for the facial bones:

   a. The MSP is parallel to the cassette
   b. The MSP is perpendicular to the cassette, the head rests on the chin, the OML forms a 53-degree angle with the plane of the film
   c. The MSP is perpendicular to the cassette, the head rests on the chin, the OML forms a 37-degree angle with the plane of the film
   d. The MSP is perpendicular to the cassette, the head rests on the nose, the OML forms a 37-degree angle with the plane of the film

77. For the unilateral tangential (May) projection of the zygomatic arches:

   a. The IOML is parallel to the plane of the film, the MSP is rotated 15 degrees away from the affected side, cassette is centered 3 inches distal to the most prominent point of the zygoma, the central ray is directed perpendicular to the IOML through the zygomatic arch, 1.5 inches posterior to the outer canthus
   b. The IOML is parallel to the plane of the film, the MSP is rotated 15 degrees towards the affected side, the cassette is centered 3 inches distal to the most prominent point of the zygoma, the central ray is directed perpendicular to the IOML through the zygomatic arch, 1.5 inches posterior to the outer canthus
   c. The IOML is parallel to the plane of the film, the MSP is rotated 15 degrees away from the affected side, the cassette is centered 3 inches distal to the most prominent point of the zygoma, the central ray is directed perpendicular to the zygomatic arch 1.5 inches posterior to the outer canthus
   d. The IOML is parallel to the plane of the film, the MSP is rotated 25 degrees away from the affected side, the cassette is centered 3 inches distal to the most prominent point of the zygoma, the central ray is directed perpendicular to the IOML through the zygomatic arch, 1.5 inches posterior to the outer canthus

78. When radiographing the mandibular body with the patient in the SMV position:

    a. Head and neck are extended and resting on chin
    b. MSP is parallel with cassette
    c. IOML is perpendicular with plane of film, head and neck are resting on vertex, and MSP is perpendicular to the cassette
    d. IOML is parallel with plane of film, head resting on vertex, and MSP is perpendicular to the cassette

79. The best survey film of the paranasal sinuses is obtained using:

    a. Lateral
    b. Parietoacanthial (Waters)
    c. PA axial
    d. SMV
    e. Upright lateral

Use the listing below to answer questions 80–84. Items may be used more than once.

    A. Annular carcinoma
    B. Crohn's disease
    C. Hiatus hernia
    D. Ileus
    E. Peptic ulcer disease

80. Condition wherein a portion of the stomach protrudes through the diaphragm

81. Intestinal obstruction

82. Chronic inflammation of portions of bowel

83. Loss of mucous membrane in a portion of the GI system

84. Shows as "apple-core" pattern on barium enema

Use the listing below to answer questions 85–89. Items may be used more than once.

    A. Diverticula
    B. Ulcerative colitis
    C. Pyloric stenosis
    D. Adynamic ileus
    E. Cholelithiasis

85. Gallstones

86. Bowel obstruction caused by immobility of bowel

87. Pouchlike herniations of the colonic wall

88. Narrowing of sphincter at distal end of stomach

89. Severe inflammation of colon and rectum with loss of mucosal lining

For the following questions, choose the single best answer.

90. For the RAO position of the esophagus:

    a. Patient is rotated obliquely by elevating right side 35 to 40 degrees, esophagus is centered to film at level of T5 or T6
    b. Patient is rotated obliquely by elevating left side 35 to 40 degrees, center film at level of T5 or T6
    c. Patient is rotated obliquely by elevating right side 55 to 60 degrees, esophagus is centered to film at level of T5 or T6
    d. Patient is rotated obliquely by elevating left side 55 to 60 degrees, esophagus is centered to film at level of T5 or T6

91. For the PA projection of the stomach:

    a. Center midway between the xiphoid process and the umbilicus
    b. Center halfway between the midline and lateral border of abdominal cavity
    c. Center midway between the manubrium and the umbilicus and halfway between the midline and lateral border of abdominal cavity
    d. Center midway between the xiphoid process and the umbilicus and halfway between the midline and lateral border of abdominal cavity

92. For the LPO or RPO positions for the colon:

    a. Patient is prone, rotated 35 to 45 degrees, central ray at level of iliac crest
    b. Patient is supine, rotated 55 to 60 degrees, central ray at level of ASIS
    c. Patient is supine, rotated 35 to 45 degrees from the AP, central ray at level of iliac crest
    d. Patient is prone, rotated 55 to 60 degrees, central ray at level of iliac crest

93. For the lateral decubitus positions of the colon:

    a. Patient lying on side, cassette centered to iliac crest, central ray horizontal to midline at level of iliac crest
    b. Patient prone, cassette centered to iliac crest, central ray horizontal to midline at level of iliac crest
    c. Patient lying on side, cassette centered 3 inches above iliac crest, central ray horizontal 3 inches above iliac crest
    d. Patient prone, cassette centered to L1, central ray horizontal to L1

94. A procedure that evaluates biliary and pancreatic pathologies using an endoscope is:

    a. Sonography
    b. MRI
    c. ERCP
    d. IVP
    e. T-tube cholangiogram

Use the listing below to answer questions 95–99. Items may be used more than once.

    A. Polycystic kidney disease
    B. Renal calculus
    C. Wilm's tumor
    D. Renal cysts
    E. Pyelonephritis

95. Fluid-filled masses in kidney

96. Malignant cancer of the kidney in children

97. Enlarged kidneys containing numerous cysts

98. Inflammation of renal pelvis and parenchyma

99. Kidney stone

For the following question, choose the single best answer.

100. For the RPO and LPO positions of the kidneys:

    a. Patient is prone, body is rotated obliquely 30 degrees, kidney farthest from film is imaged in profile and kidney nearest film is imaged in its entirety, central ray is perpendicular
    b. Patient is supine, body is rotated obliquely 45 degrees, kidney farthest from film is imaged in profile and kidney nearest film is imaged in its entirety, central ray is perpendicular
    c. Patient is supine, body is rotated obliqued 30 degrees, kidney farthest from film is imaged parallel to film and kidney nearest film is imaged perpendicular to film, central ray is perpendicular to film
    d. Patient is supine, body is rotated obliqued 30 degrees, kidney nearest the film is imaged in profile and kidney farthest from film is imaged in its entirety, central ray is perpendicular

Chapter 6

Review of Patient Care and Management

▲ Scheduling of Radiographic Examinations

A. General considerations
1. Schedule in an appropriate and timely sequence to ensure patient comfort and fiscal responsibility
2. Sequence so that exams do not interfere with one another
3. Barium studies are scheduled last
4. Several exams are scheduled in one day, if the patient is able to tolerate them
5. Seriously ill or weak patients may be able to tolerate only one exam per day or must have a rest between examinations
6. If sedation is used, patient must be given time to recover from sedation before beginning fluoroscopic studies
7. Thyroid assessment must precede any examinations involving iodinated contrast media
8. Radiographic exams not requiring contrast agents are scheduled first
9. Total doses of iodinated contrast media should be calculated, if a series of examinations using it will be performed
10. Patients who have been held NPO should be scheduled first
11. Pediatric and geriatric patients should be scheduled early
12. Diabetic patients must be scheduled early because of their need for insulin

B. Sequencing
1. Fiber-optic (endoscopy) studies are conducted first in a series
2. Radiography of the urinary tract
3. Radiography of the biliary system
4. CT studies should be scheduled before examinations involving the use of barium sulfate
5. Lower GI series
6. Upper GI series

▲ Patient Preparation

A. Gastrointestinal system or urinary system
1. Low-residue diet
2. NPO for 8 to 12 hours before the procedure
3. Cathartics and enemas are used to cleanse the GI system
4. If scheduled as an outpatient:
   a. Patient must clearly understand the routine for proper preparation
   b. Patient should be asked to explain the procedure back to the radiographer to verify understanding
B. All procedures
1. Clothing removed from area to be radiographed, replaced by patient gown when appropriate
2. All radiopaque objects removed from area of interest

▲ Patient History

A. Assists the radiographer in knowing the extent of injury and the range of motion the patient will tolerate
B. Assists the radiologist during interpretation of the radiographs
C. History should begin with radiographer introduction and verification of the patient's name
D. Questions for use in taking a patient's history, depending upon type and site of injury include:
1. How did injury occur?
2. When did injury occur?
3. Where is your pain?
4. Do you have tingling or numbness?

5. Do you have any weakness?
6. Were you unconscious following your injury?
7. Why did your doctor order this exam?
8. Have you experienced shortness of breath or coughing?
9. Have you experienced a fever or heart problems?
10. Have you experienced any nausea, vomiting, or diarrhea?

▲ *Medicolegal Aspects of Practice*

A. Torts
 1. Violations of civil law
 2. Also known as *personal injury law*
 3. Injured parties have a right to compensation for injury
B. Intentional misconduct
 1. Assault
  a. Patient is apprehensive about being injured
  b. Imprudent conduct of radiographer that causes fear in patient is grounds for an allegation of civil assault
 2. Battery
  a. Unlawful touching or touching without consent
  b. Harm resulting from physical contact with radiographer
  c. May also include radiographing the wrong patient, the wrong body part, or performing radiography against a patient's will
 3. False imprisonment
  a. Unjustified restraint of a person
  b. Care must be taken when using restraint straps or other individuals to hold a patient still
 4. Invasion of privacy
  a. Violation of confidentiality of information
  b. Unnecessarily, or improperly, exposing the patient's body
  c. Unnecessarily, or improperly, touching a patient's body
  d. Photographing patients without their permission
 5. Libel—written information that results in defamation of character or loss of reputation
 6. Slander—verbally spreading false information that results in defamation of character or loss of reputation
C. Unintentional misconduct (negligence)
 1. Neglect or omission of reasonable care
 2. Based on doctrine of the reasonably prudent person
 3. Reasonably prudent person—based on how a reasonable person with similar education and experience would perform under similar circumstances
 4. Gross negligence-acts that demonstrate reckless disregard for life or limb
 5. Contributory negligence—instance in which the injured person is a contributing party to the injury

D. Four conditions needed to establish malpractice:
 1. Establishment of the standard of care
 2. Demonstration that standard of care was violated by the radiographer
 3. Demonstration that loss or injury was caused by radiographer who is being sued
 4. Loss or injury actually occurred and is a result of the negligence
E. Respondeat superior
 1. Literally, "let the master answer"
 2. Legal doctrine stating that an employer will be held liable for an employee's negligent act
F. Rule of personal responsibility—each individual is responsible for own actions
G. Res ipsa loquitur
 1. Literally, "the thing speaks for itself"
 2. Legal doctrine stating that cause of the negligence is obvious (e.g., forceps left inside a patient during surgery is not an arguable fact)
H. Charting
 1. Writing on the patient's chart by radiographer
 2. Varies by institution
 3. Radiographer's responsibilities in this regard must be carefully outlined during new employee orientation
 4. Write clear statements regarding patient's condition, reaction to contrast agents, amount of contrast material injected, etc.
 5. Must be clearly stated on the chart
 6. Information must also include the date and time of the occurrence
 7. Radiographer must sign such entries using full name and credentials
I. Radiographs
 1. Radiographs are legal documents
 2. Radiographs must include:
  a. Patient identification
  b. Anatomical markings including left and right markers
  c. Markings must be carefully placed on each radiograph using lead markers
  d. Date of exposure
  e. Other markings (using stickers, grease pencils, etc.) applied to the radiograph after processing may not be legally admissible
 3. Retention of radiographs
  a. Varies according to state law
  b. Normally maintained for a period of five to seven years after the date of the last radiographic examination
  c. Film folders on minors are normally retained for five to seven years after the minor reaches the age 18 or 21, depending on the state of residence
 4. Careful documentation must be maintained when radiographs are checked out for use by physicians, students, or other health care practitioners

J. Patient consent
  1. Patient bill of rights provides for patient consent or refusal of any procedure
  2. Implied consent
     a. Provides for care when patient is unconscious
     b. Based on assumption that patient would approve care if conscious
  3. Valid consent
     a. Patient must be of legal age
     b. Patient must be mentally competent
     c. Consent must be offered voluntarily
     d. Patient must be adequately informed
     e. Also called *informed consent*
     f. Requires radiographer and radiologist to carefully explain all aspects of procedure and risks involved
     g. Requires that explanation be provided in lay terms that the patient understands

▲ Patient Transfer

A. Check identification bracelet to determine correct patient
B. Ask patient to state name to double check identity; ask date of birth as a backup
C. Explain transfer procedure to patient to gain cooperation and alleviate fear
D. Radiographer must always use proper body mechanics for patient transfer:
  1. Keep knees slightly bent
  2. Keep back straight
  3. Perform all lifting using legs, not back

Transfer from Wheelchair to X-ray Table

A. Wheelchair parallel to the table
B. Brakes applied with step stool nearby
C. Using face-to-face method, assist the patient to a standing position
D. Have patient place hand on footstool handle, the other arm on your shoulder, and step up onto the stool
E. Patient pivots with back against the table into a sitting position on the edge of the table
F. Place one arm around patient's shoulder and the other arm under the knees
G. Assist patient to a supine position

Transfer from X-ray Table to Wheelchair

A. Check to see that brakes of wheelchair have been applied
B. Assist patient to a sitting position
C. Allow patient to sit up for a short time to regain sense of balance
D. If patient is ambulatory,
  1. Assist to a standing position and pivot

2. Have patient reach back with both hands and grab arms of wheelchair
3. Assist patient to sit in the wheelchair
E. If patient is nonambulatory,
  1. Stand facing the patient
  2. Reach around the patient and place your hands on each scapula
  3. Lift the patient upward to a standing position
  4. Pivot so that the back of the patient's leg is touching the edge of the wheelchair
  5. Ease the patient down to a sitting position
  6. Position foot and leg rests into place
  7. Cover patient's lap with a sheet

Cart Transfer

A. Place cart near and parallel to the x-ray table
B. Do not attempt patient transfer from cart to x-ray table without assistance
C. One person supports the neck and shoulders at the head of the cart; the second individual lifts the pelvis and knees; other individuals, if available, support patient at both sides
D. Transfer sheet or draw sheet should be used under the patient
E. On signal, all involved in transfer move the patient in one fluid motion to the x-ray table

▲ Patient Comfort

A. Taking into account the patient's physical condition, carefully position pillows or radiolucent sponges so that they will not interfere with the examination
B. Evaluate patient's condition
  1. Ability to breathe
  2. Presence of nausea
  3. Allow the patient to remain semi-upright when possible
  4. Special care must be given elderly patients who may have decubitus ulcers or particularly sensitive or thin skin

▲ Infection Control

Routes of Transmission

A. Direct contact
  1. Infected person touches the susceptible host, allowing the infectious organisms to come in contact with susceptible tissues
B. Indirect contact
  1. Fomite—an object containing pathogenic organisms which is placed in contact with a susceptible person
  2. Vector—an animal that contains and transmits an infectious organism to humans

3. Airborne contamination—droplets and dust
4. Droplets—primarily transmitted by coughs, sneezes, or other methods of spraying on to a nearby host

Universal Precautions

A. Also known as *body substance precautions (BSP)*
B. System that uses barriers between infected individuals and susceptible persons
C. Assumes all body fluids are sources of infection
D. Assumes all patients are infected
E. Guidelines:
  1. Always wear gloves when there is any chance of being in contact with body substances
  2. Protect clothing by wearing a protective gown or plastic apron if there is a chance of coming in contact with body substances
  3. Masks and/or eye protection must be worn if there is a chance of body substances splashing
  4. Handwashing is the most effective method to prevent the spread of infection
  5. Uncapped needle syringe units and all sharps must be discarded in biohazard containers
  6. If any contact is made with body substances, the entire area must be washed completely with bleach
  7. Needles should never be recapped but should be placed along with the syringe in a sharps container
  8. Use protective masks and/or mouth pieces when performing CPR

Medical Asepsis

A. Microorganisms have been eliminated as much as possible by the use of water and chemical disinfectants

Surgical Asepsis

A. Complete removal of all organisms from equipment and the environment in which patient care is conducted
B. Includes complete sterilization of equipment and appropriate skin preparation
  1. Chemical sterilization—soaking objects in germicidal solution
  2. Boiling—sterilization with moist heat
  3. Dry heat—placing objects in an oven at temperatures in excess of 300° F
  4. Gas sterilization—items are exposed to a mixture of gases that will not harm the materials
  5. Autoclaving—steam sterilization under pressure; most convenient way to sterilize materials

Sterile Technique

A. Steps to follow in opening sterile packs
  1. Place pack on a clean surface
  2. Break the seal and open the pack
  3. Unfold first corner of the pack away from you
  4. Unfold both sides
  5. Pull front portion of the wrap toward you and drop it
  6. Inner surface must never be touched
  7. If there is an inner wrap, it is opened using the same method
  8. Separately wrapped sterile items may be added to the sterile field by opening the pack and allowing them to drop onto the sterile field
  9. Container must never touch the sterile field
B. Pouring liquids into containers in a sterile field
  1. Carefully determine the contents of the container
  2. Pour a small amount into a waste receptacle to cleanse the lip of the bottle
  3. Pour the medium into the receptacle, being careful not to touch the sterile field in the process
C. Sterile objects or fields touched by unsterile objects or persons are immediately contaminated
D. Avoid reaching across sterile fields
E. If there is suspicion about an object being contaminated, assume that it is contaminated
F. Damp items are always assumed to be contaminated
G. Do not invade the space between a physician and the sterile field
H. Never abandon a sterile field; it must be under direct observation at all times
I. Never turn back on a sterile field

Gloving

A. Wash hands thoroughly
B. Open outer package containing gloves
C. Open inner package exposing gloves
D. Approach glove from the open end, touch only inner surface with opposite hand
E. Put on glove, touching only the folded cuff
F. Pick up other glove with gloved hand under the cuff
G. Place second glove on other hand and unfold cuff
H. Carefully unfold the cuff on both gloves
I. Always keep hands in front of the body without touching body covering or placing hands under arms

Isolation Technique: Types

A. Category specific
  1. Strict isolation
    a. Masks, gowns, and gloves are required for all individuals entering the patient's room
    b. Careful handwashing must be performed
    c. Contaminated articles must be carefully bagged and discarded

2. Contact isolation
   a. Masks, gowns, and gloves are indicated for persons coming in contact with the patient
   b. Careful handwashing must be performed
   c. Contaminated articles must be carefully bagged and discarded
3. Respiratory isolation
   a. Masks required for individuals coming in close contact with the patient
   b. Gowns and gloves are not required
   c. Careful handwashing must be performed
   d. Contaminated articles must be carefully bagged and discarded
4. AFB (acid-fast bacilli) isolation
   a. Mask required for patients who cough
   b. Gowns used to prevent clothing contamination
   c. Gloves not required
   d. Careful handwashing must be performed
   e. Contaminated articles must be carefully bagged and discarded
5. Enteric isolation
   a. Masks not required
   b. Gowns and gloves used if there is any chance of coming in contact with products of the gastrointestinal system
   c. Careful handwashing must be performed
   d. Contaminated articles must be carefully bagged and discarded
6. Drainage/secretion precautions
   a. Masks not required
   b. Gowns and gloves used if there is any chance of coming in contact with drainage
   c. Careful handwashing must be performed
   d. Contaminated articles must be carefully bagged and discarded
7. Body substance precautions
   a. Masks not required
   b. Gowns and gloves required if there is a chance of coming in contact with blood or body fluids
   c. Careful handwashing must be performed
   d. Contaminated articles must be carefully bagged and discarded
   e. Extra care is needed to avoid needle-stick injuries
   f. Blood spills must be carefully cleaned up with gloved hands and appropriate cleaning solution (bleach 10:1)
B. Disease specific
   1. Each patient condition is evaluated
   2. Appropriate isolation technique is put in place

Isolation Technique: Mobile Radiography

A. If protective cap is indicated, it should be put on and all hair tucked inside

B. Mask should be put on next, completely covering nose and mouth
C. Gown should be put on and tied securely at the back and at the neck
D. Gloves should be put on and pulled over the end of the sleeve on the gown
E. Radiographic cassette should be placed in a protective cover
F. Enter patient's room and follow all isolation guidelines that have been posted
G. When possible, have a second radiographer handle the portable x-ray machine and controls while the first radiographer touches only the patient
H. After the radiographic exposure is made:
   1. Remove cassette from the vicinity of the patient
   2. End of the protective covering is opened
   3. Radiographer handling the equipment should remove cassette from the open end of the cover
I. When leaving the patient's isolation room, carefully remove attire:
   1. Untie waist belt of protective gown
   2. Remove gloves
      a. Pull off one glove by grasping the cuff and invert it as it is pulled off
      b. Remove second glove by inserting clean fingers inside the cuff and inverting it as it is removed
   3. Untie neck and back strings from gown
   4. Remove mask by using strings only
   5. Remove gown by holding it away from the body as it is removed
   6. Carefully wash hands
   7. Use paper towels to touch faucet handles
   8. Once portable x-ray unit is safely outside the room, it should be cleaned thoroughly before returning to the radiology department

Isolation Technique: Patients in Radiology Department

A. Identify isolation category and follow guidelines
B. Isolation patients should never spend time waiting in the hallway
C. Carefully cover x-ray table with a sheet
D. Work in pairs so that only one radiographer is in contact with the patient, while the other manipulates the equipment
E. When returning patient to the wheelchair or cart, carefully cover with protective sheets and blanket
F. All contaminated materials must be placed in an appropriate discard bag
G. Carefully clean off the x-ray table and any other equipment with which the patient came in contact
H. Remove gloves and carefully wash hands

Reverse (Protective) Isolation

A. Used for patients who are:
1. Immunosuppressed
2. Severely burned
3. Neonates
B. Used to protect the patient from the health care worker
C. Equipment must be cleaned extensively before entering the patient's room
D. Extensive handwashing is required before touching the patient, the bed, or any articles handled by the patient
E. Masks, gowns, gloves, and caps must be worn
F. Cassettes must be placed in protective coverings before coming into contact with the patient
G. Portable radiography of patients in reverse isolation should be performed by radiographers working in pairs so that one remains totally clean while the other handles the portable x-ray machine and other equipment

▲ Assessment of Changing Patient Conditions

A. Visual observation of patient
B. Changes in skin color to cyanotic or waxen pallor
C. Patient verbalizes discomfort or dizziness
D. Cyanosis of lips or nail beds
E. Patient is cool and diaphoretic to the touch

Vital Signs

A. Temperature—normal oral temperature 98° to 99° F
B. Pulse
1. Taken at radial artery or carotid artery
2. More than 100 beats per minute—tachycardia
3. Fewer than 60 beats per minute—bradycardia
C. Respiration—normal rate of respiration 12 to 16 breaths per minute
D. Blood pressure
1. Measured using sphygmomanometer
2. Systolic pressure—measurement of the pumping action of the heart
3. Diastolic pressure—measures the blood pressure of the heart at rest
4. Diastolic pressure over 90 indicates increasing level of hypertension
5. Diastolic pressure less than 50 gives some indication of shock
6. Always expressed as systolic pressure over diastolic pressure, e.g., 120/80

Medical Emergencies

A. Oxygen administration
1. Generally administered using mask or nasal cannula
2. Usual oxygen flow rate is 3 to 5 liters per minute
3. Care must be taken in radiographing patients who are on portable oxygen support so that oxygen tubing is not pinched or kinked
4. Radiographer must know how to operate oxygen tank or wall oxygen outlet so as to administer oxygen to a patient in the event of an emergency
B. Suction unit
1. Used to maintain patient's airway
2. Must be used any time the airway becomes obstructed by fluids
3. If working alone and patient needs suctioning, call for help before beginning procedure
C. Cardiac arrest
1. Cessation of heart function
2. Specific routine for announcing cardiac arrest must be followed
3. Emergency medical assistance must be called immediately
4. Cardiopulmonary resuscitation must commence immediately
5. Radiographer must be familiar with location and contents of "crash cart"
   a. Medications
   b. Airways
   c. Sphygmomanometers
   d. Stethoscopes
   e. Defibrillators
   f. Cardiac monitors
   g. Medications
D. Respiratory arrest
1. Cessation of breathing
2. Respiratory arrest may be caused by:
   a. Upper respiratory tract swelling
   b. Failure of the central nervous system
   c. Choking
2. Tracheolaryngeal edema may necessitate an emergency tracheotomy
3. Tracheolaryngeal edema may follow injection of iodinated contrast material
   a. Radiographer should be aware of location of tracheotomy tray
4. Respiratory arrest secondary to CNS failure necessitates calling a respiratory arrest
5. Respiratory arrest secondary to choking necessitates the use of suction or the Heimlich maneuver
E. Shock
1. Failure of circulation in which blood pressure is inadequate to oxygenate tissues and remove by-products of metabolism
2. Hypovolemic shock—follows the loss of a large amount of blood or plasma
3. Septic shock—occurs when toxins produced during massive infection cause a dramatic drop in blood pressure

4. Neurogenic shock—causes blood to pool in peripheral vessels
5. Cardiogenic shock—secondary to cardiac failure or other interference with heart function
6. Allergic shock (*anaphylaxis*)
   a. Allergic reaction to foreign proteins following injections
   b. Marked by extremely low pressure, dyspnea, and possible death
   c. May follow injection of iodinated contrast media
7. Symptoms of shock
   a. Restlessness, apprehension
   b. Accelerated pulse
   c. Pale skin
   d. Weakness
   e. Alteration in ability to think
   f. Cool, clammy skin
   g. Systolic blood pressure below 30
8. Radiographer's response to shock
   a. Stop procedure
   b. Place patient in a recumbent (Trendelenburg) position
   c. Immediately obtain help, calling a code if necessary
   d. Determine blood pressure
   e. Administer oxygen
   f. Carefully document the time and occurrence of each symptom
F. Trauma
   1. Serious potential life-threatening injuries
   2. Radiographer must be careful to do no additional harm to the patient
   3. Be prepared to work with other health care professionals present in the radiographic room
   4. Be prepared to perform a lateral crosstable cervical spine as soon as possible
   5. Regardless of which area of the body is to be radiographed, assume a serious internal injury is present
   6. Patient will be at one of four levels of consciousness
      a. Alert and conscious
      b. Drowsy
      c. Unconscious but reactive to stimuli
      d. Comatose
   7. Carefully observe the condition of the patient when first brought to the radiographic room
   8. Note any changes in patient's condition during the course of the radiographic procedures
   9. Under no circumstances should trauma patients be left alone
   10. Until otherwise informed by a physician, assume the presence of serious spinal injuries
   11. Slight movement of patient with spinal injuries may result in paralysis or death
   12. Immobilization devices such as cervical collars or splints must never be removed without the permission of a physician
   13. Be prepared to alter routine positions and projections because of the inability of the anatomical part to be moved
   14. Adjust radiographic technique to compensate for the presence of splints, spine boards, and other immobilization devices
   15. Work carefully with patients who have wounds
   16. Observe condition of wound when patient is brought for radiography and immediately notify emergency room personnel of any changes in the wound, including fresh bleeding
   17. Patients with severe burns will require protective isolation
      a. Such patients either experience no sensation at all or extreme pain
      b. Care must be exercised in working with burn patients under either condition

Patient Monitoring/Support Equipment

A. Ventilators
   1. Mechanical respirators attached to tracheostomies
   2. Patient with a ventilator has been intubated (a tube inserted into the trachea)
   3. Care must be taken not to dislodge the tubing connected to the tracheostomy
B. Nasogastric tubes
   1. Tube inserted through the nose and down the esophagus into the stomach
   2. Used to feed the patient or to conduct gastric suction
   3. Care must be taken by the radiographer not to pull on the nasogastric tube while moving the patient or performing the examination
C. Chest tube
   1. In place to remove fluid or air from the pleural space
   2. May be connected to a suction device
   3. Radiographer must be careful not to disturb the chest tube or suction devices or bottles to which the tube may be attached
   4. Bottle must never be raised above chest level
   5. Tubing must not be pinched
D. Venous catheters
   1. May be kept in place for patients requiring long-term chemotherapy or nutrition
   2. Must not be disturbed or pulled upon in any way
E. Urinary catheters (both Foley and suprapubic)
   1. Care must be taken during the transfer and radiography of patients with urinary catheters in place
   2. Attention must be given to urinary catheter tubing so that it is not bent, pinched, or caught on other equipment
   3. Bag attached to urinary catheters must always be kept below the level of the bladder

4. Allowing urine to flow retrograde into the urethra and bladder can cause urinary tract infections
   a. Urinary tract infections are the number one cause of nosocomial infections (infections acquired in the hospital)

F. Oxygen
1. Oxygen should not be removed during radiographic examinations
2. Oxygen may only be removed with a physician's order
3. Care should be taken so that tubing is not pinched

▲ Contrast Media

A. Negative contrast agent
1. Most commonly used is air
2. Requires fewer x-rays and produces a higher density on the radiograph
3. Air may be used in combination with a positive contrast agent on double-contrast studies
4. Most common exam performed using a negative contrast agent is the routine chest radiograph

B. Positive contrast agents
1. Examples are:
   a. Iodine (atomic number 53)
   b. Barium (atomic number 56)
2. Relatively high atomic numbers
   a. Result in greater attenuation of x-rays
   b. Provide lower density on the radiograph
   c. Provide an increase in contrast between the structure to be visualized and surrounding structures

C. Barium
1. Is administered to the patient in the form of barium sulfate, an inert salt
2. For upper GI series and esophagram, the barium is most palatable when mixed with very cold water
3. For barium enema, the barium powder is mixed with water at a temperature of approximately 100° F
4. For some studies of the esophagus, a barium sulfate paste may be administered which is much thicker and more difficult to swallow
5. Barium tends to absorb water
6. Patients must be given careful instructions regarding fluid intake following barium studies so that the barium does not cause an impaction
7. Barium sulfate escaping into the peritoneal cavity can cause peritonitis

D. Aqueous iodine compounds
1. Used for contrast studies of the GI tract
2. Used in cases where barium could prove to be a surgical contaminant
   a. Perforated ulcers
   b. Ruptured appendix
3. Aqueous iodine compounds may also be used in patients with a high risk for impactions

5. These compounds may cause significant dehydration

E. Iodinated contrast media
1. Ionic contrast agents
   a. Salts of organic iodine compounds
   b. Composed of positively and negatively charged ions
2. Nonionic contrast agents
   a. Similar to ionic contrast agents
   b. Do not ionize into separate positive and negative charges, which is their primary advantage over ionic contrast agents
   c. Provide far lower incidence of contrast agent reactions
3. Contraindications to the use of iodinated contrast media
   a. Previous sensitivity to contrast agents
   b. Known sensitivity to iodine
4. It should be noted that both ionic and nonionic contrast agents are iodinated, that is, both contain various concentrations of iodine (nonionic does not mean noniodinated)

Contrast Media Reactions

A. Overdose—may occur in infants or adults with renal, cardiac, or hepatic failure
B. Anaphylactic reactions—flushing, hives, nausea
C. Cardiovascular reactions—hypotension, tachycardia, cardiac arrest
D. Psychogenic factors—may be caused by patient anxiety or may be suggested by the possible reactions described during the informed consent process
E. Other symptoms of contrast agent reactions
1. Nausea and vomiting
2. Sneezing
3. Sensation of heat
4. Itching
5. Hoarseness (or change in pitch of voice during conversation)
6. Coughing
7. Urticaria
8. Dyspnea
9. Loss of consciousness
10. Convulsions
11. Cardiac arrest
12. Paralysis
13. Any change in level of orientation
F. Complications may occur at the site of injection
1. Local irritation may occur if the contrast material extravasates
2. Phlebitis may occur in the vein in which the contrast material was injected

Patient Care Preceding Injection of Iodinated Contrast Media

A. Determine history of allergies or previous hypersensitivity to contrast media
B. Determine extent of patient's medical problems
C. Review possible reactions to the contrast medium being used
D. Know the location of all emergency equipment
E. Carefully observe and evaluate the patient, noting color of skin, tone and pitch of voice, presence of apprehension or anxiety so that changes from these baselines may be noted after injection

Patient Care Following Injection of Iodinated Contrast Media

A. Continue conversation with patient
   1. Encourage patient to speak
   2. Laryngeal swelling as a contrast agent reaction will first manifest itself as a change in the tone and pitch of the patient's voice
B. Continue to observe the patient for early signs of urticaria, profuse sweating, or extreme anxiety
C. If patient becomes overanxious, take patient's pulse and determine if tachycardia is present
D. If patient becomes faint, immediately check respirations, pulse, and blood pressure and observe for signs of cyanosis
E. Be aware of the location of a physician in the event of an emergency
F. Remain with the patient
   1. Except when at the control panel to make exposures
   2. Patient should never be left alone following injection or at any time during the procedure
   3. Though most contrast media reactions are noticeable, and may even by violent, others are more difficult to observe
      a. A patient who appears to be resting comfortably or sleeping may have experienced cardiac arrest
   4. Summon help immediately upon observing the onset of a contrast agent reaction
      a. Though a calm response is required to avoid alarming the patient, urgency is important because a mild contrast agent reaction may quickly accelerate into a more serious reaction

▲ *Venipuncture*

A. Use of hypodermic needle
   1. May be used for small injections
   2. Described by gauge
      a. Unit of measurement that indicates diameter
      b. The larger the gauge, the smaller the diameter of the needle opening
      c. Higher gauge needles are useful for IV injection of contrast agents because they make a smaller hole and limit bleeding at the site
      d. Higher gauge needles limit the rate at which contrast material may be injected and consequently limit the size of the bolus that may be injected
   3. If a hypodermic is used, the contrast medium must fill the needle before venipuncture so that air is not injected
B. Butterfly set
   1. Smaller and sometimes easier to handle
   2. Plastic projections make the needle easier to hold during venipuncture and during injection
   3. Radiographer must remember to fill plastic tubing and needle with contrast medium before venipuncture so that air is not injected
   4. Butterfly may also be taped to the patient's arm so that the radiographer's hands are free to hold syringe and plunger
C. IV catheter
      a. Combination unit with a needle inside a flexible plastic catheter
      b. Combined unit is inserted into the vein, needle first
      c. Once in place, the catheter is pushed in over the needle
      d. Afterward, the needle is withdrawn
      e. Catheter may then be connected to the syringe containing contrast medium
      f. Entire system is more flexible than a hypodermic needle or butterfly
      g. Also allows for attachment to IV tubing leading to bag or bottle that can be used in the event of a serious contrast agent reaction
D. Procedure for performing venipuncture
   1. Wash hands
   2. Always wear gloves
   3. Secure tourniquet in place
   4. Select vein
   5. Thoroughly cleanse the skin observing departmental protocol
   6. Insert needle into vein
   7. Observe blood return into catheter, plastic tubing, or syringe depending upon equipment used; remove tourniquet
   8. Tape catheter or butterfly in place and begin injection

   9. If using hypodermic needle, begin injection immediately
   10. If using hypodermic needle, remove needle at conclusion of injection
      a. Place small piece of gauze or alcohol wipe on puncture site and bend patient's arm
   11. If using catheter or butterfly, continue until all contrast medium has been injected, then disconnect syringe and observe site for swelling

▲ Review Questions

Read the following paragraph. Determine the accuracy of each underlined word or phrase. Then refer to questions 1–6 below the paragraph and choose the one statement that best completes and corrects it.

When scheduling radiography examinations, it is important to (1) schedule barium studies first, because these are the most difficult for the patient to tolerate. Several (2) nonconflicting exams should be scheduled the same day, if possible.(3) Elderly patients should be scheduled later in the day to give them time to get up their strength for the exam(s).(4) Patients who have been held NPO should be scheduled first so they may eat or drink as allowed once the exam is over. It is important for (5) patients with diabetes to be scheduled later in the morning so they may take their insulin and have a higher energy level for the exam. (6) Endoscopic procedures should be scheduled after ingestion of barium for increased contrast.

1.
  a. The underlined word or phrase is accurate as written
  b. True; barium hardens quickly and must be used first thing in the morning
  c. True; fluoroscopy must be done first so the radiologists have time to dictate reports
  ✓d. False; barium may interfere with the visibility of anatomical structures; non-barium studies should be performed first

2.
  a. The underlined word or phrase is accurate as written
  b. False; exams should be spread out so patients and staff are under less stress
  ✓c. True; it is generally easier, more convenient, and possibly less costly for the patient to make one trip to radiology either as an inpatient or outpatient
  d. True; discounts are given when all exams can be combined and films on the same patient can be interpreted all at once; further, it aids in the determination of a diagnosis if the radiologist can see the images from all the exams on one view box

3.
  a. The underlined word or phrase is accurate as written
  b. True; radiography exams can be exhausting to the elderly
  c. False; radiography exams must be scheduled at the convenience of the radiology department
  ✓d. False; elderly patients should be scheduled early when they are the strongest, especially if they have been held NPO

4.
  ✓a. The underlined word or phrase is accurate as written
  b. False; trauma cases should be scheduled first
  c. False; it is important that the GI system be as empty as possible; scheduling these cases last ensures the GI system will be totally empty
  d. True; NPO all night is sufficient time; further, patients are extremely hungry and may be weak if the exam is postponed

5.
  a. The underlined word or phrase is accurate as written
  ✓b. False; patients with diabetes should be scheduled first because of their need for insulin
  c. False; patients with diabetes may experience hyperglycemia if they have taken their insulin but have not eaten
  d. True; the need for insulin is great and the diabetic patient needs the extra sugar from the insulin to be alert and cooperative

6.
  a. The underlined word or phrase is accurate as written
  ✓b. False; barium will interfere with most endoscopic procedures
  c. True; barium is an excellent contrast medium
  d. False; barium may harden and damage the fiber optics

For the following questions, choose the single best answer.

7. Torts:
  a. Are violations of civil law
  b. Considered part of personal injury law
  c. May be committed by radiographers
  d. Provide for compensation for injury
  ✓e. All of the above

8. Which of the following may be considered an example of battery?
  a. Touching the patient without consent
  b. Threatening the patient
  c. Radiographing the wrong patient
  d. Radiographing the wrong part
  ✓e. More than one but not all of the above

9. Assault means:

   ✓a. Threatening the patient with harm or causing the patient to be apprehensive
   b. Striking the patient
   c. Touching the patient without consent
   d. Performing radiography against the patient's will
   e. More than one but not all of the above

10. Which of the following is false concerning invasion of privacy?

   a. Violation of confidentiality, such as discussing the patient's case in public
   ✓b. Unjustified restraint of patient
   c. Improperly exposing the patient's body
   d. Improperly touching the patient's body
   e. Photographing the patient without consent

11. Unintentional misconduct is also called:

   ✓a. Negligence
   ✓b. An accident
   c. Libel
   d. Slander
   e. Defamation of character

12. The concept of reasonably prudent person is interpreted as:

   a. How a reasonable jury member would perform the act
   b. How a professional with similar education, training, and experience would perform the act
   c. How a prudent attorney would interpret the act
   d. How a reasonable and prudent judge will rule on the act
   ✓e. None of the above

13. The notion of respondeat superior means:

   a. "The thing speaks for itself"
   b. A radiographer has no need to carry malpractice insurance
   c. The reasonable and prudent person should make the decision
   ✓d. "Let the master answer"
   e. None of the above

14. Gross negligence is:

   a. A case that includes the injured person as a contributing party to the injury
   b. Loss of life or limb
   ✓c. An act that shows reckless disregard for life or limb
   d. Found in criminal cases only
   e. All of the above

15. Which of the following conditions must be met to prove malpractice?

   a. The injury actually occurred and is a result of negligence
   b. The standard of care was violated
   c. The injury was caused by the person being sued
   d. The standard of care has been established
   ✓e. All of the above

16. A case involving obvious negligence would be defined by the doctrine of:

   a. Respondeat superior
   b. Slander
   c. Libel
   ✓d. Res ipsa loquitur
   e. All of the above

17. Which of the following is (are) true concerning valid (informed) consent?

   (1) Patient must be of legal age
   (2) Patient must be provided a brochure describing the procedure's risks in lay terms
   (3) Consent must be offered voluntarily
   (4) Patient must be mentally competent
   (5) Patient must completely understand all aspects of the procedure

   a. 1, 3, 4
   b. 1, 2, 3, 4, 5
   ✓c. 1, 2, 3, 4
   d. 1, 2, 3, 5

18. Patient transfers from cart to x-ray table, and back, should be performed:

    a. By the radiographer alone, when the patient is ambulatory

    √b. By two or more radiographers, to ensure patient and radiographer safety

    c. By the radiographer alone, when the department is short-staffed

    d. By the radiographer alone, so as not to frighten the patient

    e. By two or more radiographers, only when the patient has IV's and catheter in place

19. A history on the patient should be taken by the radiographer:

    a. To secure the patient's confidence in the radiographer

    b. To assist the radiologist with interpretation of the radiographs

    c. To verify patient name and condition

    d. To assist the radiographer in understanding the patient's injury and range of motion

    e. All of the above

Read the following paragraph. Determine the accuracy of each underlined word or phrase. Then refer to questions 20–26 below the paragraph and choose the one statement that best completes and corrects it.

The most obvious route of infection transmission is direct contact. (20) <u>Direct contact allows the infectious organism to move from the susceptible host directly to the infected person</u>. The other route of transmission is called (21) <u>indirect contact</u>. There are several routes of indirect contact. (22) <u>A fomite is an animal that contains and transmits an infectious organism to a human</u>. Such (23) <u>fomites may be rabid dogs, bats, etc</u>. (24) <u>A vector is an object that contains an infectious organism; when the vector is touched by a human, the infection is spread</u>. (25) <u>Airborne transmission of infection may take the form of bird droppings, acid rain, air pollution etc</u>. Finally, (26) <u>droplets such as those from coughs or sneezes also spread infections</u>.

20.

    a. The underlined word or phrase is accurate as written

    b. False; infectious organisms do not move easily

    √c. False; the organism moves from the infected person to the susceptible host

    d. False; this type of transmission is called indirect contact

21.

    √a. The underlined word or phrase is accurate as written

    b. False; the other route is called direct contact

    c. Droplet transmission

    d. Infectious transmission

22.

    a. The underlined word or phrase is accurate as written

    √b. False; a vector is an animal in which infectious disease develops and is transmitted to humans

    c. False; a fomite is another term for an infected person

    d. False; a bacterium is an animal that contains an infectious organism and that transmits the infection to a human

23.

    a. The underlined word or phrase is accurate as written

    b. False; fomites are bacteria

    c. False; fomites live only on the scalp of humans

    √d. False; fomites are objects containing pathogenic organisms

24.

    a. The underlined word or phrase is accurate as written

    b. False; vectors cannot sustain infectious organisms

    √c. False; a vector is an animal that contains and transmits an infectious organism to a human

    d. False; a human cannot become infected just by touching a vector; the vector must be ingested

25.

    a. The underlined word or phrase is accurate as written

    √b. False

    c. False; airborne infections are only contracted on long airplane trips

    d. False; only acid rain has been shown to transmit infection

26.

    √a. The underlined word or phrase is accurate as written

    b. False; there is no scientific evidence to support this concept

    c. Partially false; infections can only be spread in this manner during cold and flu season

    d. False; such infection can only be spread if the exposed person has low resistance to droplet infections

Read the following paragraph. Determine the accuracy of each underlined word or phrase. Then refer to questions 27–34 below the paragraph and choose the one statement that best corrects and completes it.

Universal precautions, also known as body substance precautions,(27) <u>is a system that emphasizes the placement of barriers between the health care worker and the patient</u>. This system assumes that (28) <u>all patients are infected with the HIV virus and that most body fluids are sources of infection</u>. Because the system of universal precautions emphasizes barriers, (29) <u>gloves are the most effective method used to prevent the spread of infection</u>. Given that barium enemas increase the possibility of contact between body substances and clothing, (30) <u>disposable gowns or surgical scrubs should be worn by the radiographer in these cases</u>. Because blood needs to enter the body to cause infection, (31) <u>there is no need to wear eye protection for any radiologic procedures</u>. In the interest of safety, (32) <u>needles should be carefully recapped following injections for IVPs so that no one else is stuck by the needle</u>.(33) <u>Any area that is touched by body fluids must be washed completely</u>. Finally, (34) <u>hands should be washed at least five times each shift to help stop the spread of infections</u>.

27.
  a. The underlined word or phrase is accurate as written
  b. False; in the interest of compassionate patient care, barriers should not come between patient and health care worker
  c. False; barriers have been shown to be quite ineffective
  d. False; universal precautions is not a system; it's the law

28.
  a. The underlined word or phrase is accurate as written
  b. False; this system assumes that all patients under the age of 50 are infected with HIV
  c. False; universal precautions apply only to patient with HIV and hepatitis
  d. False; the system of universal precautions assumes that all patients are infectious, regardless of diagnosis

29.
  a. the underlined word or phrase is accurate as written
  b. False; gloves are permeable
  c. False; handwashing is the most effective method
  d. False; as with radiation, the most effective method is distance

30.
  a. The underlined word or phrase is accurate as written
  b. False; the use of disposable gowns or surgical scrubs is against the dress code
  c. False; the use of disposable gowns or surgical scrubs is too expensive
  d. False; there is little chance of disease transmission during barium enemas because most patients are not infected

31.
  a. The underlined word or phrase is accurate as written
  b. False; any radiologic procedure, such as angiography, that may involve blood splashing requires eye protection,
  c. False; eye protection should be worn for all exams requiring venous injection
  d. False; eye protection should be worn for all radiologic exams

32.
  a. The underlined word or phrase is accurate as written
  b. False; needles should be recapped after all injections
  c. False; all sharps should be disposed of in appropriate containers, never recapped
  d. False; following injection for an IVP, the needle should be kept nearby in the event of a contrast medium reaction

33.
  a. The underlined word or phrase is accurate as written
  b. False; the radiographer does not have time to perform housekeeping duties
  c. False; not all body fluids are infectious
  d. False; this is an expensive process and it is not justified by scientific research

34.
  a. The underlined word or phrase is accurate as written
  b. False; hands should be washed after each patient and before touching equipment and other patients
  c. False; the Centers for Disease Control determined that handwashing has little effect on the spread of infection
  d. False; handwashing should be done only at the start and end of the shift

For the following questions, choose the single best answer.

35. The process of eliminating as many organisms as possible by the use of water and chemical disinfectants is called:

    a. Surgical asepsis
    b. Sterilization
    c. Medical asepsis
    e. Boiling

36. The process of eliminating all organisms from the environment by methods such as gas sterilization, use of germicides, or use of dry heat is called:

    a. Surgical asepsis
    b. Sterilization
    c. Medical asepsis
    d. Autoclaving
    e. Boiling

37. When gloving for a procedure, which of the following should take place first?

    a. Carefully open glove package, and avoid touching outside of gloves
    b. Wash hands
    c. Place glove package in center of sterile field in preparation for the procedure
    d. Put on one glove immediately so one hand is protected and the other is free
    e. None of the above takes place first

38. Once gowned and gloved for a procedure, hands may NOT be placed:

    a. Anywhere on the body because the gown and gloves are sterile
    b. Anywhere on the front or sides of the gown
    c. Anywhere on the table containing the sterile field
    d. Under the arms or on the sides or back of the gown
    e. In the sterile field

39. The radiographer who is assisting with a sterile procedure but is not gloved and gowned,

    a. Should never step between the physician and the sterile field
    b. Should carefully place all utensils needed in the center of the sterile field by dropping them from above from their packages
    c. Should not come in contact with the sterile field under any circumstances
    d. Should assist the physician with gowning
    e. All of the above

40. The two types of isolation technique are called:

    a. Universal precautions and body substance precautions
    b. Disease specific and category specific
    c. Direct and indirect
    d. Respiratory and gastrointestinal
    e. Strict and lenient

41. Reverse isolation does NOT mean:

    a. The patient must be protected from the health care worker
    b. Gown and gloves should be taken off in reverse order from the way they were put on
    c. Patients who are severely burned, immunosuppressed, or neonates must be protected
    d. Equipment must also be cleaned before exposing the patient to it
    e. None of the above describe reverse isolation

42. The one action that is common to all category-specific isolation is:

    a. Gloves must be worn
    b. Gowns must be worn
    c. Patient must not have any direct contact with the health care worker
    d. Handwashing must be performed
    e. All are common to all category-specific isolation

Use the listing below to answer questions 43–50. Items may be used more than once.

A. Strict isolation
B. Respiratory isolation
C. Enteric isolation
D. Body substance precautions
E. Reverse isolation

43. Does not require the use of gloves

44. All equipment and personnel must be carefully covered

45. Used to totally protect the health care worker from every method of transmission possible in the work setting

46. Used if there is any chance of coming in contact primarily with products of GI system of infected person

47. Gowns and gloves not required

48. Masks not required, needle stick injuries must be avoided

49. Used to protect the worker from airborn droplets

50. Used with patients who are not infectious

For the following questions, choose the single best answer.

51. Assessment of changing patient conditions includes observing for:

   a. Skin temperature becoming cool and diaphoretic
   b. Patient expression of discomfort or dizziness
   c. Changes in skin color to waxen pallor
   d. Cyanosis of lips or nail beds
   e. All of the above indicate changing patient conditions

52. The normal adult body temperature taken orally is:

   a. 98.6° C
   b. 98° to 99° C
   c. 99.6° F
   d. 98° to 99° F
   e. 95° to 99° F

53. Which of the following are true concerning the pulse?

   a. All of these are true
   b. Normally taken at the radial artery
   c. Normal range of values is 60 to 72 beats per minute
   d. May be counted at the carotid artery
   e. More than 100 beats per minute indicates tachycardia

54. Normal respiration is:

   a. 30 breaths per minute
   b. 12 to 16 breaths per minute
   c. 10 to 12 breaths per minute
   d. 60 to 72 breaths per minute
   e. 15 to 20 breaths per minute

55. A sphygmomanometer is used to:

   a. Hear the heart beat
   b. Hear the blood pressure
   c. Measure blood pressure
   d. Measure body temperature
   e. Measure the pulse

56. With blood pressure of 120/80, one knows that:

   a. The pressure is 120 when the heart is at rest
   b. The diastolic pressure is 120
   c. The systolic pressure is 80
   d. The pressure is 80 when the heart is at rest
   e. The pressure is 80 when the ventricles contract

57. When administering oxygen the usual rate is:

   a. 3 to 5 pounds per minute
   b. 3 to 5 liters per hour
   c. 3 to 5 liters per second
   d. 5 to 7 liters per minute
   e. 3 to 5 liters per minute

58. A mechanical method used to clear the patient's airway is called:

   a. Heimlich maneuver
   b. CPR
   c. Suctioning
   d. NG tube insertion
   e. Respiratory massage

59. A device that contains all the instruments and medications necessary for dealing with cardiac or respiratory arrest is called:

   a. Crash cart
   b. Tackle box
   c. IVP cabinet
   d. Code blue cabinet
   e. CPR cart

Use the listing below to answer questions 60–65. Items may be used more than once.

A. Anaphylaxis
B. Cardiogenic shock
C. Hypovolemic shock
D. Septic shock
E. Neurogenic shock

60. Caused by loss of a large amount of blood or plasma *C*

61. Causes blood to pool in peripheral vessels *B*

62. Allergic reaction to foreign proteins *A*

63. Caused by infection that results in extremely low blood pressure *D*

64. Occurs secondary to heart failure or interference with heart function *E*

65. May occur after injection of iodinated contrast agent *A*

For questions 66-68, choose the best answer.

66. Which of the following is a symptom of shock?

    a. Accelerated pulse
    b. Restlessness, apprehension, alteration in ability to think
    c. Cool, clammy, pale skin
    d. Systolic pressure below 30
    e. All of the above

67. Of the following, which should the radiographer first perform when a patient is suspected of going into shock?

    a. Call for assistance
    b. Place patient in Trendelenburg position
    c. Take patient's blood pressure to confirm shock status
    d. Administer oxygen
    e. Call a code

68. Which of the following are true when radiographing trauma patients?

    (1) Work quickly and efficiently ✓
    (2) Patient may be left alone if unconscious
    (3) Spinal injury may be ruled out if patient is not on spine board or wearing a cervical collar
    (4) Observe for changes in wound dressing while performing radiography ✓
    (5) Document, in writing, changes in patient condition ✓

    a. 1, 3, 4
    b. 1, 2, 3
    c. 1, 4, 5
    d. All of the above

Use the listing below to answer questions 69–73. Items may be used more than once.

A. Urinary catheter
B. Chest tube
C. Ventilator
D. Nasogastric tube
E. Venous catheter

69. Used to feed patient or to conduct gastric suction *D*

70. Used to administer nutrition or long-term chemotherapy *E*

71. Site of most nosocomial infections *A*

72. Helps to remove fluid or air from pleural space *B*

73. Mechanical respirator *C*

For the following questions, choose the single best answer.

74. The most frequently performed exam using a contrast medium is:

    a. Small bowel study
    b. IVP
    c. Barium enema
    d. Upper GI
    e. Chest x-ray

75. Which of the following are true concerning positive contrast media?

    (1) Air is the most commonly used
    (2) Aqueous iodine compounds may be used if perforations are suspected
    (3) Barium should be mixed with cold water for retrograde administration
    (4) Nonionic contrast media are ideal for injection because they do not contain iodine, reducing the risk of reactions
    (5) Barium is an inert substance
    (6) Aqueous iodine compounds may cause serious dehydration
    (7) Barium is a surgical contaminant

    a. 2, 5, 6, 7
    b. 1, 2, 3, 4, 5, 6, 7
    c. 1, 2, 3, 4, 7
    d. 1, 2, 4, 5, 6, 7
    e. 2, 4, 5, 7

76. Which of the following are legitimate contraindications to the use of iodinated contrast media?

    a. Allergy to seafood
    b. Known sensitivity to iodine
    c. Previous sensitivity to contrast agents
    d. All of the above
    e. b and c only

77. Reaction at the site of injection of iodinated contrast media may be caused by:

    a. Patient fear and anxiety
    b. Extravasation of contrast agent
    c. Anaphylaxis
    d. Phlebitis
    e. b and d

78. Which of the following is NOT a symptom of a contrast agent reaction?

    a. Hoarseness
    b. Sneezing
    c. Urticaria
    d. Coughing
    e. All are symptoms

79. Following injection of iodinated contrast media, the radiographer should:

    a. Leave the room so the patient may remain quiet
    b. Remain with the patient
    c. Tell the patient about his or her previous weekend as a means of allaying anxiety about the procedure
    d. Converse with the patient, listening for signs of laryngeal swelling
    e. b and d

80. At the first indication of a contrast agent reaction, the radiographer should:

    a. Immediately shout for help
    b. Stop exam and obtain help so as not to alarm the patient
    c. Continue with exam, because most reactions turn out to be minor
    d. Call a code blue
    e. Leave the patient to get the radiologist

81. Hypodermic needles are described by their gauge. Gauge:

    a. Is a listing of the uses of the needle
    b. Is a measure of the length of the needle
    c. Is a measure of the diameter of the needle
    d. Is a measure of the diameter of the syringe used with the needle
    e. Is a measure of the diameter of the needle opening; the larger the gauge, the smaller the diameter

82. Air must not be injected when performing venipuncture because:

    a. An air embolus will form which may be fatal to the patient
    b. Most exams requiring injection are not air contrast studies
    c. It will interfere with the iodine
    d. It will prevent the iodine from visualizing
    e. None of the above

83. A smaller, easier to handle injection set, which includes plastic projections on both sides of the needle, may be used for venipuncture . This is called a:

    a. Venous catheter
    b. Butterfly
    c. Hypodermic needle
    d. Single-injection needle
    e. None of the above

84. A venous catheter:

    a. Consists of a long plastic tube which is inserted into the artery during angiography

    b. Is more flexible and easier to use than a needle or butterfly

    c. Is a combination unit with a needle inside a flexible plastic catheter; both the needle and the catheter are inserted into the vein, after which the needle is withdrawn

    d. All of the above

    e. b and c

85. Place the following steps for performing venipuncture in the proper order.

    (1) Secure tourniquet in place
    (2) Thoroughly cleanse the skin
    (3) Wash hands
    (4) Select vein
    (5) Put on gloves
    (6) Perform puncture
    (7) Cover wound and compress site
    (8) Inject contrast agent
    (9) Check wound for swelling
   (10) Observe blood return

    a. 5, 4, 1, 6, 8, 7
    b. 3, 1, 4, 5, 2, 6, 10, 8, 7, 9
    c. 3, 5, 1, 4, 2, 6, 10, 8, 7, 9
    d. 4, 1, 3, 5, 2, 6, 8, 9, 10, 7

86. Venipuncture:

    a. May be performed only where allowed by state law
    b. May be performed by a nurse only
    c. May be performed by a radiology supervisor only
    d. a and c
    e. b and c

87. A contrast medium overdose:

    a. Cannot occur because it is not a drug
    b. May occur in infants
    c. May occur if contrast material was injected during the week before the exam
    d. May occur in infants or adults with renal, cardiac, or hepatic failure
    e. Is a common occurrence

88. Barium and iodine are excellent contrast media because:

    a. They are inert substances
    b. Both are high atomic number elements, resulting in low attenuation of x-ray photons
    c. Both are high atomic number elements, resulting in high attenuation of x-ray photons
    d. Both are negative contrast media, the most commonly used
    e. None of the above

89. When performing patient care following the injection of an iodinated contrast medium, the radiographer must make full use of which senses?

    a. Visual
    b. Hearing
    c. Touch
    d. Speech
    e. All of the above

Use the listing below to answer questions 90–100. Items may be used more than once.

    A. Mild to moderate reaction to contrast agent
    B. Severe reaction to contrast agent
    C. Not considered a reaction to contrast agent

90. Intermittent sneezing

91. Vomiting

92. Constipation

93. Dyspnea

94. Sensation of heat

95. Cardiac arrest

96. Loss of consciousness

97. Nausea

98. Disorientation

99. Hoarseness

100. Convulsions

Chapter 7

Practice Radiography Exam

Choose the *one best* answer for each item in this exam. Questions are written to challenge your critical thinking skills and overall knowledge of the subject matter. Read each question and the answer choices carefully. Refer to the appropriate chapter in this book for review of questions you miss.

For questions 1–14, based on the following real-life drama at a major metropolitan medical center, choose the answer which best completes the sentence.

You have been chosen as the student representative to the advisory committee that is planning a new radiology department at your place of employment. It is your task to assist in developing the radiation protection policies in the new department. Your conversation with the department head and the chief of radiology, Dr. Raydee Ologist, goes something like this:

"I think it is very important for each room to be constructed properly right from the start. First, we must consider several factors that determine selection of protective barriers: (1). As you both know, we need a primary protective barrier of (2). The secondary protective barrier must be installed to extend from the primary barrier to the (3)."

"Very good," says Dr. Ologist. "I am glad you learned your structural requirements so well. It's time to move on to the equipment in the room. Can you help us out on this too?"

"I sure can!" you begin happily. "Let's talk about fluoroscopic facilities first." The department head and Dr. Ologist nod in agreement.

"As you know, each x-ray tube must have total filtration of at least (4). The fluoroscopic source-to-tabletop distance must be (5). The x-ray intensity during fluoroscopy may not exceed (6) at the tabletop. We must install two protective devices for Dr. Ologist and her colleagues. The Bucky slot cover and the protective curtain each must be at least (7)."

"Golly, these second-year students are sure on the ball. I'm glad we have them around!" Dr. Ologist says, excitedly.

"You're right," says the department head. "I hope they can help us with personnel radiation protection policies also."

"I sure can," you begin. "I have a list here of some things

we will need to consider."
"Go right ahead!" (Isn't it nice to see everyone working so well together?)

"We want to be sure we have the right lead aprons available. Different thicknesses of lead provide different levels of protection, but we must ensure that the minimum thickness available is (8). If the staff will combine the use of the lead apron with the inverse square law, their total dose will remain very, very low."

"Just a minute," interrupts Dr. Ologist. "I think you will need to refresh my memory of the inverse square law."

"Gladly," you begin. "My instructor taught me well! Let's say the exposure measured is 10 R per minute at a distance of 2 feet from the x-ray table. If the radiographer will step back to a distance of 4 feet, the new exposure measured will only be (9). It's really quite simple and shows how effective distance can be. Also, remember that the x-ray tube may put out some leakage radiation, which should (10)."

"Now, about mobile units," you continue. "The minimum distances are as follows: (11)."

"Finally, we need to review our personnel monitoring policies. Traditionally, we have used film badges. Among the advantages and disadvantages are (12). Also available are thermoluminescent dosimeters which the nuclear medicine technologists wear on their fingers but which can be worn as badges. Their advantages and disadvantages are (13). Of course, we could always issue everyone a pocket ionization chamber."

"Wait a minute," declared the department head. "Those are expensive; besides, a reading of 200 mR concerns me because (14)."

"Well, this has been a very productive committee meeting! I am happy to be able to help," you finish. "I'm sure we all agree that it is important to keep the dose to the patients and staff ALARA!"

1.
   a. Distance, occupancy, workload, use factor
   b. Fluoroscopy, radiography, CT, tomography
   c. Inverse square law, lead thickness, total fluoroscopy time, number of patients
   d. Distance, occupancy (divided between controlled and uncontrolled area), workload (measure in mA minutes per week), use (amount of time beam is on and directed at a barrier
   e. mA, time, kVp, distance, focal spot size

2.
   a. $\frac{1}{16}$ inch aluminum equivalent
   b. 0.25 mm lead equivalent
   c. $\frac{1}{16}$ inch lead equivalent
   d. $\frac{1}{32}$ inch lead equivalent
   e. $\frac{1}{32}$ inch aluminum equivalent

3.
   a. Ceiling, $\frac{1}{32}$ inch aluminum equivalent, with a $\frac{1}{2}$-inch overlap
   b. Ceiling, $\frac{1}{32}$ inch aluminum equivalent, with a 1-inch overlap
   c. Ceiling, $\frac{1}{16}$ inch lead equivalent, with a $\frac{1}{2}$-inch overlap
   d. Ceiling, $\frac{1}{16}$ inch aluminum equivalent, with a 2-inch overlap
   e. Ceiling, $\frac{1}{32}$ inch lead equivalent, with a $\frac{1}{2}$-inch overlap

4.
   a. 2.5 mm lead equivalent
   b. 2.5 mm aluminum equivalent
   c. 1.5 mm lead equivalent
   d. 1.5 mm aluminum equivalent
   e. .25 mm lead equivalent

5.
   a. No less than 5 inches
   b. No less than 12 inches
   c. No less than 12 inches should be 15 inches
   d. No less than 15 inches should be 20 inches
   e. No less than 15 inches

6.
   a. 10 roentgens per minute
   b. 10 rads per minute
   c. 10 roentgens per hour of fluoroscopy
   d. 10 rem per minute
   e. 10 mR per minute

7.
   a. 0.50 mm aluminum equivalent
   b. 2.50 mm aluminum equivalent
   c. 0.25 mm lead equivalent
   d. 0.50 lead equivalent
   e. 2.50 lead equivalent

8.
   a. 0.25 mm lead equivalent
   b. 0.50 mm lead equivalent but 0.25 mm lead equivalent preferred
   c. 0.50 mm lead equivalent preferred
   d. 1.0 mm lead equivalent preferred
   e. 2.5 mm lead equivalent preferred

9.
   a. 5 R per minute
   b. 2 R per minute
   c. 2.5 rads per minute
   d. 2.5 rem per minute
   e. 2.5 R per minute

10.
   a. Not exceed 100 R per hour, 1 meter from the housing
   b. Not exceed 100 mR per hour, 1 meter from the housing
   c. Not exceed 100 mR per hour
   d. Not exceed 100 R per hour
   e. None of the above

11.
   a. Radiography (minimum source-to-skin distance = 12 inches); fluoroscopy (minimum source-to-skin distance = not less than 12 inches, 15 inches preferred)
   b. Radiography (minimum source-to-skin distance = 15 inches); fluoroscopy (minimum source-to-skin distance = not less than 15 inches)
   c. Radiography (minimum source-to-skin distance = 12 inches); fluoroscopy (minimum source-to-skin distance = not less than 12 inches)
   d. Radiography (minimum source-to-skin distance = 10 inches); fluoroscopy (minimum source-to-skin distance = not less than 10 inches , 15 inches preferred)
   e. Radiography (minimum source-to-skin distance = 12 inches); fluoroscopy (minimum source-to-skin distance = must be 12 inches)

12.
 a. Advantages—accurate as low as 5 mrem; disadvantages—costly, sensitive to temperature extremes
 b. Advantages—accurate as low as 10 mrem; disadvantages—may not be used longer than one month
 c. Advantages—inexpensive, accurate as low as 10 mrem, simple to use; disadvantages—sensitive to temperature and humidity extremes, not accurate at extremely low doses
 d. Advantages—inexpensive; disadvantages—none

13.
 a. Advantages—accurate as low as 5 mrem, dilithium crystals may be reused, may be worn up to 3 months; disadvantages—expensive
 b. Advantages—accurate as low as 5 mrem, lithium fluoride chips may be reused, may be worn up to 3 months; disadvantages—expensive
 c. Advantages—accurate as low as 1 mrem, lithium fluoride chips may be reused, may be worn up to 6 months; disadvantages—expensive
 d. Advantages—accurate as low as 10 mrem, dilithium crystals may be reused, may be worn up to 3 months; disadvantages—expensive

14.
 a. It is the maximum dose
 b. 200 mR is beyond the monthly absorbed dose equivalent limit
 c. Work must stop at that reading while the unit is charged
 d. The maximum reading is 200 mR; one does not know how much over that amount the dose is

For the following questions, choose the single best answer.

15. The amount of radiation deposited per unit length of tissue traversed by incoming photons is called:

 a. Tissue exposure
 b. Linear deposition of energy
 c. Linear energy transfer
 d. Absorbed dose equivalent limit
 e. Photon energy deposit

16. Cataractogenesis, life span shortening, embryological effects, and carcinogenesis are examples of:

 a. Short-term somatic effects
 b. Genetic effects
 c. Acute radiation syndrome
 d. Long-term somatic effects
 e. b and d

17. Compton's interaction:

 a. Produces contrast in the radiographic image
 b. Results in scattering of the incident photon
 c. May produce a fog on the radiograph
 d. Results in displacement of an inner-shell electron
 e. More than one but not all of the above

18. Rem multiplied by a quality factor equals:

 a. Rads
 b. Roentgens
 c. Grays
 d. Curies
 e. No such equation is used

19. Effective absorbed dose equivalent limit:

 a. Is the level of radiation that an organism can receive and probably sustain no appreciable damage
 b. Is a safe level of radiation that can be received with no effects
 c. Should be absorbed annually to maintain proper immunity to radiation
 d. Is 5000 mrem per year for the general public
 e. All of the above

20. Radiation with a high LET:

 a. Has low ionization
 b. Is highly ionizing
 c. Carries a low quality factor
 d. Equates with a low RBE
 e. Always causes a direct effect on the irradiated cells

21. Radiation protection is based on which dose-response relationship?

 a. Linear-threshold
 b. Nonlinear-nonthreshold
 c. Linear-nonthreshold
 d. Nonlinear-threshold
 e. None of the above

22. Which of the following states that the radiosensitivity of cells is directly proportional to their reproductive activity and inversely proportional to their degree of differentiation?

 a. Inverse square law
 b. Law of Bergonié and Tribondeau
 c. Reciprocity law
 d. Ohm's law
 e. Radiosensitivity law

23. Which of the following causes about 95% of the cellular response to radiation?

   a. Direct effect
   b. Law of Bergonié and Tribondeau
   c. Target theory
   d. Indirect effect
   e. None of the above causes that much damage

24. When radiation strikes deoxyribonucleic acid which of the following will occur?

   a. Direct effect
   b. Law of Bergonié and Tribondeau
   c. Target theory
   d. Indirect effect
   e. None of the above occurs when such acid is struck

25. The amount of radiation that causes the number of genetic mutations in a population to double is called:

   a. Threshold dose
   b. Doubling dose
   c. Mutagenic dose
   d. Genetic dose
   e. Carcinogenic dose

26. The units of dose equivalency, activity, in-air exposure, and absorbed dose are, respectively:

   a. Roentgen, rad, rem, curie
   b. Rad, coulomb per kilogram, curie, becquerel
   c. Rem, curie, roentgen, rad
   d. Sievert, becquerel, gray, coulomb per kilogram
   e. None of the above

27. Medical x-rays are an example of:

   a. Natural background radiation
   b. Artificial radiation
   c. Nonionizing radiation
   d. Ionizing, natural background radiation

28. The absorbed dose equivalent limit for the embryofetus is:

   a. 500 mrem per year
   b. 5 rem per year
   c. 0.5 rem per month
   d. 50 mrem per year
   e. 500 mrem during gestation

29. The photoelectric effect:

   a. Results in absorption of the incident photon
   b. Results in absorption of the incident electron
   c. Produces contrast in the radiographic image
   d. Is the same as brems radiation
   e. a and c

30. The effective absorbed dose equivalent limit for radiographers is:

   a. 3 rem per quarter
   b. 500 mrem per year
   c. 5000 mrem per year
   d. 100 mrem per month
   e. None of the above

31. Voltage ripple of 100% is characteristic of:

   a. Single-phase power
   b. Three-phase, six-pulse power
   c. Three-phase, twelve-pulse power
   d. High-frequency power
   e. None of the above

32. Which of the following is true regarding frequency and wavelength of electromagnetic radiation?

   a. Frequency and wavelength are proportional to one another
   b. Frequency and wavelength are unrelated to one another
   c. Wavelength and frequency are inversely proportional to the square of the distance between wave crests
   d. Wavelength and frequency are inversely proportional to one another
   e. None of the above

33. The smallest particle of a compound that retains the characteristics of the compound is a(n):

   a. Element
   b. Atom
   c. Molecule
   d. Neutron
   e. Electron

34. Which of the following does not belong in the definition of matter?

   a. Travels at the speed of light
   b. Has shape
   c. Has form
   d. Occupies space
   e. None of the above describes matter

35. A step-up transformer:

    a. Has more turns in the primary coil than in the secondary coil
    b. Has more turns in the secondary coil than in the primary coil
    c. Steps down voltage
    d. Steps up current
    e. None of the above

36. An ionization chamber circuit places:

    a. A photomultiplier tube between the film and the patient
    b. An ionization chamber beneath or behind the film
    c. An ionization chamber between the patient and the x-ray tube
    d. An ionization chamber in front of a photomultiplier tube
    e. An ionization chamber between the film and the patient

37. Full-wave rectification uses:

    a. A single semiconductor
    b. Four silicone-based semiconductors
    c. The x-ray tube as a semiconductor
    d. Four silicon-based semiconductors
    e. None of the above

38. Which of the following is (are) false?

    a. The octet rule states that no more than eight electrons may occupy the *K* shell at any time
    b. Falling load generators are extremely efficient and should be used when breathing techniques are required, such as lateral thoracic spines and oblique sternums
    c. The nucleus of an atom contains protons and electrons
    d. All are true
    e. All are false

39. A full-wave rectified, three-phase twelve-pulse x-ray machine produces approximately _____ % more average photon energy than a full-wave rectified, single-phase x-ray machine.

    a. 35
    b. 50
    c. 41
    d. 100
    e. Average photon energy is the same

40. According to the anode heel effect, the intensity of radiation is greater at the _____ side of the x-ray tube.

    a. Anode
    b. Central ray
    c. Neither side; the beam is of uniform intensity
    d. Cathode
    e. Positive

41. The amount of time needed for an AEC to terminate the exposure is called:

    a. Exposure latitude
    b. Minimum reaction time
    c. Chamber response time
    d. Electronic time
    e. Semiconductor response time

42. A tube rating chart is used to determine:

    a. The safety of a single exposure
    b. The safety of a series of exposures such as would take place in tomography
    c. Patient dose per mAs
    d. The number of exposures made on the anode
    e. The amount of time needed for the x-ray tube to cool before making additional exposures

Use the listing below to answer questions 43–48. Items may be used more than once.

    A. Characteristic radiation
    B. Photoelectric effect
    C. Pair production
    D. Bremsstrahlung
    E. Compton's interaction

43. Occurs when an incident electron interacts with the force field of an atomic nucleus

44. Occurs when an incident photon interacts with an outer-shell electron producing a scatter photon and a recoil electron

45. Occurs when an incident electron dislodges a *K*-shell electron

46. Produces contrast in the radiographic image

47. Occurs when an incident photon interacts with an atomic nucleus, above 1.02 meV

48. Primary source of diagnostic x-rays

Use the following diagram (Fig. 7-1) to answer questions 49–52.

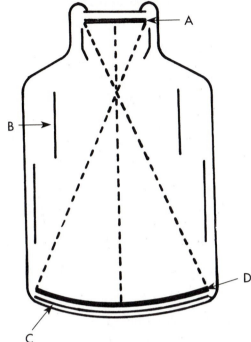

Figure 7-1 Use this figure to answer questions 49–52. (From Malott, JC and Fodor III, J: The art and science of medical radiography, ed 7, St. Louis, 1993, Mosby.

49. Electron beam is focused here *B*

50. Electronic image is produced here

51. Visible image is distributed to viewing and/or recording media from here *A*

52. X-ray energy is converted to visible light here

For the following questions, choose the single best answer.

53. A particular x-ray room is "shooting dark." The problem arises when changing from 200 mA to 300 mA using fixed kVp techniques at 0.16 seconds. Which of the following would lead to an accurate diagnosis of the problem?

  a. Wire mesh test
  b. Pinhole camera test
  c. Use of a digital dosimeter to determine HVL
  d. Use of digital dosimeter to determine exposure linearity
  e. Use of digital dosimeter to determine exposure reproducibility

54. An outpatient radiographic room is used primarily for tabletop radiography of the extremities. On a particularly busy afternoon, the radiographers find that similar exposure techniques on successive patients result in substantially different radiographs. Which of the following would lead to an accurate diagnosis of the problem?

  a. Wire mesh test
  b. Pinhole camera test
  c. Use of a digital dosimeter to determine HVL
  d. Use of a digital dosimeter to determine exposure linearity
  e. Use of a digital dosimeter to determine exposure reproducibility

55. Localized unsharpness on a radiograph may be diagnosed using which of the following tests?

  a. Wire mesh test
  b. Pinhole camera test
  c. Use of a digital dosimeter to determine HVL
  d. Use of a digital dosimeter to determine exposure linearity
  e. Use of a digital dosimeter to determine exposure reproducibility

56. X-ray beam quality is expressed in terms of:

  a. Half-value layer
  b. Exposure linearity
  c. Exposure reproducibility
  d. mAs
  e. Size of focal spot

57. The accuracy of collimation at a 40-inch SID must be:

  a. ± 4 inches
  b. ± 8/10 inch
  c. ± 1 inch
  d. ± 1/10 inch
  e. ± 2 inches

58. The accuracy of kVp at 80 kVp must be:

  a. No lower than 75 kVp and no higher than 85 kVp
  b. No lower than 79kVP and no higher than 81 kVp
  c. No lower than 76 kVp and no higher than 84 kVp
  d. No lower than 78 kVp and no higher than 82 kVp
  e. None of the above

59. The apparent size of the focal spot as viewed by the image receptor is called the:

   a. Actual focal spot
   b. Target angle spot
   c. Anode heel effect
   d. Effective focal spot
   e. Star test pattern

60. As the angle of the anode decreases,

   a. The actual focal spot decreases
   b. The effective focal spot increases
   c. The actual focal spot increases
   d. The effective focal spot remains the same
   e. The effective focal spot decreases

For questions 61 and 62 indicate which set of exposure factors would produce the greatest density.

61.
   a. 100 mAs, 70 kVp, 0.5 mm focal spot, 60-inch SID
   b. 200 mAs, 60 kVp, 1.2 mm focal spot, 60-inch SID
   c. 100 mAs, 70 kVp, 1.2 mm focal spot, 60-inch SID
   d. 50 mAs, 90 kVp, 0.5 mm focal spot, 60-inch SID

62.
   a. 80 mAs, 85 kVp, 40-inch SID, 1.2 mm focal spot
   b. 40 mAs, 80 kVp, 40-inch SID, 0.5 mm focal spot
   c. 160 mAs, 70 kVp, 40-inch SID, 1.2 mm focal spot
   d. 160 mAs, 60 kVp, 40-inch SID, 0.5 mm focal spot

For questions 63–68, choose the best answer.

63. The components of a grid are:

   a. Pb strips and Pb interspacers
   b. Al strips and Pb interspacers
   c. Pb strips and Al interspacers
   d. Pb strips and cardboard interspacers
   e. None of the above

64. What is the purpose of a grid?

   a. To remove scatter radiation from the exit beam
   b. To increase radiographic contrast
   c. To decrease dose to the patient
   d. All of the above
   e. More than one but not all of the above

65. Of the following substances that compose the human body, which listing places them in increasing order of density?

   a. Air, fat, water, muscle, bone
   b. Bone, muscle, water, fat, air
   c. Air, fat, muscle, water, bone
   d. Air, fat, water, muscle, bone, tooth enamel
   e. None of the above

66. The solution filtered through the Ag recovery unit is:

   a. Developer
   b. Fixer
   c. Water
   d. Replenishment solution
   e. None of the above

67. The action of the developer solution on the film is controlled by:

   a. Chemical activity
   b. Solution temperature
   c. Film immersion time
   d. All of the above
   e. More than one but not all of the above

68. If it is necessary to reduce radiographic density by one-half, and it is not possible to do so by changing mAs, the radiographer may:

   a. Reduce SID by one-half
   b. Double SID
   c. Decrease kVp by 10
   d. Reduce time a "step"
   e. Reduce kVp by 15 %

Use the listing below to answer questions 69–74. Items may be used more than once.

   A. Replenishment system
   B. Transport system
   C. Recirculation system
   D. Dryer system
   E. Starter solution

69. Controls immersion time   B

70. Seals the film's emulsion   D

71. Moves film through the processor   B

72. "Seasons" fresh developer solution   E

73. Replaces developer and fixer   A

74. Filters reaction particles from developer   C

For questions 75–84, relating to intensifying screens, indicate what effect the change has on the item in parentheses. Answer *A* if it increases, *B* if it decreases, *C* if it has no effect.

75. Increase phosphor size (speed)

76. Increase active layer thickness (resolution)

77. Decrease phosphor layer thickness (IF)

78. Decrease film-screen contact (resolution)

79. Decrease phosphor size (resolution)

80. Increase kVp (speed)

81. Decrease phosphor size (speed)

82. Decrease active layer thickness (resolution)

83. Increase active layer thickness (speed)

84. Increase light-absorbing dye in active layer (speed)

Use the accompanying graph (Fig. 7-2) for questions 85–92. Then choose your answer from the list.

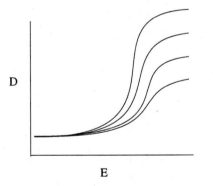

Figure 7-2 Use this figure to answer questions 85–92.

Which film:

85. Has the largest AgBr crystals?

86. Demonstrates the least number of gray tones?

87. Results in the patient being exposed to the least amount of radiation?

88. Has the ability to image the greatest number of LP/MM?

89. Is the least sensitive to x rays and light?

90. Has the lowest number of sensitivity specks?

91. Demonstrates the narrowest range of OD numbers?

92. Has the ability to cause radiographers the most trouble?

For questions 93–110, relating to radiographic quality, indicate what effect the change has on the item in parentheses. Answer *A* if it increases, *B* if it decreases, *C* if it has no effect.

93. Decrease anode angle (recorded detail)

94. Increase mAs (contrast)

95. Increase SID (density)

96. Decrease OID (recorded detail)

97. Decrease developer temperature (density)

98. Increase kVp (contrast)

99. Decrease film-screen system speed (recorded detail)

100. Conversion from nongrid to 12:1 grid (contrast)

101. Decrease SID from 60 inches to 30 inches (magnification)

102. Decrease kVp (recorded detail)

103. Move film from tabletop to Bucky (recorded detail)

104. Decrease source-to-object distance (recorded detail)

105. Increase film immersion time (recorded detail)

106. Increase added filtration (contrast)

107. Tighten collimation (density)

108. Use cylinder cone (contrast)

109. Switch large focal spot to small focal spot (density)

110. Change kVp when using AEC (density)

For the following questions, choose the single best answer.

111. The carpal bones are arranged in two rows as follows:

    a. Proximal row (scaphoid, lunate, triquetrum, pisiform) and distal row (trapezium, trapezoid, capitate, hamate)
    b. Distal row (scaphoid, lunate, triquetrum, pisiform) and proximal row (trapezium, trapezoid, capitate, hamate)
    c. Proximal row (scaphoid, triquetrum, capitate, pisiform) and distal row (trapezium, trapezoid, lunate, hamate)
    d. The carpals are not arranged in rows
    e. Proximal row (scaphoid, lunate, triquetrum) and distal row (trapezium, trapezoid, capitate, pisiform, hamate)

112. The prominent point of the elbow:

    a. Is called the olecranon, part of the radius
    b. Is called the semilunar notch
    c. Is called the trochlea
    d. Is called the olecranon, part of the ulna
    e. Is called the styloid process

Use the following list to answer questions 113–117. Items may be used more than once or not at all.

    A. Talipes
    B. Colles' fracture
    C. Boxer's fracture
    D. Jefferson fracture
    E. Ankylosing spondylitis

113. Imaging of this pathology would require radiography of the cervical spine

114. Imaging of this pathology would require radiography of the hand

115. Imaging of this pathology would require radiography of the distal forearm

116. Imaging of this pathology would require radiography of the feet

117. Imaging of this pathology would require radiography of the entire spine

Use the following diagram (Fig. 7-3) to answer questions 118–123.

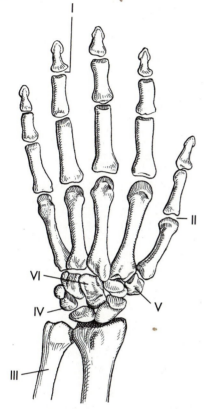

Figure 7-3 Use this figure to answer questions 118–123. (From Ballinger, P: Merrill's atlas of radiographic positions and radiologic procedures, ed 8, St. Louis, 1995, Mosby.)

118. The structure designated as I is the:

    a. Carpometacarpal joint
    b. Interphalangeal joint
    c. Proximal phalanx
    d. Distal interphalangeal joint
    e. Metacarpophalangeal joint

119. The structure designated as II is the:

    a. Carpometacarpal joint
    b. Interphalangeal joint
    c. Proximal phalanx
    d. Distal interphalangeal joint
    e. Metacarpophalangeal joint

120. The structure designated as III is the:

    a. Ulna
    b. Metacarpal
    c. Radius
    d. Humerus
    e. Carpal

121. The structure designated as IV is the:

    a. Lunate
    b. Triquetrum
    c. Capitate
    d. Scaphoid
    e. Pisiform

122. The structure designated as V is the:

    a. Lunate
    b. Scaphoid
    c. Trapezium
    d. Trapezoid
    e. Triquetrum

123. The structure designated as VI is the:

    a. Lunate
    b. Triquetrum
    c. Capitate
    d. Scaphoid
    e. Pisiform

Use the following diagram (Fig. 7-4) to answer questions 124–128.

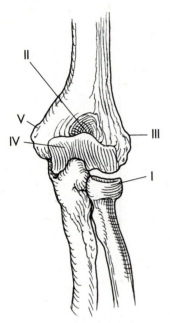

Figure 7-4 Use this figure to answer questions 124–128. (From Ballinger, P: Merrill's atlas of radiographic positions and radiologic procedures, ed 8, St. Louis, 1995, Mosby.)

124. The structure designated as I is the:

   a. Head of ulna
   b. Radial head
   c. Medial epicondyle
   d. Lateral epicondyle
   e. Humeral head

125. The structure designated as II is the:

   a. Coronoid fossa
   b. Olecranon
   c. Semilunar notch
   d. Radial head
   e. Medial epicondyle

126. The structure designated as III is the:

   a. Head of the ulna
   b. Radial head
   c. Medial epicondyle
   d. Lateral epicondyle
   e. Humeral head

127. The structure designated as IV is the:

   a. Medial epicondyle
   b. Trochlea
   c. Lateral epicondyle
   d. Ulnar head
   e. Olecranon

128. The structure designated as V is the:

   a. Medial epicondyle
   b. Trochlea
   c. Lateral epicondyle
   d. Ulnar head
   e. Olecranon

Use the following diagram (Fig. 7-5) to answer questions 129–133.

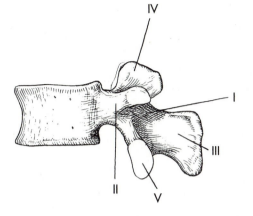

Figure 7-5 Use this figure to answer questions 129-133. (From Ballinger, P: Merrill's atlas of radiographic positions and radiologic procedures, ed 8, St. Louis, 1995, Mosby.)

129. The structure designated as I is the:

   a. Pedicle
   b. Superior vertebral notch
   c. Interior vertebral notch
   d. Spinous process
   e. Lamina

130. The structure designated as II is the:

   a. Pedicle
   b. Superior vertebral notch
   c. Interior vertebral notch
   d. Spinous process
   e. Lamina

131. The structure designated as III is the:

   a. Lamina
   b. Spinous process
   c. Superior articular process
   d. Pedicle
   e. Inferior articular process

132. The structure designated as IV is the:

   a. Superior vertebral notch
   b. Superior articular process
   c. Transverse process
   d. Spinous process
   e. Lamina

133. The structure designated as V is the:

   a. Lamina
   b. Spinous process
   c. Inferior vertebral notch
   d. Pedicle
   e. Inferior articular process

Use the following diagram (Fig. 7-6) to answer questions 134–137.

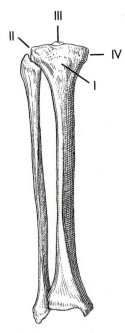

Figure 7-6 Use this figure to answer questions 134–137. (From Ballinger, P: Merrill's atlas of radiographic positions and radiologic procedures, ed 8, St. Louis, 1995, Mosby.)

134. The structure designated as I is the:

    a. Head of the fibula
    b. Head of the tibia
    c. Tuberosity
    d. Styloid process
    e. Lateral condyle

135. The structure designated as II is the:

    a. Medial condyle
    b. Lateral condyle
    c. Intercondylar eminence
    d. Head of the fibula
    e. Trochlea

136. The structure designated as III is the:

    a. Tubercle
    b. Lateral condyle
    c. Medial condyle
    d. Intercondylar eminence
    e. Olecranon

137. The structure designated as IV is the:

    a. Tubercle
    b. Lateral condyle
    c. Medial condyle
    d. Intercondylar eminence
    e. Olecranon

Use the following diagram (Fig. 7-7) to answer questions 138–143.

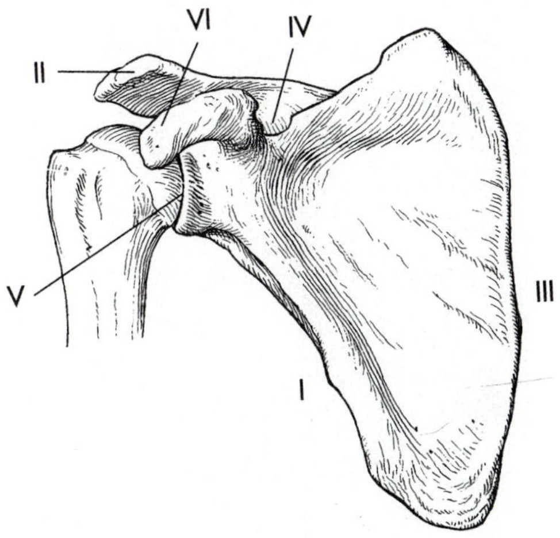

Figure 7-7 Use this figure to answer questions 138–143. (From Ballinger, P: Merrill's atlas of radiographic positions and radiologic procedures, ed 8, St. Louis, 1995, Mosby.)

138. The structure designated as I is the:

a. Vertebral border
b. Scapular notch
c. Body
d. Subscapular fossa
✓e. Axillary border

139. The structure designated as II is the:

a. Humeral head
✓b. Acromion
c. Coracoid process
d. Coronoid process
e. Superior angle

140. The structure designated as III is the:

a. Vertebral border
b. Scapular notch
c. Body
d. Subscapular fossa
e. Axillary border

141. The structure designated as IV is the:

✓a. Coracoid process
b. Coronoid process
c. Scapular notch
d. Glenoid fossa
e. Superior angle

142. The structure designated as V is the:

a. Glenoid fossa
b. Acromion
c. Coronoid process
d. Coracoid process
e. Scapular notch

143. The structure designated as VI is the:

a. Glenoid fossa
b. Acromion
c. Coronoid process
d. Coracoid process
✓e. Scapular notch

Use the following diagram (Fig. 7-8) to answer question 144.

Use the following diagram (Fig. 7-9) to answer question 145.

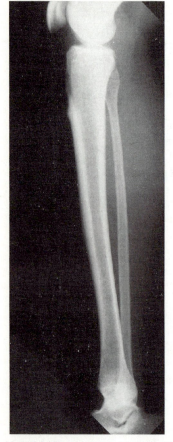

Figure 7-8 Use this figure to answer question 144. (From Ballinger, P: Merrill's atlas of radiographic positions and radiologic procedures, ed 8, St. Louis, 1995, Mosby.)

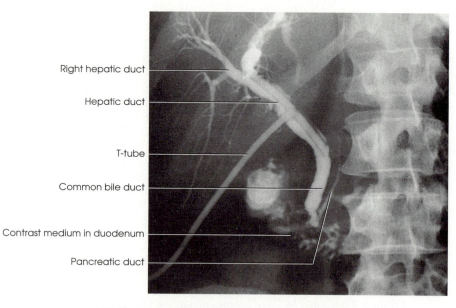

Right hepatic duct

Hepatic duct

T-tube

Common bile duct

Contrast medium in duodenum

Pancreatic duct

Figure 7-9 Use this figure to answer question 145. (From Ballinger, P: Merrill's atlas of positions radiographic and radiologic procedures, ed 8, St. Louis, 1995, Mosby.)

144. Critique the radiograph (Fig. 7-8):

   a. Radiograph is not acceptable; radius and ulna should be superimposed
   b. Radiograph is not acceptable; tibia and fibula should be superimposed
   c. Radiograph is acceptable, but only one joint needed
   d. Radiograph is acceptable
   e. Radiograph is not acceptable; entire ankle needed

145. Critique the radiograph (Fig. 7-9):

   a. Radiograph taken during surgery; acceptable
   b. Radiograph taken during surgery; unacceptable
   c. Radiograph taken post-op; unacceptable
   d. Radiograph taken post-op; need contrast agent added
   e. Radiograph taken post-op; acceptable

Use the following diagram (Fig. 7-10) to answer question
146.

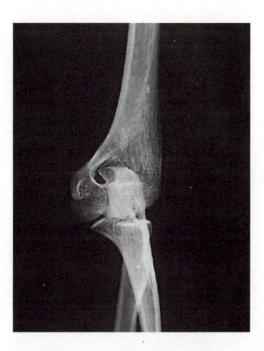

Figure 7-10 Use this figure to answer question 146. (From Ballinger, P: Merrill's atlas of
radiographic positions and radiologic procedures, ed 8, St. Louis, 1995, Mosby.)

146. Critique the radiograph (Fig. 7-10):

    a. Radiograph unacceptable; arm rotated
    b. Radiograph acceptable for medial oblique
    c. Radiograph acceptable for lateral oblique
    d. Radiograph unacceptable; humerus and forearm
       must be in same plane
    e. Radiograph unacceptable; elbow must be in flexion

Use the following diagram (Fig. 7-11) to answer question 147.

Use the following diagram (Fig. 7-12) to answer question 148.

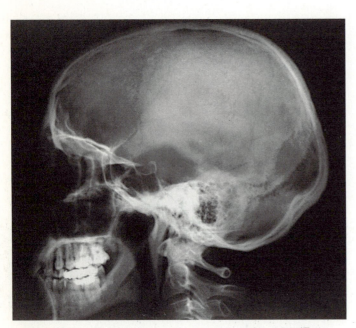

Figure 7-11 Use this figure to answer question 147. (From Ballinger, P: Merrill's atlas of radiographic positions and radiologic procedures, ed 8, St. Louis, 1995, Mosby.)

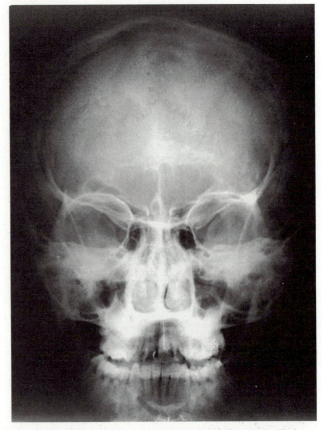

Figure 7-12 Use this figure to answer question 148. (From Ballinger, P: Merrill's atlas of radiographic positions and radiologic procedures, ed 8, St. Louis, 1995, Mosby.)

147. Critique the radiograph (Fig. 7-11):

   a. Radiograph was taken with interpupillary line parallel to film
   b. Radiograph was taken with MSP perpendicular to film
   c. Radiograph was taken with interpupillary line perpendicular to film
   d. Radiograph was taken with MSP parallel to central ray
   e. None of the above is accurate

148. Critique the radiograph (Fig. 7-12):

   a. Radiograph was taken with central ray angled 15 degrees caudad
   b. Radiograph was taken with central ray angled 0 degrees
   c. Radiograph was taken with central ray angled 15 degrees cephalad
   d. Radiograph was taken with MSP perpendicular to central ray
   e. Radiograph was taken with MSP parallel to film

Use the following diagram (Fig. 7-13) to answer questions 149–153.

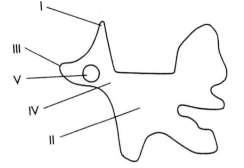

Figure 7-13 Use this figure to answer questions 149-153. (From Ballinger, P: Merrill's atlas of radiographic positions and radiologic procedures, ed 8, St. Louis, 1995, Mosby.)

149. The structure designated as I is the:
    a. Pars interarticularis
    b. Superior articular process
    c. Pedicle
    d. Lamina
    e. Spinous process

150. The structure designated as II is the:
    a. Pars interarticularis
    b. Superior articular process
    c. Pedicle
    d. Lamina
    e. Spinous process

151. The structure designated as III is the:

    a. Spinous process
    b. Transverse process
    c. Pedicle
    d. Inferior articular process
    e. Pars interarticularis

152. The structure designated as IV is the:

    a. Spinous process
    b. Transverse process
    c. Pedicle
    d. Inferior articular process
    e. Pars interarticularis

153. The structure designated as V is the:

    a. Spinous process
    b. Transverse process
    c. Pedicle
    d. Inferior articular process
    e. Pars interarticularis

For the following questions, choose the single best answer.

154. The lateral transthoracic humerus, oblique sternum, and lateral thoracic spine may be imaged best by using a technique called:

    a. Tomography
    b. Zonography
    c. Autotomography
    d. Computed tomography
    e. Falling load

155. A patient unable to supinate the hand for an AP projection of the forearm:

    a. Should be made to do so in order to provide a diagnostic radiograph
    b. Probably has a fracture of the radial head and must be handled carefully
    c. Probably has a low pain tolerance and must be handled carefully
    d. May require radiographs with and without weights
    e. May require the use of sandbags to hold the hand and forearm in the supinated position

156. When performing a PA axial projection of the clavicle, the central ray should be angled:

    a. 15 degrees cephalad
    b. 15 degrees caudad
    c. 25 to 30 degrees cephalad
    d. 25 to 30 degrees caudad
    e. 0 degrees

157. When performing a lateral projection of the knee, the knee should be:

    a. extended 20 to 30 degrees
    b. flexed to a 90-degree angle
    c. flexed 20 to 30 degrees
    d. fully extended
    e. flexed 5 to 10 degrees

158. When performing a tangential projection of the patella with the patient prone, the central ray should be angled:

    a. 15 degrees cephalad
    b. 15 degrees caudad
    c. 25 degrees cephalad
    d. 45 degrees caudad
    e. 45 degrees cephalad

159. Use of which of the following would provide an improved image of the femur?

    a. Trough filter
    b. Anode heel effect
    c. Short SID
    d. Long OID
    e. Large focal spot

160. When performing an AP projection of the hip, the central ray is directed:

    a. Perpendicular to a point 2 inches medial to the a.s.i.s. at the level of the superior margin of the greater trochanter
    b. Parallel to a point 2 inches medial to the a.s.i.s. at the level of the superior margin of the greater trochanter
    c. At a 15-degree cephalad angle
    d. To the level of the a.s.i.s.
    e. To the level of the greater trochanter

161. When performing the AP oblique projection for the cervical vertebrae, the central ray is directed:

    a. 25 to 30 degrees cephalad
    b. 15 to 20 degrees caudad
    c. 5 to 10 degrees cephalad
    d. 25 to 30 degrees caudad
    e. 15 to 20 degrees cephalad

162. When performing the AP oblique projection for the lumbar vertebrae, the side of interest is:

    a. Farthest from the film
    b. Nearest the film
    c. Rotated 30 degrees
    d. Rotated 20 degrees
    e. Rotated 90 degrees

163. When performing the PA oblique projection for the sacroiliac joints, the side of interest is:

    a. Farthest from the film
    b. Nearest the film
    c. Rotated 10 degrees
    d. Rotated 45 degrees
    e. Rotated 90 degrees

164. Routine chest radiography is performed:

    a. At the end of full inspiration
    b. At the end of full expiration
    c. At the end of the second full inspiration
    d. With the patient supine or upright
    e. Routinely upon admission

165. The primary purpose of performing the oblique projections of the ribs is:

    a. To image the axillary portion of the ribs
    b. To image the ribs above the diaphragm
    c. To image the ribs below the diaphragm
    d. To determine the extent of the patient's pain tolerance
    e. To image dislocations

166. When performing the PA projection of the skull to image the frontal bone,

    (1) The central ray is directed perpendicular to the cassette
    (2) The OML is perpendicular to the cassette
    (3) The central ray exits at the glabella
    (4) MSP is parallel to cassette

    a. 1, 2, 3, 4
    b. 1, 2
    c. 1, 3, 4
    d. 1, 3
    e. Neither a, b, c, nor d is correct

167. When performing the AP axial projection of the skull,

    (1) The OML is parallel to cassette
    (2) The central ray is directed through the foramen magnum 37 degrees to the OML
    (3) The central ray is directed through the foramen magnum 30 degrees to the IOML
    (4) The MSP is parallel to the plane of the film

    a. 1, 2, 3, 4
    b. 1, 2
    c. 1, 3, 4
    d. 1, 3
    e. Neither a, b, c, nor d is correct

168. When performing the SMV projection of the skull, the IOML is placed:

    a. Perpendicular to the plane of the cassette
    b. Is not used in positioning for the SMV
    c. Parallel to the plane of the cassette
    d. Parallel to the central ray
    e. None of the above

169. When performing the parietoorbital oblique projection of the optic foramen, the MSP is placed:

    a. 53 degrees from the central ray
    b. 37 degrees from the cassette
    c. 37 degrees from the perpendicular
    d. 12 degrees cephalad
    e. 12 degrees caudad

170. For the parietoacanthial projection of the facial bones, the OML:

    a. forms a 37-degree angle with the plane of the film
    b. forms a 53-degree angle with the plane of the film
    c. forms a 37-degree angle with the central ray
    d. is not used, but the IOML forms a 37-degree angle with the plane of the film
    e. is not used, but the IOML forms a 53-degree angle with the plane of the film

171. The radiographer must be proficient in the use of which medical instruments?

    a. Angiography catheter
    b. Sphygmomanometer
    c. Thermometer
    d. Oxygen administration equipment
    e. b, c, and d

172. A tube used to feed the patient or to perform gastric suction is called:

    a. Tracheostomy tube
    b. Tracheotomy tube
    c. Nasogastric tube
    d. Ventilator tube
    e. Suction tube

173. Nosocomial infections are:

    a. Infections acquired in radiology
    b. Infections acquired through the nose
    c. Infections acquired during cold and flu season
    d. Infections acquired during surgery
    e. Infections acquired in the hospital

174. During movement and transfer of patients, urinary catheter bags should be:

    a. Safely placed on the patient's abdomen
    b. Kept below the level of the urinary bladder
    c. Kept below the level of the x-ray table
    d. Kept on the cart or wheelchair
    e. Disconnected and emptied

175. The first task that must be performed when beginning a radiographic examination on a patient is:

    a. Verify patient identity
    b. Determine accuracy of physician's orders
    c. Verify exam to be performed
    d. Remove radiopaque objects from area of interest
    e. Identify oneself

176. Which of the following is NOT required for valid consent?

    a. Patient must be of legal age
    b. Patient must be adequately informed and sign consent form
    c. Patient must be mentally competent
    d. Consent must be offered voluntarily
    e. Patient must be adequately informed

177. The most common site of radiographer injury incurred in the performance of patient care is:

    a. Head
    b. Arms and shoulders
    c. Lumbosacral spine
    d. Lower leg
    e. Cervical spine

178. When taking a patient's history, which of the following questions is inappropriate?

    a. Why did your doctor order this exam?
    b. Have you experienced any difficulty breathing or shortness of breath?
    c. Have you experienced nausea or vomiting?
    d. How long ago was your cancer diagnosed?
    e. All are inappropriate

179. A system that uses barriers between individuals and assumes all patients are infectious is called:

    a. Universal precautions
    b. Whole body isolation
    c. Sterile technique
    d. Body substance precautions
    e. More than one of the above

180. When performing patient care in radiology,

a. Hands should be washed after each procedure
b. Gowns and gloves should always be worn
c. Hands should be washed only after caring for obviously infectious patients
d. Gloves should be worn only when performing GI procedures or performing venipuncture
e. None of the above

181. Patient transfer from cart to x-ray table should be performed:

a. Alone when working evenings or nights
b. By radiographers working in pairs at all times
c. Alone when the department is busy or short-staffed
d. In pairs only when other radiographers are available to assist
e. With the patient and radiographer working together

182. When seeking the latest information regarding universal precautions, the best source is:

a. The radiology administrator
b. The radiology purchasing manager
c. The infection control department
d. The radiologist
e. The attending physician

183. Following all radiographic or fluoroscopic procedures, the radiographer should clean surfaces with which the patient was in contact using:

a. Alcohol
b. Surgical asepsis
c. Soap and water
d. Medical asepsis
e. Autoclaving

184. When preparing sterile fields, damp packages:

a. Are always considered contaminated
b. Are always considered sterile, because the dampness confirms they were cleaned
c. Should be unwrapped first and placed in the center of the sterile field
d. Are always considered sterile; the dampness is only a remnant of the gassing process
e. None of the above

185. When performing mobile radiography,

a. The mobile unit does not have to be cleaned because it is never in contact with sterile fields
b. The mobile unit must be cleaned before and after each use
c. The mobile unit must be cleaned before entering surgical areas or reverse isolation units
d. The mobile unit should be cleaned only before entering surgery
e. The mobile unit must be cleaned before entering surgical areas or reverse isolation units and after leaving most isolation units

186. When performing radiography on patients in isolation:

a. The cassette needs to be placed in a protective covering only if the patient is in reverse isolation
b. The cassette must always be placed in a protective covering
c. The cassette needs to be placed in a protective covering to keep it free of microbes
d. The cassette needs to be placed in a protective covering so that no microbes leave the room
e. None of the above

187. A radiographer should be prepared to assist with which of the following procedures at any time?

a. CPR
b. Intubation
c. Suctioning
d. Tracheotomy
e. All of the above

188. In addition to performing radiography on a trauma victim, the radiographer should be:

(1) Continually assessing the patient's condition
(2) Interpreting the radiographs for the ER physician
(3) Taking additional projections as indicated by the patient's condition or preliminary radiographs
(4) Keeping all other health care workers out of the room because of radiation protection standards
(5) Providing comfort and communicating quietly with the patient, whether the patient is conscious or unconscious

a. 1, 3
b. 1, 2, 3, 4, 5
c. 1, 3, 5
d. 1, 3, 4, 5
e. 1, 2, 3

189. For a barium enema, the contrast agent should be:

    a. Mixed with cold water
    b. Mixed with water at or below body temperature
    c. Mixed with water at approximately 120° F
    d. Mixed with water at approximately 100° F
    e. Mixed with water and air at room temperature

190. All iodinated contrast media used today:

    a. Contain iodine and free ions
    b. Contain free ions
    c. Contain only iodine
    d. Contain salts of organic iodine compounds
    e. Are nonionic

191. The highest incidence of contrast agent reactions occur when using:

    a. Negative contrast media
    b. Ionic iodinated contrast media
    c. Nonionic iodinated contrast media
    d. Barium sulfate
    e. Oily iodinated contrast media

192. It is important for the radiographer to obtain the recent history of radiographic examinations on a patient so that:

    a. An overdose of iodinated contrast media does not occur from exams performed in the past week
    b. An overdose of radiation is not administered
    c. A pattern of unnecessary exams may be established
    d. Examinations may be tracked for departmental quality assurance
    e. None of the above

193. For patients with a history of intravenous urography and no contrast agent reactions:

    a. The radiographer may assume there will be no reaction on subsequent intravenous urograms
    b. The radiographer must assume there is a chance of a reaction on other contrast examinations
    c. The radiographer must assume there is a chance of a reaction on subsequent intravenous urograms
    d. There is no chance of reactions on subsequent intravenous urograms
    e. None of the above is accurate

194. When performing venipuncture

    a. The radiographer is not responsible for obtaining patient history because the exam was ordered by a physician
    b. The contrast agent should be flushed through the syringe, any tubing used, and the needle before injection
    c. The contrast agent must be cooled to make it easier to inject
    d. The use of high-gauge needles is indicated for injecting oily iodinated contrast agents
    e. The contrast agent must always be flushed through the syringe, any tubing used, and needle before injection

195. After cleansing the injection site, before performing venipuncture, the radiographer should:

    a. Immediately perform the puncture
    b. Palpate the vein once more just before the puncture to make certain of the site
    c. Apply a tourniquet
    d. If using a butterfly, tape the tubing to the patient's arm

196. Factors that contribute to contrast media reactions caused by patient anxiety or suggestibility (e.g., resulting from the informed consent process) are called:

    a. Psychosomatic factors
    b. Psychogenic factors
    c. Psychological factors
    d. Anxiety factors
    e. None of the above

197. Contrast agent reactions such as flushing, hives, and nausea are called:

    a. Psychosomatic
    b. Cardiovascular
    c. Anaphylactic
    d. Nonsystemic
    e. None of the above

198. Aqueous iodine compounds are used as contrast media when radiographing the:

    a. Urinary system
    b. GI system
    c. Reproductive system
    d. CNS
    e. Joints

199. When entering data on a patient's chart, the radiographer must:

    a. Sign and date the entry
    b. Date the entry and sign with name and credentials RT(R), which means radiologic technologist (radiography)
    c. Date the entry and sign with name and credentials RT(R), which means registered technician (radiography)
    d. Date the entry and sign with name and credentials RT(R), which means registered technologist (radiography)
    e. Date the entry and sign with name and credentials RT(R), which means registered radiologic technologist

200. In an attempt to maintain the quality of patient care at the highest level possible over time, proof of continuing education is mandatory for renewal of certification with the:

    a. State licensing board in all fifty states
    b. American Society of Radiologic Technologists
    c. Joint Commission on Accreditation of Healthcare Organizations
    d. Continuing Education Board
    e. American Registry of Radiologic Technologists

Chapter 8

Examination Procedure

▲ *Application Process*

At the appropriate point in your educational program, your program director will provide you with a booklet published by The American Registry of Radiologic Technologists entitled *Examinee Handbook*. Read everything in the handbook that pertains to the radiography exam. Also pay close attention to the ARRT Rules and Regulations as well as to the Standards of Ethics. Though your program director may highlight certain portions of the booklet, it remains your responsibility to understand everything contained in it. This is probably the most important examination you have taken up to this point in your life, so be sure to read the materials provided.

After reading the entire booklet, you should concentrate on several key points. The first is to be aware of the application deadlines. Note that the application for examination in radiography must be postmarked no later than May 1 for the July exam; no later than August 1 for the October exam; and no later than January 1 for the March exam. The ARRT strictly adheres to these deadlines, and it is your responsibility to abide by them. Any applications postmarked after these dates will not be considered for the next administration of the exam. Once you have missed the deadline, no program director, attorney, or congressperson can get your application accepted.

Next, it is important to fill out the application providing all of the information requested. Be sure to fill in all information and dates accurately, printing legibly. Note that your signature on the application must be witnessed by a notary public. Do not sign the application until you are with the notary public. Be sure to observe the rules that require you to attach a photograph to the application.

Once you have signed the application in the presence of a notary public, attach the check or money order for the application fee and insert these documents into the envelope that is provided in the *Examinee Handbook*. It is important for you to mail the envelope yourself. Don't include it in a large envelope with applications from other members of your class and don't trust anyone else to mail the application for you.

When you mail your application, be sure to send it certified and request a return receipt. Although this will cost more than regular mail, it will ensure that you receive verification of your application's delivery. You will also have proof of the postmark. Should any question arise about whether you met the deadline for application, you will have proof that your application was received and proof of postmark. Be sure to save the return receipt until after you receive your exam results.

Some time after your application is received, a written acknowledgment will be sent to you at the address you provided on your application. Several weeks later you will receive an admission ticket to the examination center. Upon receiving the admission ticket you should immediately check it to verify the date, the exam you are taking, and the location of the test center. If any of this information is in error, or if you fail to receive an admission ticket at least one week before the test, it is your responsibility to immediately contact the Registry office at (612) 687-0048. Once you've received the admission ticket, put it in a safe place until the day of the exam.

During this period, your program director will also receive a listing of all of the individuals from your program who have applied to take the examination. The program director will verify the date of completion of the program, sign the form, and return it to the ARRT to prove that you have, in fact, completed the educational program and are eligible to take the examination.

You must have completed all of the educational requirements of your program in order to take the test. This may be particularly significant if your program requires you to make up missed time after graduation. If missed time must be made up as a condition of program completion, you must fulfill this requirement before sitting for the exam. If, for any reason, the program's requirements are not satisfied in time for the exam, and you have received your admission ticket and taken the exam, your scores may be canceled. Your program director will be happy to explain this policy to you, if necessary.

▲ Materials Needed for Exam

You should take very few items with you to the examination center. No papers or books of any kind may be taken into the examination room. The items that you will want to bring include several sharpened #2 pencils, a calculator, your admission ticket, a watch, a photo ID (such as a driver's license), and another picture of yourself similar to the one attached to the examination application. This second photograph should be recent (i.e., taken within six months of the exam) and should have your signature on the back.

Be sure to have all of your pencils sharpened before arriving at the examination center. There is no guarantee that a pencil sharpener will be available and sharing of pencils during the exam is not allowed.

Though you may use a calculator on the exam, make certain that you are able to perform all calculations with pencil and paper. Do not rely on a calculator. Should your calculator malfunction or fall to the floor and break, you will not be allowed to share someone else's calculator. It would be foolish to miss most of the questions on the examination involving calculations simply because your calculator failed to operate. Again, be sure you can perform all calculations manually.

Also, make certain that you have placed fresh batteries in your calculator and tested it ahead of time. Solar-powered calculators are not recommended because your test center may have high ceilings with room lights that are too far away to activate the solar cells on your calculator. Don't leave anything to chance regarding power for your calculator. Note that using AC cords to plug in the calculator is not allowed.

It is wise to use your own watch to pace yourself, if necessary. There is no guarantee that the test room will have a clock available. Though the test proctor may write times for all to see, do not rely on this possibility. You will be more at ease if you are able to check your own time as you progress through the test. As a reminder, be sure to set your watch to the starting time announced by the proctor so that your timing will be accurate.

▲ Test Dates, Times, and Conditions

The radiography examination is administered on the third Thursday of March, July, and October. By now you probably know the date of your examination or your program director will advise you of it shortly. The examination is administered at 4 p.m. on those three test dates. Because many of the examination centers are located in high schools or colleges, it is necessary to schedule the examination in the late afternoon when such facilities are available. Actually, your examination will probably begin closer to 4:30 by the time everyone is processed and the necessary information is filled out on your answer sheet. You will still be given three hours, from the time you open your test booklet, to take the exam.

It is important to note that the testing conditions can vary from one examination center to the next. The type of desks or tables that are used will determine your physical comfort. In addition, temperature conditions can be very difficult to stabilize in many large rooms. As a result, the testing room may be warmer or cooler than you would prefer. If being too cool is a concern for you, consider taking a sweater into the examination room. A good way to prepare for a less than ideal testing situation is to study and take practice examinations under different conditions. By doing so, you will be able to adapt more easily to the variations in temperature and to the seating arrangements that you may face when you take the real exam.

Careful attention to the details contained in this chapter, as well as to those in the *Examinee Handbook,* will ensure that you have everything you need for the test day. Addressing these issues well ahead of time will free your mind for the more important task, that of passing the exam.

▲ Awaiting Test Results

Many graduates have commented that the most difficult period in this entire process is waiting for the results. You should plan on receiving your results five to six weeks after taking the exam. The most frequently asked question is "Why does it take so long?" As explained in the *Educator's Handbook*, published by the American Registry of Radiologic Technologists, the first week allows time for the test booklets and answer sheets to be mailed from all the test centers to the ARRT office in St. Paul, Minnesota. Once these are received, the computer file of examinees is updated to reflect those who did or did not take the test. Next, all of the answer sheets are placed in numerical order and inspected for stray markings or damage.

During the next work week, the answer sheets are scanned. The raw data provided by this scanning are the basis for the statistical analysis and scoring that follows.

The data then are analyzed to equate the current test with the tests previously administered throughout the year. This ensures that the scores are valid and that the items have been consistently weighted across administrations. This equating process eliminates differences in the scores that reflect variations, from one exam to another, in the level of difficulty. At this point in the process, the raw scores are translated into scaled scores for your final test results.

Individual answer sheets, with final scores just below the passing scaled score of 75, are hand corrected to ensure accuracy. This helps eliminate mistakes in scoring caused by stray marks or other problems not detectable by the scanner.

Approximately four weeks will now have elapsed since you took the exam. At this stage, materials are about to be printed for mailing. The examinees' score reports, together with reports for certain licensing states, summary reports for program directors, and reports indicating no-shows and failures must be printed. Those individuals who have passed the examination will now have their certificates and pocket cards printed and mailing labels will be prepared.

Before the materials are taken to the St. Paul post office, they must be enclosed in envelopes, the envelopes must be sealed, and mailing labels affixed. Those who have passed will receive their results in a large mailing envelope because ARRT certificates (8.5 x 11 inches) are included with their score reports. Those receiving failing scores will be sent their report in a regular business-sized envelope.

Problems outside the control of the ARRT may delay your receipt of the test results. Weather or labor problems may cause delays in the delivery of the mail, either in its arrival from the examination centers or as it is forwarded from the ARRT office. Energy or weather problems may delay the scoring of the exams or printing of results. Unforeseen computer glitches may cause additional delays. Be aware that neither test results nor explanations for delay are given over the telephone. The ARRT insists on quality control at all stages of the process to ensure that you receive excellent service and accurate results and credentials.

Finally, do not be surprised when members of your class receive their results on different days. Though the results were all mailed on the same day, variations in mail routing and urban and rural delivery will affect their arrival. Sometimes students living a few blocks apart in the same city will receive their scores on different days. There in no correlation between day of receipt and whether you passed or failed. Your time to open the large envelope will finally arrive!

Chapter 9

Test Taking Skills

> *Do not fear the winds of adversity. Remember, a kite rises against the wind rather than with it.*

▼

▲ Physically and Mentally Preparing for Test Day

While most of your preparation for the exam centers on reviewing your course work, the physical and mental preparation must be taken into account as well. The question of when, in relation to the test date, to discontinue your review has no definitive answer. It is a very individual decision based on how lengthy and thorough a review you have done and how comfortable you are with the material. Consulting your instructors to clarify your specific needs will prove most helpful in answering this question. A brief discussion of the points involved may assist you in deciding how long to study.

If you are the type of student who conducts a well-thought-out, carefully planned review of all of the material, as suggested in Chapter 1, then it is reasonable to expect that studying will taper off within two to three weeks before the examination. If you use this review book effectively and cover all of the content areas over a period of at least six months, then you should be well prepared for the examination and can draw your review to a close several weeks before the exam.

On the other hand, if you have not allowed yourself sufficient time and are attempting to compress your review into a few weeks, you may wish to study to a point nearer the exam. Be aware that anxiety, which tends to increase as the exam approaches, may interfere with learning and recalling even the most basic information as you continue to review. It may also be true that if you haven't learned the material over a period of time, there is little that you can learn in the last few weeks. Trying to cram for the exam is futile. If you have waited too long to begin studying, limit your review to the key points in all of the major subject areas.

As you prepare mentally for the day of the test, realize that apprehension about the exam may surface in unexpected ways; it is not unusual for students to report having strange dreams about the exam. The content of these dreams involves arriving too late at the test center and not being admitted; starting the exam, falling asleep and waking up with only five minutes left and nearly 200 questions to answer; and answering the final question on the examination and finding that you have room for three more answers. These are all normal responses to your anticipation of a major event. They may also serve as a motivation to continue reviewing and preparing for the exam. You may wish to share your dream experiences with other students in your class. You will come to realize that most of them are having this response, and that it is perfectly normal.

Another important aspect of preparation for the exam involves your physical readiness, which means having gathered all of the materials you will need for the test as well as having prepared your body physically to take an exam of this type. Having the appropriate materials ready well in advance of the test has been discussed previously. Again, do not wait until the day before or the day of the exam to acquire your pencils, prepare your calculator, and get your paperwork in order to take with you. Allowing several days to accomplish these tasks will ensure that you are prepared for any emergency that arises.

In preparing your body to take the exam, the basic rule of thumb is to treat exam day much as you would any other day. This phase of your preparation should actually begin the evening before the test. Intake of alcohol or large amounts of food should be avoided. You should get approximately the same amount of sleep as usual, waking at your normally scheduled time.

On the day of the exam, use the hours before the test is administered to enhance your mental and physical readiness. Start the day by eating a substantial and healthy breakfast. While you should do this every day, it is particularly important on test day. As the hour of the exam nears, you may feel less like eating. If you have eaten a substantial breakfast, it will help carry you into the afternoon. You should also plan to eat a light lunch. Remember, you will be in the middle of the exam during what is probably your dinner hour. Having a light snack in the early afternoon is a good idea; however, avoid high sugar snacks so that you do not experience a blood sugar drop as you go in to take the exam.

If you have an exercise regimen that you follow daily, you should do that on test day as well. For many, exercise helps to relieve stress and anxiety. You will likely find that trips to the restroom will increase in number on test day. This is a normal physiological response to the stress associated with the anticipation of a major event.

Is such physical preparation really necessary? Why should you be attentive to this aspect of test taking? With all of the time and effort expended during your two years of education in medical radiography and during the review process, you want to be certain that fatigue and physical stress don't impede your ability to sit for the examination.

Your instructors probably gave you a series of review examinations in the last few months of the program. One reason for this was to help assess your strengths and weaknesses in the various subject areas. Another reason was to help you acclimate to sitting for two or three hours to take an examination. It is important not to let the physical aspect of test taking hamper your ability to pass the exam.

The final aspect of preparation for the exam involves traveling to and arriving at the test center. The accessibility of test centers around the United States varies, requiring some students to travel for hours to reach a site, while others take the test in their home town. Whatever your situation, it is important to allow ample time to travel to the test center to ensure that potential delays (e.g., heavy traffic, road construction, accidents that may impede the flow of traffic, or problems with your own automobile) are avoided.

It is better to arrive at the test center early than to pull into the parking lot with barely a minute or two to spare. Arriving early will give you time to relax after your drive and to become accustomed to the new surroundings. It will also allow for the possibility that there has been a building or room change at the last minute. If you have arrived with spare time you will have no problem locating the building and the room in which you will take the examination. Of course, arriving at the test center early will also afford you the opportunity to visit the restroom again before entering the exam room. While you may be excused during the exam to use the restroom, it is best to allow time, should the need arise, before the exam begins.

The writing of this book is grounded in many years of experience in preparing students to take the ARRT exam. Attention to the details in this section will help relieve your anxiety about the exam and allow you to focus on the more important aspects of reviewing and writing the exam.

▲ *The Answer Sheet*

A sample of the answer sheet is included in your *Examinee Handbook*. Look at it carefully and note how the sheet is laid out. Notice whether answers progress vertically down the page or horizontally across the page. This will prevent confusion about placement of your answers. Though you may have taken many standardized tests in the past, do not take anything for granted. Be sure you are familiar with the answer sheet. Notice that you will be asked to sign it twice. One signature will verify that you are the person taking the test; the second signature will authorize or withhold authorization for your scores to be sent to your program director.

From the perspective of a program director, it is most helpful to receive the scores of all of the students taking the exam from one's program. This information may be used to assess strengths and weaknesses in the program itself and to evaluate the review process. Releasing your scores is a valuable aid in the ongoing effort to improve the quality of the radiography program from which you have just graduated. Your scores will not be shown to others but will be used as part of the program's outcomes assessment and planning process. Please consider signing the release so that your total score and section scores will be reported to your program director.

Provide all of the requested information, carefully ensuring that the circles are filled in fully and with sufficient density to be read by the computer. As you probably know from taking past examinations that use scanned test blanks, it is very important not to make any stray marks on the answer sheet. For example, do not put a mark next to an item on the answer sheet to remind yourself to come back and reread that question. Make such a mark in the test booklet. Stray marks on the answer sheet may be misread by the scanning equipment and may result in that item being scored as incorrect, even though you have the correct answer filled in. Also, be sure that erasures are clean and that they completely remove your unwanted choices from the page. One way to prevent insufficient erasures is to answer all of the questions in the test booklet and, afterward, to transfer the answers to the answer sheet. That way, if any changes are to be made, you can do so before transferring the answers to the answer sheet.

Though the Registry office personnel screen the answer sheets for stray marks, you cannot be certain that each one will be found. As with so many other aspects of this process, do not rely on someone else for something that is your responsibility.

▲ The Test Booklet

The radiography examination is in booklet form. Though you will not be given extra sheets of paper on which to write, you may write in the margins of the test booklet once you begin the examination. It is also important to remember NOT to open the test booklet until you are instructed to begin the exam. Once you enter the examination room be sure to follow the directions of the individual administering the test.

Understand that the person proctoring the examination cannot answer any of your questions pertaining to the exam content. The proctor is neither a radiologic technologist nor an employee of the ARRT.

▲ Strategies for Taking the Exam

Everyone tends to have a preferred system for taking a lengthy, multiple-choice format examination. If you have a method that has worked well in the past, then continue to use it. However, if you seem to lose focus when taking such a test, consider the following suggestions for structuring your approach to this exam.

Just getting started may be difficult for some individuals and cause them to experience discomfort. Many graduates have reported that, upon opening the test booklet, they were very uneasy. This is usually the result of the apprehension and stress surrounding this important event. Such an initial response should not be viewed as abnormal, and you can rest assured that several of your peers are experiencing that same discomfort. Should this occur, close the test booklet, close your eyes, breathe deeply several times, and reopen the booklet. Unless you have severe test anxiety, or failed to review and prepare carefully ahead of time, you will be ready to begin answering the questions.

There are 200 test items on the exam. A test item includes the stem, or question, and the set of possible answers. The stem will ask a question or make an incomplete statement. Of the possible answers, one will be correct. The others are called distracters. Distracters are choices designed to make you think they are the correct answer. They will usually consist of the most common incorrect response or will include all but a small portion of the correct answer. There can be only one correct answer to the question.

Those who construct the exam attempt to include only those items for which there is a broad consensus regarding the correct response. Questions about specific departmental routines and information drawn from only one textbook are not used. Several sources are consulted when screening questions for the exam, and only the information common to most sources is used. There are no textbooks officially endorsed by the ARRT to screen or write test items, so you may be assured that you will not be penalized on the exam because you did not use a certain textbook as a student.

As you begin taking the exam, be sure to read each question carefully. It is extremely important to comprehend what is being asked. Do not attempt to read more into the question than is printed. Do not assume that it is a "trick" question. The exam is a carefully written, well-constructed document. There should be nothing on the test that you have not seen before in your studies and during your review. Be careful not to read the question the way you want it to be asked. Take the question at face value. Beware of words such as *none*, *every*, *always*, *never*, and *all*. These are qualifiers that usually indicate a false statement.

Further, be aware of the different types of items that may be asked. One type, called completion or open-ended, will simply give you a statement to complete, as in the following example:

The negative electrode in the x-ray tube is called the:

a. Cathode
b. Rotor
c. Anode
d. Focusing cup
e. Target

Another type of item that may be used is the question. Here a complete question will be asked and you will need to choose the answer. An example of such an item follows:

Which interaction results in complete absorption of the energy of the incoming photon?

a. Compton's
b. Pair production
c. Coherent scattering
d. Photoelectric effect
e. Brems

The third form of test question—called a negative-type item—can cause problems for many students. This item will measure your knowledge of exceptions to the data you have learned. Following is an example of a negative-type item:

Which of the following is not part of an image intensifier tube?

a. Rotor
b. Photocathode
c. Input phosphor
d. Cesium iodide
e. Output phosphor

Becoming familiar with the types of items that may be used will help you to anticipate what the test will be like and will assist you in studying and preparing for the exam. There is a wide variety of question types used in this book. Some will be found on the exam, whereas others are included only to encourage use of your critical thinking skills. Being aware of all of the types of questions will aid in your exam preparation.

After determining the type of item and reading the stem of the item, read each answer choice. Be certain to read all of the answers! While choice *A* may appear to be correct, choice *D* may be a more complete answer. Further, the correct answer may be choice *E* ("all of the above"), as in the following item:

An example of natural background radiation is:

a. Radon gas
b. The sun
c. Radioactive elements in the earth
d. Radioactive substances in air, food, and water
e. All of the above

Reading the question and the first answer, "radon gas" might lead you to fill in *A* and move to the next question. After all, you learned that radon gas is a type of natural background radiation. However, taking the time to read all of the answers leads you to choices *B*, *C*, and *D*. You remember that they are all types of natural background radiation, making choice *E* the correct answer. This is not a trick question; it is assessing whether you know the different sources of natural background radiation.

Be particularly careful of answer choices that may include several correct answers, such as "more than one but not all of the above' "or "A and C above", or "B and D above." In such cases, take your time. Read each possible choice and determine if it is a correct answer on its own. One method used is to reread the question, complete it with

each possible answer, and determine if the resulting statement is true or false. A previous question has been rewritten below to provide an example:

"An example of natural background radiation is"

(1) Cosmic radiation
(2) Medical and dental x rays
(3) Radon gas
(4) Radioactive elements in the earth
(5) Radioactive substances in food, water, and air
(6) Nuclear weapons testing

a. 1, 2, and 3 above
b. 4, 5, and 6 above
c. 1, 3, 5, and 6 above
d. 1, 3, 4, and 5 above
e. All of the above

First, take your time with a question of this type. You will have plenty of time to complete the exam, even if you spend extra time on these items. Read the question, then look at choice *A*. Check to see if every item in this choice makes a true statement when it is used to complete the test question. Ask yourself, "An example of natural background radiation is cosmic radiation, true or false?" The answer is true. Next, "An example of natural background radiation is medical and dental x rays, true or false?" The answer is false. You know that medical and dental x rays are a source of artificial or human-made radiation. This single false statement rules out choice *A* as a possible answer. Continue in this fashion until you have found a choice in which all of the possible statements are true. Using this example, that would be choice *D*.

Not all such questions will require you to take as much time to answer. However, having a specific method to use will reduce your anxiety when you're presented with a multiple-choice question which has several correct answers. Remember that after reading the question and all of the choices, the first answer you choose will usually be correct. Be careful not to begin second-guessing your choice of an answer. In addition, do not watch for patterns of answers. For example, resist choosing *A* because you haven't used it in a while, but don't be surprised if another choice is used for several consecutive questions.

If you have no idea what the answer is, guess. There is no guessing penalty on the exam. However, even when guessing, have a strategy. Do not choose an answer that includes terms that are unfamiliar to you. Students sometimes reason that such a choice must be the answer, because they have never heard of it before. Most often, this is not the case. Make an educated guess by ruling out answers you are sure are wrong. Then choose from among those containing familiar terminology. Do not mark more than one answer on the answer sheet for that item, hoping that the machine will count one of your choices correct. Such a marking will be scored as incorrect even if one selection is the right answer.

Alternatives for recording your responses on the answer sheet were briefly mentioned earlier. Some students fill in their choice as each question is answered, while others prefer to circle their responses in the test booklet and then transfer them to the answer sheet after they've answered all of the questions. There is no right or wrong way. Let's consider both methods.

If you fill in your choice as you answer each question, you will find it easier to track your answers for proper placement on the answer sheet. Unless you choose to skip an item and return to it later, it is unlikely that you will fill in a circle after the wrong item number. However, should you wish to change your answer, you will need to erase completely. While changing answers is something you should not do often, it may be necessary if you are certain you have entered a wrong answer the first time. If you tend to change answers when you shouldn't, recording them in this way may reduce the number of changes. Remember, most of the time you will change a correct response to an incorrect one.

You may choose to answer all of the questions first, circling your selections in the test booklet and, afterward, transferring them to the answer sheet. The advantage here is that it is easier to change answers if necessary. There is also less risk of error if you decide to skip certain questions and come back to them later. Markings in the test booklet are allowed and have no bearing on the final answers or your score. A disadvantage to this method is that you will be filling in two hundred answers at the conclusion of the test when you are likely to be fatigued. It may then be easy to make a mistake transferring answers from the test booklet to the answer sheet. Only you know for sure which method will work best for you. You may wish to try both during practice tests.

In summary, the certification exam is nothing to fear if you review and prepare properly. Be sure to consider the suggestions and strategies presented here and those identified by your instructors. If you have practiced, studied, and have your strategy ready, the exam will be just another quiz!

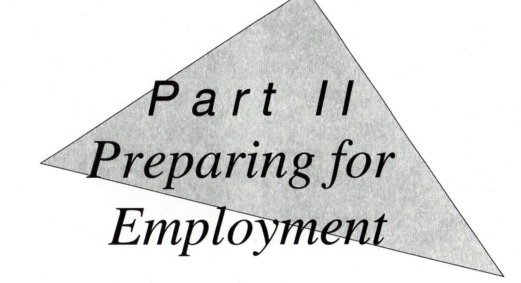

Part II
Preparing for
Employment

Chapter 10

Career Planning

> *Do it now. You become successful the moment you start moving toward a worthwhile goal.*

▼

▲ *Motivation*

Individuals pursue chosen careers for a variety of reasons. Sources of motivation for enrolling in an educational program and satisfying all of the graduation requirements may include the need for a stable income, the desire to establish oneself in a career, or an interest in expanding one's horizons. Incentives to undertake such a process are unique to each individual and may clearly distinguish a forty-five year old from an eighteen-year old. It is also true that incentives can change as you move toward a goal, so that the circumstances that led you to select this educational program may differ considerably from those influencing you to establish a career in this field.

As the requirements for graduation from the educational program are met, it would be wise to examine your motivation for seeking employment and actually establishing a career in radiologic technology. You should reexamine your motivation and adjust your goals on a regular basis, perhaps annually. The questions listed below will help with that process and assist you in establishing career goals.

1. Based upon my studies and clinical education so far, what aspects of this profession am I really excited about?

2. Which aspects of patient care have I found the most satisfying?

Rationale: Questions 1 and 2 attempt to help you focus on what has brought you true satisfaction so far in the educational program. Being excited about what you do is critical to your longevity in the field. It is a daily reinforcement to your motivation. It helps you bring a positive attitude to class and to the clinical environment. Many individuals have certain aspects of patient care that they find particularly satisfying. Identifying yours will help you to set goals for job placement or for continuing your education. For example, if you find great satisfaction working with children, pediatric radiography may be an excellent choice for a career. You would want to examine job possibilities at children's hospitals. Perhaps trauma radiography is particularly challenging and satisfying for you. Pursuing employment at an institution with a trauma center, and on a shift with a high trauma case load, would be a wise choice. Maybe teaching and working with students appeal to you. If so, your goals may include completing advanced academic degrees and finding a clinical job in a teaching institution.

Take time now to answer questions 1 and 2 in the space provided. Remember, you are examining situations you find motivating and exciting. You will have an opportunity to set your goals later in this chapter.

I am really excited about:

_____

_____

_____

The aspects of patient that have been most satisfying are:

_____

_____

_____

3. Of the people with whom I have worked in clinical education, who has been most helpful?

4. Which characteristics do I want to emulate most ?

Rationale: As a radiography student, you may be profoundly influenced by the personnel in the clinical department. It is important to identify those people who have been particularly helpful to you as you have acquired your clinical skills. All too often, it is tempting to think about, talk about, and remember only those who have been hindrances to your education or who simply did not enjoy working with students. Concentrate instead on the positive people and prepare a list of their names. Describe the personal and professional characteristics they possess. Explain why you enjoy working with them. Everyone benefits from role models. Describe why you wish to emulate, or pattern your professional attitudes and demeanor after, certain people with whom you have worked.

The most helpful individuals in clinical education have been:

_____

_____

_____

They have been great to work with because:

_____

_____

_____

I will emulate these positive behaviors (also explain why):

_____

_____

_____

5. When during the educational process have I been happiest?

6. When during the educational process have I been least happy?

Rationale: An awareness of events, people, or situations that have caused you to feel happy or unhappy will be helpful in setting goals for employment. While it is not possible to be happy on the job all of the time or always to avoid unpleasant situations, being aware of such times can help you to decide where you may or may not wish to work. Also, by addressing these issues now, you can gain an understanding of how you respond to positive and negative situations and how to alter your responses, if necessary. You may also wish to consider ways in which you can retain a positive outlook when dealing with unpleasant situations or individuals by recalling successful self-motivating strategies from the past. The mark of a true professional is the ability to summon the highest level of performance from yourself and those around you, even during difficult times.

I have been happiest during my education when:

_____

_____

_____

I have been most dissatisified during my education when:

_____

_____

_____

7. What employment needs will I have upon graduation?

8. What financial needs will I have upon graduation?

9. What housing needs and living conditions will I seek to meet upon graduation?

10. Do I want or need to stay in this geographical area or do I want or need to relocate?

Rationale: It is, unfortunately, too often the case that individuals do little or no planning for their employment, financial needs, or living conditions and, consequently, are buffeted about by the winds of change and quirks of chance.

Consider what your needs will be for employment when you graduate. Decide whether you will need to begin work immediately and to accept the first job offer you receive or wish to wait a short time to scout the job market more thoroughly. It is crucial to have some idea of what your financial needs will be. Be aware of the cost of setting up your own living arrangements, paying back school loans, or providing for your family's well-being. If you are not currently responsible for your own housing, decide how you want to arrange that. With a fluctuating job market, you must consider whether you will remain rooted where you are or will relocate to find the type of position you desire. Perhaps relocating is something you have wanted to do all along. Maybe relocating is simply not possible at this point in your life.

Answer each question in the space below; describe what your needs and wants will be after graduation.

Employment:

_____

_____

_____

Financial:

_____

_____

_____

Housing:

_____

_____

_____

Location:

_____

_____

_____

11. Am I more excited about working with the high-touch (people-oriented) aspects of this profession or the high-tech (equipment) aspects of the field?

Rationale: There are individuals who work in this field because they truly love working with people and assisting with the diagnosis of their conditions. There are others who much prefer working with complex electronic and computerized equipment and would rather not be involved in direct patient care. There is room for both types in this profession. Identifying the aspects of the field that excite you will help with your career planning.

Perhaps you wish to remain in direct patient care. Maybe you would rather work with equipment, such as in quality control, medical physics, or the sale and service of equipment. Nothing will cause you to become more dissatisfied with your career choice than to be working in an area of radiologic technology to which you are not suited. Develop an awareness now of what you most enjoy doing. There is no right or wrong answer nor are you good or bad for what you prefer. Most important, be honest with yourself. You have much to contribute to this field if you are working where you are happiest and most productive.

Take some time and write below your honest preferences based on your experiences so far. Remember, you are not setting a goal at this point and your answer may change over time.

High tech vs. high touch, my preference and why:

_____

_____

_____

_____

_____

12. Do I enjoy learning all that I can about this field or do I want to learn only what I need to graduate?

Rationale: Your answer to this question is very important. The field you have chosen changes rapidly. You must be honest with yourself about your desire to study and learn. The equipment currently used in clinical education was not even invented just a few years ago. You will use equipment a few years after you graduate that does not exist today! If you are content to learn only what you need to graduate, you will soon possess skills that are outdated. Also, consider whether you truly enjoy learning or tend to regard it as a burden. Your education in this field will have barely begun by the time you graduate. Be aware that you will need to set a course for lifelong learning. Understanding this reality now will assist you in developing your professional attitude and in planning for continuing education. Realizing the importance of a commitment to learning may also serve to motivate you through the remainder of your educational program.

Take time to assess your motivation for learning. In the space below, describe your honest feelings and attitudes about the enjoyment of learning for its own sake as opposed to learning just enough to perform your job.

I want to learn all that I can or just enough to get by. Here are my reasons and motivations:

_____

_____

_____

_____

_____

_____

13. Which aspect(s) of the specialty of radiography do I enjoy the most (general radiography, fluoroscopy, mobile radiography, surgical radiography, trauma, pediatric)?

14. Are there any other radiologic specialties I have particularly enjoyed (angiography, mammography, computed tomography, magnetic resonance imaging, sonography, nuclear medicine, radiation therapy, quality control)?

Rationale: You may not yet realize that radiography is a specialty within which are areas of further specialization (e.g., general, fluoroscopy, mobile). You are probably already familiar with the other specialties listed in question 14. By being aware of what you enjoy, you will have little difficulty later setting goals for employment or education. If you have not yet had the opportunity to spend clinical time in some of the above areas, you may need to postpone answering this question. When such an opportunity arises, however, prepare yourself for the clinical experience by reading about the specialty area in your textbook and by taking careful notes about your experiences. This field has countless opportunities for you in the practice of radiography or any of the other special imaging or therapy modalities.

List below the areas in which you are particularly interested and describe why you have enjoyed them. Also list the areas that you look forward to visiting and explain why they are important to you.

I particularly enjoy working in the following area(s):

_____

_____

_____

I want to explore the following areas further:

_____

_____

_____

15. Are there any special projects that I have done that brought me satisfaction (research papers, exhibits, in-class presentations, participation in radiography college bowls)?

16. Am I interested in pursuing positions of leadership or membership in local, state, or national radiologic technology organizations?

Rationale: This profession needs you! It needs what you have to offer. It needs your fresh ideas and observations. It needs your leadership, motivation, talents, and abilities. By considering the issues raised in questions 15 and 16, you will be able to set goals for your postgraduation involvement.

Perhaps you have already written a research paper, constructed an exhibit, or participated in college bowl competition. Don't stop now! You have momentum working in your favor. Consider how these projects may have brought you satisfaction and served to motivate you further. Think about how you may set goals for doing additional projects as a radiographer for state or national presentations.

Local, state, and national professional organizations in radiologic technology need the involvement of motivated, committed professionals. Gauge your interest in becoming involved. Don't let fear of the unknown deter you. Remember that those who are currently active were, at one time, attending their first meeting, serving on a committee for the first time, or holding their first office. Think about how such involvement may add to your career and personal satisfaction.

In the space provided, write your thoughts and feelings about pursuing these activities. Describe how you would feel if you became involved at this level of the profession.

The special projects that brought me the most satisfaction were:

_____

_____

_____

I wish to become involved in the following organization(s) in this capacity:

_____

_____

_____

17. Do I believe I will have an interest in working with students when I am employed?

Rationale: You will need to assess your interest in working with students. Many of us truly enjoy helping students acquire skills, while others would prefer to avoid the responsibility of educating. If you believe you would enjoy teaching, then seeking employment in an academic environment is a reasonable goal. If you would prefer not to work with students, then it would be better for you and for the students to seek employment in another setting. Many otherwise excellent radiographers find frustration on the job because they are not suited to the clinical teaching role. Do not take this issue lightly. Having a student assigned to you every day of work can be exhilarating or burdensome, depending upon your professional preferences.

In the space below, state whether you prefer to work with students or to find employment in a nonteaching institution.

I would or would not like to work with students after graduation. Here are my reasons:

_____

_____

_____

_____

_____

_____

18. In what type of clinical setting am I most comfortable (hospital, small clinic, physician's office, urgent care)?

Rationale: Health care assumes many forms depending, in part, on the environment in which it is delivered. If you have had the opportunity to spend clinical time in more than one of the settings mentioned above, decide which you found most to your liking. If you have not had this opportunity, check with your program director about the availability of clinical rotations. If none are available in the program, consider spending time outside of school, in one or more of these clinical settings, to gain some idea of how they operate and to observe the radiographer at work.

Each clinical setting has qualities that will appeal to you as a radiographer and others that make it a less attractive choice. You may also be guided by a strong personal preference about where you would like to work. Consider these factors carefully when setting goals for employment.

I have had experience in the following clinical settings. Here is what I liked and disliked:

_____

_____

_____

_____

_____

_____

19. What particular talents do I possess about which I feel proud?

Rationale: Identify your talents and all that you have to offer a potential employer. Consider how you may use these talents to pursue your personal and professional goals. Think of how your strengths may benefit the patients you serve. Understand the impact you may have on coworkers. It is important to be proud of your talents and to use them to the greatest benefit. It is not conceited to list them or to use them. You must concentrate on being the best you can be by developing your abilities and acquiring others. Use them to enhance your practice of radiography and your personal life.

My particular talents and positive attributes are listed below. Here is how I have used them and why I am excited about them:

_____

_____

_____

_____

_____

_____

▲ *Goal Setting*

By carefully answering the questions listed above, you should now have a fairly good idea of the things that motivate you in this field. The choice of a career is important and you should be intent upon doing those things you particularly enjoy.

Individuals who have been successful in the field of radiologic technology are those who have set goals for themselves and have worked hard to achieve them. Goal setting is not an easy task, particularly in view of the fact that it is seldom taught in school. However, all of the great motivational speakers and career planners indicate that goal setting should be a priority, not only when beginning a career, but throughout your working lifetime.

Goals are not meant to be etched in granite, never to be changed or updated. Rather, goal statements should be flexible and fluid. As was mentioned earlier, goals should be updated as needed, at least annually.

The wording of goal statements can be as important as setting the goals themselves. Phrases such as "I want to be a nuclear medicine technologist within three years" are not powerful enough. "I will be a registered nuclear medicine technologist by the end of (specify year)" is more specific. It is action-oriented. It says you will do something and you will direct your energies toward achieving that goal within a specific time frame. It is not merely a wish, but a statement that you expect to realize.

Post your goals where you can see them daily and share them with those who are significant in your life. These individuals, with their encouragement and moral support, can help you achieve your goals. It is well documented that shared goals are more likely to be met because of the increased sense of accountability to others who are aware of them.

Listed below are a series of questions to consider as you write your goal statements. Sample goal statements are provided. Note that they are specific, have time frames, and use the words "I will." You may be thinking that you lack some of the information needed to write your goal statements. Recognize, however, that by writing goals and planning your future you are in the process of bringing that future about. This helps you to direct your energies toward pursuing and accomplishing your goals.

Setting goals should not be taken lightly, but should not be so arduous a task that it becomes a burden. Be excited about setting your goals and beginning to map out your future! Also, don't get discouraged if your goals seem simple at first. They are there to provide you with direction.

It will be up to you to adjust them and to direct the course you plan to follow.

1. What deadline have I set for completion of my goal statements? In other words, how soon will I have thought about them and written them down?

Goal:
I will list my goals along with a timetable by the following date:

_____

2. What kind of review schedule have I established to prepare for the radiography certification exam?

Goal:
I will review the subjects included on the exam according to the following schedule:

Radiation Protection:

_____

Equipment Operation and Maintenance:

_____

Image Production and Evaluation:

_____

Radiographic Procedures:

_____

Patient Care and Management:

_____

3. Do I want to pursue additional education in radiologic technology or seek an advanced degree?

Goal:
I will write for information on baccalaureate degrees by the following date:

_____

Goal:
I will take _____ number of credit hours per semester

beginning on _____ so

that I will complete my degree on

_____

Goal:
I will write for information on educational programs in (sonography, nuclear medicine, radiation therapy)

by _____

Goal:
I will attend an educational program in (sonography, nuclear medicine, radiation therapy) beginning

_____ and will graduate

from the program in _____

4. Do my regular study habits need to be examined and fine-tuned?

Goal:
I will examine my current study habits on

_____

Goal:
I am modifying my current study habits as follows:

_____

_____

Goal:
I will begin my new study habits on

_____

5. Do I need to examine my lifestyle choices regarding diet, exercise, sleep requirements, etc.?

Goal:
I will evaluate my lifestyle choices in diet, exercise, sleep, and recreation on

_____

Goal:
I am modifying my diet as follows (be specific):

_____

_____

_____

_____

Goal:
I am modifying my exercise routine as follows (be specific):

_____

_____

_____

_____

Goal:
I am modifying my sleep routine as follows:

_____

_____

_____

Goal:
I am taking time for recreation as follows:

_____

_____

_____

6. Have I taken into account the needs of my family or significant others?

Goal:
I will consult with my significant others regarding these goals on

_____

Goal:
I will list below the needs of my significant others in view of the goals I have set on

_____

_____

_____

_____

7. What do I want to accomplish in the next 30, 60, and 90 days related to my career?

Goal:
By 30 days from now, on

_____ ,

I will have accomplished the following to advance my career goals:

_____

_____

_____

_____

Goal:
By 60 days from now, on

_____ , *I will have accomplished the following to advance my career goals, built on my 30-day objectives:*

_____

_____

_____

_____

Goal:
By 90 days from now, on

_____ , *I will have accomplished the following to advance my career goals, built on my 30- and 60-day objectives:*

_____

_____

_____

_____

8. To reinforce my positive attitude, I will need to avail myself of motivational materials.

Goal:
By _____ , I will read the following motivational books:

_____

_____

_____

_____

9. Postgraduation needs that I must consider:

Goal:
I will begin work by _____

Goal:
I will make the following hourly salary to maintain the lifestyle I have chosen: _____

Goal:
I will live in the following type of house or apartment:

_____

Goal:
I will live in the following city or geographical area:

_____

10. High-tech versus high-touch aspects of radiography:

Goal:
I will work in the following direct patient care area of medical radiography:

_____

Goal:
I will work in the following non-patient care area:

_____

11. Continuing education in radiography:

Goal:
I will follow this schedule for remaining current in my chosen field:

Type of meetings or conferences I will attend on a regular basis:

Local _____

State _____

National _____

12. Other radiologic specialties:

Goal:
I will do extra reading and clinical observation in the following radiologic specialties (e.g., angiography, mammography, computed tomography, magnetic resonance imaging, sonography, nuclear medicine, radiation therapy, quality control) by the dates I have listed:

_____

_____

_____

_____

_____

13. Special projects to pursue after graduation:

Goal:
I will write a research paper and submit it for competition at the state or national level on

_____. *The possible subjects for this paper are:*

_____

_____

_____

Goal:
I will prepare an exhibit for presentation at a state or national meeting on _____.
The possible subjects for this exhibit are:

_____

_____

_____

Goal:
I will assist with planning the following local or state meeting

_____

on _____

Goal:
I will run for the office of

_____ *of my local, state, or national professional organization on*

_____

14. Working with students:

Goal:
I will work in a department that (is, is not) in a teaching institution.

15. Work setting:

Goal:
I will work in the following type of institution: hospital, clinic, physician's office, urgent care.

16. Professional attributes:

Goal:
I will work to maintain the attributes that I admire most in the professionals who have helped in clinical education. Those attributes are:

_____

_____

_____

_____

_____

17. Other goals I am setting for myself:

Goal:

_____

_____

_____

Goal:

_____

_____

_____

Goal:

_____

_____

_____

Goal:

_____

_____

_____

By now you have had considerable experience in describing the aspects of this field that you find motivating. You have also listed specific career goals that you have the ability to achieve. Performing this type of personal inventory has gotten you off to a great start. In addition to reading your goal statements daily, revisit these goals at regular intervals over the next 6 to 12 months. There will be no stopping you now!

Chapter 11

Writing a Professional Résumé

▲ Purpose of a Résumé

Your résumé is, in effect, your professional calling card. It is a summary of your academic and work history, along with relevant accomplishments and credentials. It should be brief (i.e., one or two pages). It is, essentially, a snapshot of your career to date. In addition to offering samples of résumés, this section will also describe ways in which to use the résumé and will provide the rationale for including or excluding certain information.

There are probably as many different styles and formats for résumés as there are instructors attempting to describe them. You may wish to take advantage of your radiography instructor's expertise in this area. In addition, if you are enrolled in a collegiate radiography program, there may be a learning resource center, a writing center, or a career counseling center from which you can obtain additional guidance. The material presented in this section was developed for courses taught by the author and has been used by his students and graduates.

The résumé may be used in three ways: 1) it may be sent as part of a mailing to prospective employers and followed with a telephone call; 2) it may be left with an interviewer after an appointment; or 3) it may be included with the job application form submitted in the human resources department.

Frequently, the student or graduate radiographer wishes to indicate availability to a large number of prospective employers in a certain geographical area. The résumé, accompanied by a cover letter, may be mailed to the directors of radiology at all facilities in the area in which the student is interested. Although this is the least effective method to use in a job search, a well-constructed résumé, with an appropriate cover letter, can produce results. Figure 11-1 shows a sample cover letter to accompany the résumé in these situations. Such a mailing should always be followed by a personal telephone call to the radiology manager as promised in the cover letter. To follow up in this way can become time-consuming, but it is one method to use when attempting to reach a large number of prospective employers.

Date

Director of Radiology
XYZ Hospital
Main Street
Anytown, USA   01234

Dear Director:

Enclosed please find my professional résumé outlining my education and work experiences. I am very interested in being considered for employment in your department of radiology in the position of staff radiographer. I appreciate whatever time and attention you are able to give to this inquiry.

I will call you in a few days to see what employment opportunities you may have available.

Sincerely,

Figure 11-1 Sample cover letter #1.

In certain situations, the student or graduate radiographer may actually have an informal interview with a radiology manager who is considering filling a position. This frequently occurs when students or graduates become aware of a job opening by word of mouth. In these situations, there may be insufficient time to mail a résumé in advance. When this occurs, the interviewee should take a copy of the résumé and give it to the radiology manager at the time of the interview. As with appropriate attire and grooming, a professional résumé can make a powerful first impression during such an interview.

▲ Contents of a Résumé

In addition to making certain that you have the appropriate writing tools available, it is also important to spend time thinking about what to include and exclude from the résumé. Though such information will be covered item by item in the next section, a few general statements are in order here. You will want to include all postsecondary (after high school) education. You should account for all of your time since high school. Be sure to enter all professional society memberships, credential numbers, awards, and accomplishments on the résumé.

The résumé should contain only information that is relevant to your accomplishments and goals as a professional. Information of a personal nature (beyond that presented in the next section), or data that could be used to discriminate, should be excluded from the résumé. Your résumé is an opportunity to advertise yourself in your absence. Construct it wisely.

▲ Writing the Résumé

Figures 11-2 and 11-3 show two résumés that could have been written by student or graduate radiographers. The résumés present applicants with slightly different backgrounds and, therefore, include different information. Your résumé is likely to be a variant of these. Keep in mind that brevity is the rule in constructing your résumé.

Personal Data
  Applicant Name
  Applicant Address
  City, State, Zip Code
  Telephone Number

Goal
  To obtain a position as an entry-level radiographer

Employment Experience
  December 19__ - Present
  Darkroom Assistant and Transporter
  Department of Radiology
  XYZ Area Hospital
  This Town, State
  Process films; clean processor; transport patients to and from radiology department

  May 19__ - October 19__
  Nursing Assistant
  Elderly Manor
  This Town, State
  Answered residents' call lights; served meals; assisted with bathing; assisted with meals

Education
  19__ - Present
  School of Radiography
  ABC Memorial Hospital
  That City, State
  Accredited program in medical radiography
  Will graduate June 19__

  19__ - 19__
  Liberal Arts Coursework
  Black Hawk Community College
  This Town, State
  Took 36 semester hours

Professional Accomplishments, Associations, and Credentials
  • Registry eligible - Taking July 19__ exam
  • Student member, American Society of Radiologic Technologists
  • Student member, This State Society of Radiologic Technologists
  • Awarded Second Place for presentation of research paper entitled "Crohn's Disease" at State Society Annual Conference

Refeerences available upon request.

Figure 11-2 Sample résumé #1.

Personal Data

Applicant Name
Applicant Address
City, State, Zip Code
Telephone Number

Goal

To obtain a position as an entry-level radiographer; willing to cross-train in angiography or mammography

Employment Experience

September 19__- Present

Front Office Clerk
Imaging Department
City Memorial Hospital
This Town, State
Greet patients; enter computer record; file radiographs

November 19__- July 19__
Serving Line Worker
Dietary Department
Saints Hospital
Our Town, State
Greeted employees and visitors in cafeteria serving line; served their choice of food; ran cash register on week-ends

Education

June 19__ - May 19__
Associate Degree Radiography Program
Our Community College
This City, State
Accredited program in medical radiography
Graduated May 19__; awarded Associate in Applied Sciences Degree

19__- 19__
Radiography program prerequisites
Our Community College
This Town, State
Took 48 semester hours in liberal arts and sciences

Professional Accomplishments, Associations, and Credentials

- Certified by the American Registry of Radiologic Technologists, #987654
- Licensed by State of __, # 123-45-6789-1-1.
- Active member, American Society of Radiologic Technologists
- Active member, This State Society of Radiologic Technologists
- Awarded Second Place for presentation of research paper entitled "Crohn's Disease" at State Society Student Conference
- Member of student team competing in annual Radiography College Bowl sponsored by State Society of Radiologic Technologists

References available upon request.

Figure 11-3 Sample résumé #2.

Personal Data

The first section should include your name, followed by the address and phone number at which you may be reached during your current job search. An address and phone number that is going to change in the very near future will cause the prospective employer to be unable to contact you and may eliminate you as a candidate for the position. If you must change your address and phone number after submitting the résumé, be sure to inform prospective employers in writing.

No additional personal information should be included on the résumé. Specific items to be excluded are date of birth, gender, race, marital status, church affiliation, number of children, disabilities, and any other data that are irrelevant to your status as a job seeker. Though such information may not be used by a prospective employer, including it on your résumé places you in the position of having raised it as an issue.

Goal Statement

As shown in the examples, the next section of the résumé should include your goal statement. The goal statement can be as simple as "To obtain a position as an entry-level radiographer" or it may include your desire to cross-train in another specialty, such as "To obtain a position as an entry- level radiographer; desire to cross-train in computed tomography." Careful consideration should be given to the goal statement. If the wording suggests that you absolutely must have the opportunity to cross-train in other modalities, you will be eliminated from consideration if the prospective employer is looking for a staff radiographer only. Wording such as "To obtain a position as an entry- level radiographer; willing to be cross-trained in other modalities" indicates your desire to expand your horizons but without the sense of urgency conveyed by the prior statement.

The goal statement may also be altered depending upon where one is seeking employment. If you know the prospective employer is seeking radiographers who definitely want to cross-train, then that interest should be included in your goal statement. If, however, one of your goals is to cross-train, and you are unwilling to accept a position that does not offer that opportunity, then you should definitely include it in your goal statement, realizing that you may be excluded from consideration if such a position is not available. Words in the goal statement that identify the strength of your interest are "desire to cross-train" or "willing to cross-train."

As you prepare to write your résumé and are setting your professional goals, give them serious consideration. The goal statement may include you in the final group of candidates for a position, or it may exclude you immediately, depending upon how it is worded. Consider, as a final example, the goal statement of an applicant to a clinic or urgent care setting. Many times the responsibilities in these positions are multifaceted. A goal statement such as "To obtain a position as a radiographer; willing to perform venipuncture, simple laboratory procedures, electrocardiograms, and take patient histories and vital signs" indicates not only a willingness to learn new procedures, but an ability to be flexible and work as a team member in a small clinic setting. Conversely, if you have no desire to perform these other functions, then you should not include such places in your job search.

Employment Experiences

Beginning with your most recent employment and working backward, you should list all employment experiences related either to health care or to working with the public. Indicate the month and year that each position began and ended, the name of the employer, the location of the employer, and a simple phrase describing your responsibilities. It is not necessary to list the names of supervisors or the salary you received. It is also not necessary to account for every job held since high school. Remember, the résumé is your statement of professional experience. Include those positions that demonstrate your ability to work with people.

Education

Your résumé should include all of the formal education you have acquired since high school, listed in reverse chronological order, beginning with the most recent. It is not necessary to provide a detailed list of the courses studied. Rather, you may wish to indicate a broad area of study; for example, "liberal arts and sciences." Some entries in this section will be self-explanatory. A radiology manager will not require explanation of an entry such as "School of Radiography." For each of your educational experiences, indicate whether you graduated or received some form of certificate or diploma. The dates in this section, along with those accompanying your employment history, should account for most of your time since high school.

Professional Accomplishments, Associations, and Credentials

It is here that you should list all professional organizations to which you belong. Be sure to include any offices you have held or other positions of responsibility, such as committee membership, etc. Examples of information for this section would include membership in local, state, or national professional societies, student radiographer associations, and any professional licenses already held. Awards for academic excellence should be included here, as well as participation in competitions, such as research paper writing, scientific exhibits, and college bowls. You may also wish to include a listing of your attendance at state or national professional society meetings.

If you have not yet taken the ARRT exam you should describe your status as "Registry Eligible - Taking July 19__ exam." If you have taken the exam but have not yet received your results, simply state "Registry Eligible - Took July 19__ exam; awaiting results." Radiology managers encounter this situation routinely and are not dissuaded from considering your application because of your transitional status. If you have received your results, you should indicate your ARRT number and expiration date. Do not include your test score.

References

References are not listed on the professional résumé. The prospective employer will provide space on the job application form for listing both work references and personal references. For the résumé itself, the statement "references available upon request" will suffice. Be sure you have obtained the permission of those individuals you wish to use as references, so they will be expecting inquiries from prospective employers.

▲ *The Cover Letter*

The résumé, if mailed, should always be accompanied by a brief and concise cover letter. Figure 11-4 shows a sample of a cover letter that you can adapt for your use.

Date

Director of Radiology
XYZ Hospital
Main Street
Anytown, USA 01234

Dear Director:

It was with great interest that I read your hospital's advertisement for the position of staff radiographer. Enclosed please find my professional résumé outlining the experiences and education that I believe qualify me for this position.

I wish to notify you of my interest in being employed in your department. I am also completing an application for employment in your Department of Human Resources and am including a copy of my résumé with it. I look forward to hearing from you regarding a personal interview so that we may discuss our mutual needs and interests.

Sincerely,

Figure 11-4 Sample cover letter #2.

▲ *Résumé and Cover Letter Cosmetics*

One of the most valuable tools for use in writing the résumé is a computer or word processor. This will allow you to work through a rough draft and, with a fair amount of ease, to refine the résumé as required. Be certain to take advantage of the "spell check" feature, if your computer is so-equipped. Handwritten, and even typewritten, résumés are no longer acceptable. For the most professional-looking résumé, you will want to print your documents using a laser or ink-jet printer.

Be aware that others who are competing with you for the same positions are preparing and printing their résumés with modern writing equipment. If you do not own such equipment, computers and word processors are available in community college writing centers and in many "quick print" retail stores. Use of these facilities and equipment, which typically are available at a modest price, is a wise investment.

There are as many different types of paper available as there are résumé formats. The résumé and cover letter should be printed on 60- to 75-pound text paper, preferably white or ivory. This type of paper will provide a positive image for your résumé. Because this paper has a heavier weight, it should not be folded. You will, therefore, wish to use a large manila envelope so that the résumé and cover letter may lie flat inside. If you are unfamiliar with paper types and weights, your writing center or retail copy shop will be happy to assist you.

Avoid the use of copier or typewriter paper; it is an inexpensive grade of paper and does not make a positive impression on the reader. In addition, many papers of this type will produce a poorer printed image when used with a laser printer.

▲ *Job Application Form*

Students are frequently dismayed that, after investing much time and effort into writing a résumé, they must still complete a job application form. This is a standard practice for many employers. Regardless of whether one is applying at several radiology facilities or just one, the applicant should always bring a copy of the résumé and make sure it is attached to the job application form. At no time should you indicate on the application form "see attached résumé." However, by bringing the résumé to the human resources office, you will have most of the information you need to fill in the job application form.

Figure 11-5 shows a typical job application form for a community hospital. Note the information you will need to completely fill out a form of this type. Make certain you bring all of the information with you (e.g., names and addresses of former employers; names, addresses, and telephone numbers of references), especially if it is not included on the résumé.

Be aware that you may request that former employers not be contacted. In addition, a detailed employment and reference check cannot be conducted without your signed authorization. Be certain to read carefully the statement you are signing at the bottom of the application form. Remember, although you've provided all of the information requested on the application form, it is still important to attach the résumé.

In conclusion, proper preparation of a professional résumé is a task not to be taken lightly. Spend the time needed to carefully construct yours and be aware of its impact on potential employers. Your résumé is a statement of your professionalism that speaks about you in your absence.

EMPLOYMENT APPLICATION

Last Name	First	Middle	Social Security Number

Present address	City	State	Zip	Telephone Number

Position applied for	Date	Salary desired

How were you referred to this facility?	Are you available for: ☐ Full-time ☐ Part-time ☐ Regular ☐ Temporary

Do you have relatives or friends employed in this facility?
☐ Yes ☐ No Department:

Date available:

Have you ever been employed by this facility? ☐ Yes ☐ No When:	Are you under 18? ☐ Yes ☐ No	Would you consider working: Weekends & holidays ☐ Yes ☐ No

Long-range occupational goals:

Rotating shifts ☐ Yes ☐ No
On call ☐ Yes ☐ No
Any shift ☐ Yes ☐ No

Are you a United States citizen or an alien legally authorized to work in the United States? ☐ Yes ☐ No

Shift preference:
☐ Days ☐ Evenings ☐ Nights
☐ 8-hour shift ☐ 12-hour shift

Have you been convicted of a felony? ☐ Yes ☐ No
If yes, explain:

After reviewing the essential functions of the job for which you are applying, are you able to perform them? ☐ Yes ☐ No If no, please explain.

School	Name & Address of School	Course of study	Did you graduate?	Diploma or degree
High				
College				
College				

Other: Business college, Other Special Courses (Include Special Military Training)

Ares of Specialization or Major Interest:

Typing: Approx. WPM _____
Shorthand: Approx. WPM _____

List healthcare, business, or industrial equipment operated:

Professional Licenses and/or Certifications

Are you currently: ☐ Registered ☐ Licensed ☐ Certified
Eligible for: ☐ Registration ☐ Licensure ☐ Certification

	Type	State Issued	Date	Number
If Licensed, Registered, or Certified	Type	State Issued	Date	Number
	Type	State Issued	Date	Number

Figure 11-5 Sample job application form.

List previous employers with most recent first	From	To	Immediate Supervisor	Last Salary
Job Title				

Employer Name _____ Phone _____
Address_____
Duties _____
Reason for leaving_____

	From	To	Immediate Supervisor	Last Salary
Job Title				

Employer Name _____ Phone _____
Address_____
Duties _____
Reason for leaving_____

	From	To	Immediate Supervisor	Last Salary
Job Title				

Employer Name _____ Phone _____
Address_____
Duties _____
Reason for leaving_____

State if you do not want us to contact any of the above listed former employers and the reasons you do not want each contacted.

Can we run a detailed employment check, including, but not limited to, a check with your previous employers? ☐ Yes ☐ No
Please sign here to authorize reference check _____

List references who are not relatives or employers:

Name	Company and Address	Present Title	Telephone #

Carefully read this section prior to providing signatures below.

I consent to any medical examination required by the facility at any time to determine my ability to perform the duties of my job or other jobs with the facility and I understand that my employment may be conditioned upon satisfactorily passing a physical examination.

I understand that my employment can be terminated at any time and for any reason, at the option of either the facility or myself. I understand that no one has any authority to enter into any agreement for employment for any specified period of time or to make any agreement contrary to the foregoing, except for a written employment agreement signed by the Chief Executive Officer of this facility.

I hearby affirm that the information provided on this application (and accompanying résumé, if any) is true and complete. I understand that any false or misleading representations or omissions may disqualify me from further consideration for employment and may result in discharge even if discovered at a later date.

I hereby authorize persons, schools, my current employer (if applicable) and previous employers and organizations named in this application (and accompanying résumé, if any) to provide this facility and all affiliates with any relavant information regarding an employment decision, and I release all such persons from any and all liability regarding the provision or use of such information.

Date _____   Signature _____

Chapter 12

Interviewing Techniques

> **D**on't wait for your ship to come in. Swim out to it.

▲ Purpose of an Interview

If your résumé is your detailed calling card, then your personal interview is your house call. It is your only opportunity to make a strong, lasting first impression with your possible future employer. Because of the many legal changes surrounding the issue of discrimination, the personal interview may not be as detailed as in the past. However, this does not diminish its significance or the importance of proper preparation.

Today, the employer may use the personal interview to verify information submitted on the résumé or on the job application. It can serve as an opportunity for the employer to show you the facilities in which you may be working, to familiarize you with the equipment, and to determine your experience with such equipment. The interviewer may also be interested in your career goals and plans you have for establishing a career ladder.

Keep in mind that another purpose of an interview is for you to become acquainted with your prospective employer. It is also a time for you to decide whether, if offered a job, you would wish to work for that department or organization. As you prepare for the interview, always consider it a two-way street.

▲ Personal Appearance

There is no substitute for making a strong first impression with the person(s) who will be conducting your interview. Like it or not, we are a very visual society, and the outward aspect you project during your initial contact with the interviewers will have a profound impact on their perception of you as a potential employee.

How you choose to present yourself for your interview says a lot about your self-image as a professional. Regardless of where you work, you represent that department or organization to the patient/customer. Appropriate professional attire begins with the interview and continues every day, once the job is begun.

Dressing for social occasions varies by age group and geographical region of the country. However, dressing for a professional job interview is fairly standard no matter the age or location. What you choose not to wear is as important as what you do wear. For the interview, do not wear your professional uniform. Casual attire and trendy clothing are also inappropriate.

By taking the time to prepare your personal appearance and to dress professionally, you are telling the interviewers that you appreciate their serious consideration of you as a job candidate. You are also making a statement about how you believe a professional should appear, not only to potential employers, but to your peers. It will be assumed that though you would be wearing a professional uniform at work, you would appear as neat and clean when performing patient care as your appearance during the interview suggests.

Pay attention to details. It does little good to wear a clean, pressed business suit only to have the interviewer see dirty fingernails. Similarly, proper grooming loses its impact when your cologne precedes you to the interview by five minutes. Because you will undoubtedly be nervous, you mouth will probably be dry. Use of a breath mint up until the interview begins will keep your mouth moist and your breath fresh.

Conservative clothing is a must. Males should always wear a business suit or sport coat, tie, and dress slacks. Female applicants should wear either a business suit or a dress. Clothing must be wrinkle-free and clean. Shoes (polished), socks, and belts should complement the clothing. Hose must be free of runs. Hair should be neatly styled and pulled back if shoulder length or longer. Jewelry should be kept to a minimum.

As your attire varies from these suggestions, the likelihood of a favorable impression on the interviewer becomes less. Under no circumstances should you wear casual slacks, jeans, shorts, walking or running shoes, etc. Applying for a professional position requires that you dress as a professional.

▲ Preparing for the Interview

To prepare for the interview, you should attempt to find out as much about your potential employer as possible. You may wish to find out why the current position is available. Is there a very high rate of turnover in this particular department? What value does this organization place on its employees? In general, is there harmony among the employees in the department? Do patients and employees speak highly of the department?

How financially secure is the organization? Have you had an opportunity to look at its most recent annual report? Such a report is available from the office of public relations at the institution. Are you aware of this employer's reputation in the community? The overall reputation in the community and the financial stability of your prospective employer are factors that you should consider before accepting a job offer.

It should not be necessary to bring anything to the interview, unless you have not previously submitted your résumé to the interviewer. In that case, bring a clean copy inside a manila folder. All of the facts pertaining to your professional preparation are on the résumé. If documentation is required for any item, it may be submitted at a later time to the department of human resources. Similarly, your list of references is probably already entered on the job application form. If not, these may also be furnished later to human resources. In most cases, individual department heads do not perform reference checks because of the legalities involved.

If you are not exactly sure where you are going, you should find the building and the office several days ahead of time. You do not want to be searching for the site on the day the interview is scheduled. You should allow plenty of time to get to your destination. If you arrive early, there is always a waiting area. Arriving late for an interview is inexcusable.

When you arrive at the site of the interview, greet everyone as if they were going to conduct the interview. Many radiology managers ask receptionists and secretaries their impressions of the individual who is being interviewed.

It is normal to feel nervous and apprehensive about an interview especially if it is for a position you greatly desire.

Try to convert your nervous energy into enthusiasm when speaking with others throughout the course of the interview.

▲ The Interview Process

When the interviewer approaches, stand and shake hands firmly. A smile and an enthusiastic, though not excessively demonstrative, attitude will create a positive first impression.

As the interview begins, try to appear as calm, comfortable, and professional as possible. Be pleasant, avoid joking, be attentive. Look at the interviewer at all times. Speak distinctly and use appropriate terminology. You may wish to bring up your career goals, as summarized in the goal statement on your résumé. Carefully indicate how you may be an asset to the department without sounding as though you are bossy or demanding. Remember to answer the interviewer's questions clearly.

There have been numerous legal challenges in recent years to what are alleged to be discriminatory interview questions and techniques. While the emphasis of such legal rulings has been to require the interviewer to ask only questions that reveal your job qualifications, it is wise for you to know what can and cannot be asked in a job interview. This will assist you in preparing for the interview. It will also make you aware of your rights so that you may recognize potentially discriminatory situations.

Following is a list of topics that may be addressed during your interview. They are relevant to the job and, therefore, are legitimate areas of inquiry. You may wish to write out your answers ahead of time in anticipation of the interview. Other interview questions, not included in this list, may also be appropriate and within current legal guidelines.

You *may* be asked:

- Any questions concerning information you entered on the application form

- Why you left your last job

- How your former employers view you

- What your job duties were on your last job

- What you liked or disliked about your prior jobs

- What job duties interest you

- The days or hours you are (or are not) available to work

- The size of the facility in which you previously worked

- What you thought of your prior supervisors, e.g., whether or not you got along, what kind of persons they were, whether they were strict or easy-going

- For what kind of supervisor would you prefer to work

- How employee problems and complaints were solved at your prior job and whether you thought is was a good procedure

- How you would prefer to have employee problems and complaints handled if hired for this job

- What wages you received at your prior job

- How frequently were pay raises given and upon what were they based, e.g., productivity, merit, etc.

- Whether pay raises were given in fixed amounts or percentages of pay

- If pay raises were based on merit, how many you received

- If you were promoted and on what criteria the promotion was based, e.g., merit, length of service, etc.

- Whether you received a shift differential, how much it was, and whether it was a fixed amount or a percentage

- What benefits you received at your prior job, including whether or not you paid part of your insurance coverage, and if the cost was deducted from your paycheck

- How you were notified about your benefits, e.g., booklets, memos, handbooks, bulletin board notices, etc.

- How much you expect an employer to communicate with you and to keep you involved in workplace activities

- What mode of communication you prefer

The interviewer will probably provide you with information about the salary structure, benefits package, sick leave, and vacation time allowed, etc. While this information is important to you, try to wait until the interviewer brings it up. In this way, you will not appear to be interested only in money and benefits.

In any interviewing situation, you should be aware of the types of questions which may NOT be asked. This is important so that you do not answer irrelevant questions that may harm your chances for securing the job. If a series of improper questions is asked, you may not wish to pursue

the position. If blatant harassment or violation of ethical interviewing guidelines occurs, you must ask yourself whether you wish to work in such an environment. If either of these situations develops, you may decide to conclude the interview with a statement such as, "Thank you for your time but I feel you are asking irrelevant questions in violation of my rights. Please remove my name from consideration for this position"; or you may opt to finish the interview and to remove your name from consideration in a follow-up letter.

Be careful not to answer questions such as those which follow. You are not required to answer them and do not want to be put in a position of volunteering such information. As a last resort, if you believe you have been discriminated against, based on questionable interview practices, you may wish to seek legal counsel. Recommendations concerning issues of a legal nature that may arise during the interview are beyond the scope of this text. Your personal attorney is best equipped to answer such questions.

You *may not* be asked:

- How old you are

- Your birth date

- How long you have resided at your present address

- What your previous address was

- What church you choose to attend (if any) or the name of your priest, minister, or rabbi

- Your father's surname

- Your maiden name, if female

- If you are married, divorced, separated, widowed, or single

- Who lives with you

- How many children you have, or intend to have

- The ages of your children

- Who will care for your children while you are working

- How you will get to work, unless owning a car is a job requirement

- Where a spouse or parent works or lives

- If you own or rent your place of residence

- The name of your bank or any information concerning outstanding loan amounts

- Whether you have ever had your wages garnished or filed bankruptcy

- Whether you have ever been arrested

- Whether you have ever served in the armed forces of another country

- How you spend your spare time or to what clubs or organizations you belong

- What foreign languages you can speak, read, or write, unless it is a job requirement

- Your position on labor unions or whether you have ever been a member of a union

- The nationality of your name

In addition, beware of other phrases, attitudes, or questions that may discriminate against you on the basis of gender. For example, you may not be referred to as "sweetie," "honey," "hunk," etc. Flirtatious behavior is not to be tolerated. Don't allow the interviewer to take advantage of your friendly nature to ask questions that should not be asked or to pry into personal aspects of your life. This is not a conversation between friends; it is a professional job interview. If you conduct yourself in such a manner, the competent interviewer will respect you and your position.

▲ Interview Outcomes and Follow-Up

Even after a good interview, you may not be hired. Among the appropriate reasons are:

1. You are unable to work the required hours.

2. You choose to reject the job offer because you are not interested in the position available.

3. You are not qualified for the position available.

4. You were obviously under the influence of drugs or alcohol during the interview.

5. Inconsistent, inaccurate, or fraudulent statements were made on your application form.

6. You are physically unable to perform the job duties (however, Americans with Disabilities Act guidelines must be considered).

A last impression can be as important as the first. At the conclusion of the interview, be sure to shake hands and thank the interviewer for the time spent with you. The interviewer will probably give some indication of when the hiring decision will be made, based upon the number of applicants and the date the position must be filled. As you leave, be sure to say good-bye to secretaries or receptionists you pass.

Immediately send a follow-up letter to the interviewer. A sample of such correspondence is shown in Figure 12-1. As with your résumé, be sure it is printed on good quality paper and reinforces the positive impression you've sought to make. Keep in mind that this is, basically, a thank-you letter and is not meant to provide additional information about yourself. Most important, be sure to send it. Many individuals fail to follow-up with a letter and, consequently, you will stand out from the rest!

Radiology Manager's Name
Imaging Center
Shepherd Road
My Town, VA 12345-9876

Date

Dear Radiology Manager's Name:

Thank you for the opportunity to interview for the position of staff radiographer. I appreciate the time you spent with me yesterday. It was a pleasure meeting you and seeing your radiology department.

I look forward to hearing from you regarding this position.

Sincerely,

Applicant, R.T.(R)

Figure 12-1 Sample interview follow-up letter.

Following the guidelines and suggestions contained in this chapter will not guarantee employment. However, it will guarantee that you will present yourself as the true professional you have studied and worked so hard to become!

Chapter 13

Employer Expectations

> *Excellence can be attained if you care more than others think is wise, risk more than others think is safe, dream more than others think is practical, expect more than others think is possible.*

▼

▲ Entering the Health Care Work Force

As you enter the workforce in medical radiography, those in charge of the facility in which you will work have expectations of you as a professional. From their standpoint, it is reasonable to expect that you will be able to fulfill the requirements of your job description. You are being hired because you have the abilities to function as an entry-level radiographer.

The task inventory conducted by the American Registry of Radiologic Technologists lists the skills expected of an entry-level radiographer. While these should coincide with the terminal competencies of your educational program, you should also be aware that your new employer will have these expectations regardless of where you attended school. The task inventory is provided below so that you may understand the technical skills expected of you as you enter the work force.

▲ Task Inventory

Completion of your educational program should enable you to:

1. Evaluate the need for and use of protective shielding.

2. Take appropriate precautions to minimize radiation exposure to patients.

3. Restrict beam to limit exposure area, improve image quality, and reduce radiation dose.

4. Set kVp, mA, and time or automated exposure system to achieve optimum image quality, safe operating conditions, and minimum radiation dose.

5. Prevent all persons not involved in the radiographic procedure from remaining in the area during x-ray exposure.

6. Take appropriate precautions to minimize occupational radiation exposure.

7. Wear a personnel monitoring device while on duty.

8. Review and evaluate individual occupational exposure charts.

9. Warm-up x-ray tube according to manufacturer's recommendations.

10. Prepare and adjust radiographic unit and accessories.

11. Prepare and adjust fluoroscopic unit and accessories.

12. Recognize and report malfunctions in the radiographic and fluoroscopic unit and ancillary accessories.

13. Perform basic evaluations of radiographic equipment and accessories (e.g., lead aprons, collimator accuracy).

14. Inspect and clean screens and cassettes.

15. Perform start-up or shutdown procedures on automatic processor.

16. Recognize and report malfunctions in the automatic processor.

17. Process exposed film.

18. Reload cassettes by selecting film of proper size and type.

19. Store film/cassette in a manner that will reduce the possibility of artifact production.

20. Select appropriate film-screen combination and/or grid.

21. Determine appropriate exposure factors using calipers, technique charts, and tube rating charts.

22. Modify exposure factors for circumstances such as involuntary motion, casts and splints, pathological conditions, or patient's inability to cooperate.

23. Use radiopaque markers to indicate anatomical side, position, or other relevant information.

24. Evaluate patient and radiographs to determine if additional projections or positions should be recommended.

25. Evaluate radiographs for diagnostic quality.

26. Determine corrective measures if radiograph is not of diagnostic quality and take appropriate action.

27. Select equipment and accessories for the examination requested.

28. Remove all radiopaque materials from patient or table that could interfere with the radiographic image.

29. Explain breathing instructions prior to making the exposure.

30. Position patient to demonstrate the desired anatomy using body landmarks.

31. Explain patient preparation (e.g., diet restrictions, preparatory medications) prior to an imaging procedure.

32. Properly sequence radiographic procedures to avoid residual contrast material affecting future exams.

33. Examine radiographic requisition to verify accuracy and completeness of information.

34. Utilize universal precautions.

35. Confirm patient's identity.

36. Question female patients of childbearing age about possible pregnancy.

37. Explain procedure to patient or patient's family.

38. Evaluate patient's ability to comply with positioning requirements for the requested exam.

39. Observe and monitor vital signs.

40. Use proper body mechanics and/or mechanical transfer devices when assisting patients.

41. Provide for patient comfort and modesty.

42. Select immobilization devices, when indicated, to prevent patient movement and/or ensure patient safety.

43. Verify accuracy of patient film identification.

44. Maintain confidentiality of patient information.

45. Use sterile or aseptic technique to prevent contamination of sterile trays, instruments, or fields.

46. Prepare contrast media for administration.

47. Prior to administration of contrast agent, gather information to determine if the patient is at increased risk of adverse reaction.

48. Perform venipuncture.

49. Observe patient after administration of contrast media to detect adverse reactions.

50. Recognize need for prompt medical attention and administer emergency care.

51. Document required information on patient's medical record.

52. Clean, disinfect or sterilize facilities and equipment, and dispose of contaminated items in preparation for next examination.

53. Follow appropriate procedures when in contact with patient in reverse/protective isolation.

54. Monitor medical equipment attached to the patient (e.g., IVs, oxygen) during the radiographic procedure.

55-121. Position patient, x-ray tube, and image receptor to produce radiographs of:

Thorax

55. Chest, routine
56. Chest, obliques, apical lordotic, decubitus

57. Ribs
58. Sternoclavicular joints
59. Sternum

Extremities

60. Toes
61. Foot
62. Os calcis
63. Ankle
64. Tibia, fibula
65. Knee
66. Patella
67. Femur
68. Fingers
69. Hand
70. Wrist
71. Forearm
72. Elbow
73. Humerus
74. Shoulder
75. Scapula
76. Clavicle
77. Acromioclavicular joints
78. Bone survey
79. Long bone measurement/scanogram
80. Bone age
81. Soft tissue

Head and Neck

82. Skull
83. Mastoids/temporal bones
84. Facial bones
85. Mandible
86. Zygoma and arches
87. Temporomandibular joints
88. Nasal bones
89. Optic foramina
90. Orbits
91. Paranasal sinuses
92. Larynx, airway

Spine and Pelvis

93. Cervical spine
94. Thoracic spine
95. Scoliosis series
96. Lumbosacral spine
97. Sacrum
98. Sacroiliac joints
99. Coccyx
100. Pelvis
101. Hip

Abdomen and GI Tract

102. Esophagus study
103. Abdomen
104. Upper GI series
105. Small bowel series
106. ERCP
107. Barium enema, single contrast
108. Barium enema, double contrast
109. Operative cholangiography
110. T-tube cholangiogram
111. Cholecystogram

Cardiovascular

112. Venogram

Other

113. Myelogram
114. Arthrogram
115. Hysterosalpingogram
116. Tomogram
117. Cystogram
118. Cystourethrogram
119. IVP
120. Retrograde pyelogram
121. Retrograde urethrogram

▲ Organizational Structure and Your Professional Responsibility

The employer has a right to expect you to use your knowledge and abilities in radiography efficiently and to provide high quality service to the patient. In return, you have a right to expect the salary and benefits to which you and your employer agreed. You should also expect to perform your job in a workplace that is free of harassment.

You are entering a dynamic and fluid sector of the national economy. Health care advances in diagnosis, treatment, and delivery are in a constant state of flux. This is the nature of the industry in which you have chosen to work and to build a career. You should expect to stay abreast of changes in the delivery of health care and to remain alert to how such changes impact your employer. Remember that issues that affect your employer will also affect you and your coworkers.

Your employer will expect you to function as part of a team, all of the members of which will be dedicated to providing efficient, accurate care to the patient in a cost-effective manner. At the same time, the employer is the coach of the team and has an obligation to maintain quality service to patients and proper accountability to payors. An examination of the expectations of your employer reveal that your job responsibilities actually fall into three distinct sets.

Expectations of Administration

The administration of the facility in which you are about to be employed expects that you are going to fulfill the job description associated with an entry-level radiographer. The administration expects you to interact with them in an honest, straightforward manner while providing excellent care and service to the patients/customers.

They trust that you will speak highly of the facility and be supportive of its efforts to provide quality patient care. You are expected to arrive for work on time and keep absenteeism to an absolute minimum. There may be times when you are expected to work extra, such as covering for other employees' vacations or sick days. Administrators are looking for employees who are willing to be strong, supportive team players.

The administration also expects that you will be willing to contribute new ideas for more efficient operation. They assume that you will work in harmony with other departments in the facility. They may request that you serve on committees, or perform other tasks not directly related to radiography. Be the type of employee that exceeds the expectations of administration and you will be well on your way toward establishing the type of reputation that will ensure your success.

Expectations of Physicians

The physicians with whom you will be working, both radiologists and referring physicians, have their own particular set of expectations. Referring physicians expect that their orders for radiologic examinations will be carried out as written. They expect that quality radiographs will be made by the radiographers and properly interpreted by the radiologists. While your interactions with these physicians may be minimal, they are nevertheless important.

Referring physicians often come to the radiology department, either to view radiographs themselves or to consult with the radiologist. They may be unfamiliar with the department and where supplies are kept. They may be there to perform a procedure. They expect to be treated as professionals. They expect to be shown where supplies are kept and to be assisted as needed. As a professional radiogra-

pher, it will be your responsibility to meet or exceed those expectations and provide high quality service to the physician as well as to the patient.

The physicians with whom you will interact most frequently are the radiologists, and most of this exchange will occur during fluoroscopy. The radiologists expect to receive the highest quality radiographs you are capable of producing. They will be providing the diagnosis from your radiographs. Radiologists do not expect to have to ask you to retake a film that you already know is unacceptable. They do not want to hear excuses for poor radiographs. Radiologists require that you keep them informed about variations from protocol. They expect you to take an adequate, but concise, patient history for their use during the interpretation of the radiographs.

As a student, there may have been radiographers to facilitate your interactions with the radiologists. As a new entry-level radiographer, it is now your responsibility to conduct yourself with the radiologist in a straightforward, professional manner. This includes not only providing the highest quality radiographs that you can but also demonstrating a willingness to resolve personality and work-related conflicts.

It is important to determine ahead of time how you wish to be regarded by the physicians. You have a right to be treated in a respectful manner and should take immediate steps to rectify a situation in which you are being mistreated. At the same time, the physicians have a right to expect that you will reciprocate in your professional conduct.

Expectations of the Radiology Manager

The person who is hiring you, the radiology manager, also has a particular set of expectations. It is this individual who is directly responsible for your on-the-job performance and overall value to the patient/customer and the administration. In research conducted by the author, radiology managers from across the United States responded to a survey regarding their expectations of new radiography graduates. Of particular interest are the traits that the radiology managers considered most important in an applicant and the areas in which radiology managers have had the most difficulty with employees once they were hired.

Forty-three percent (43%) of radiology managers said that knowledge of the technical aspects of radiography was the most important factor to them when hiring a new graduate radiographer. Thirty-three (33%) percent responded that customer service skills and interpersonal communication skills were most important to them when hiring the recent graduate. It would seem from this research that radiology managers have high expectations of you. They expect you to know the practice of radiography, to deliver quality service to patients, and to be capable of establishing positive relationships with your coworkers.

A second question inquired about problems radiology managers encountered with radiographers on the job. Thirty-seven percent (37%) identified poor communication skills as the most significant problem and the usual cause for a reprimand or termination of the employee. Thirty-six percent (36%) cited lack of knowledge of the technical aspects of the job as the primary reason for reprimand or termination. In handwritten comments on the survey forms, many radiology managers mentioned attendance, tardiness, lack of dependability, and substance abuse as problems in the workplace which have led to reprimands and terminations. Once again, the need for balance between the high-touch and high-tech aspects of radiography is evident. It is no surprise that radiology managers have high expectations of new employees. Be certain that you are prepared to exceed those expectations.

Another survey question asked the managers what areas should be most strongly emphasized with student radiographers as they prepare to enter the work force. Handwritten comments stressed the following:

1. Ongoing technical training
2. Knowledge of basic nursing skills, such as IV pumps, taking vital signs, performing venipuncture
3. Ability to work alone without constant supervision
4. Awareness of the customer's/patient's viewpoint
5. Stronger communication skills
6. Provision of quality service with a smile
7. Professionalism in dealing with the public
8. Loyalty to the employer
9. Efforts to maintain clinical skills

Since you are about ready to enter the work force you must determine how many of these traits are present in your practice already and which ones need additional attention. The managers have carefully described what they need and expect. Are you prepared to enter their workplace?

Finally, the radiology managers were asked to rank factors they viewed as most important to customer service in their department. Not surprising, the most important factor, cited by sixty percent (60%), was a pleasant and courteous staff.

As can be seen from the statistics just cited, radiology managers have fairly high expectations of the people whom they hire. Like the administrators to whom they report, they expect you to be ready to begin work on time and to keep absenteeism to a minimum. The radiology manager is counting on you to be there to provide the highest quality patient care each day you are assigned to work.

The radiology manager also expects that you will conduct yourself as a professional in your dealings with the patient/customer, the physicians, and your coworkers. You are expected to be a reliable member of the radiology team. You must be flexible and have a positive attitude about handling all of the different assignments that you may be given in a typical work day.

Other areas of concern raised by the radiology managers include bringing personal problems to work, substance abuse by employees, and overall lack of initiative. These are all areas you want to keep out of your radiography practice. Should any of these issues become matters of personal concern for you, seek counseling immediately toward the goal of bringing such problems under control. Your employer and your patients deserve no less.

Your radiology manager will expect you to remain busy throughout the day. In addition to performing your primary job duties, you may be asked to complete assignments that don't involve patient care. Quality control and cleaning of the automatic processor or x-ray equipment may be requested. You may be assigned to assist with filing or patient transportation or to clean radiographic and fluoroscopic rooms; stock supplies; clean cassettes, intensifying screens, and lead aprons; and to perform other housekeeping chores around the radiology department.

If you come to view your work area as an integral part of your practice, that sense of ownership will motivate you to care for it. Slow periods at work may be few and far between and should be taken advantage of whenever they occur. Your attitude toward the aspects of your work that don't involve patient care may determine whether the radiology manager gives you other assignments that you prefer. If you consider lounge areas off-limits and keep busy throughout the day, you will find great fulfillment in your work and will likely exceed the radiology manager's expectations.

In a field that changes as rapidly as radiologic technology, your radiology manager will expect you to be knowledgeable about the newest types of equipment and advances in imaging techniques. You are also expected to keep your skills at a level such that you can perform all of the different types of radiologic procedures required in your radiology department. On a regular basis, you should review your favorite radiographic positioning and procedures text to refresh your memory and maintain your skills.

You have become accustomed to studying and, throughout the course of your radiography program, you have had to learn how to learn. This process does not end with graduation or passing the certification exam. It is important to keep abreast of events in the field by reading the latest radiologic technology journals and textbooks. Textbooks are not written solely for students. As a practicing radiographer, you will want to keep your personal library up to date with the best resources available.

Another way to remain current in the field and to exceed your manager's expectations is to become an active member of your national and state professional organizations. Both have publications that will bring you the latest news in the profession. In addition, these organizations need your talents to continue to succeed. As a student, you have acquired a store of information and have developed skill at communicating it. Take advantage of that momentum and continue to do research in the field.

Most radiology managers will expect you to give something back to your profession, thereby increasing your level of knowledge. Present research papers at state or national meetings, hold office in one of the organizations, or offer to help out in the planning and conducting of a continuing education meeting. Organizing and conducting an in-service education program for your department is a great place to begin. If you've never taken part in such activities, this is a great time to begin. It doesn't matter whether you are sure about what you are doing, just offer to help or do that first research paper as a graduate.

Meeting and exceeding the radiology manager's expectations are sure ways to set a course for success in your chosen field. Those who follow this path derive the most satisfaction from their job and are held in the highest esteem by their employers. Most important, a commitment to excellence in your profession results in healthy self-esteem and this is reflected in the care and service provided to the patients.

Part III
Continuing Education Opportunities

Chapter 14

Continuing Education Requirements

> *The quality of a person's life is in direct proportion to their commitment to excellence regardless of their chosen field of endeavor. - Vincent Lombardi*

▲ Meeting Professional and Governmental Requirements

The purpose of certification is to assure the public that you are competent to practice in your chosen field. However, even though you pass a certification exam to enter the profession, there is no assurance that you will remain competent. It is of the utmost importance that you remain current in the knowledge and skills needed to practice radiologic technology.

Mandatory continuing education has been established in an attempt to ensure the continued competence of clinicians. Even though research indicates that mandatory continuing education in any field of study is not necessarily a guarantee of competence, it is the route that has been chosen for many of the health professions, including radiologic technology.

After you've received your initial registration upon successful completion of the certification exam, the American Registry of Radiologic Technologists requires documentation of continuing education in order for you to renew it. Participating in continuing education and documenting your participation is your responsibility as a registered technologist. While acquiring continuing education credits is not difficult for the vast majority of technologists, knowledge of the applicable rules and regulations is of paramount importance. This section includes the information published by the American Registry of Radiologic Technologists pertinent to the acquisition of continuing education credits.

In addition to certification, many states require those practicing medical radiography to hold licensure or accreditation issued by the state. Because legislation regulating state licensure may be subject to the addition or revision of statutes at any time, a listing of the requirements specific to each state is not included here. Most states accept the ARRT certification as proof of the applicant's competency. In those states, you will need to apply to the appropriate agency, supply a copy of your ARRT credentials, and pay the proper fee. Be sure to obtain the rules and regulations pertaining to licensure in the state or states in which you will be employed. Such rules will advise you of the application process, any testing or fees involved, and continuing education requirements. Educators or radiology managers should be consulted for the name and address of the specific state agency responsible for such credentialing.

It is important to keep in mind that state and national continuing education requirements may differ. Once again, it is the individual technologist's responsibility to keep abreast of the current requirements for continuing education. Neither the state nor the national agencies accept a lack of knowledge of the rules and regulations as an excuse for failure to meet the requirements. An insufficient number of continuing education credits may result in the issuance of probationary status, the levy of fines by the state, or loss of the ability to work.

Be sure to take time to review the following ARRT continuing education requirements. Your instructors will be happy to answer any questions you may have. You may also contact the ARRT office at (612) 687-0048.

▲ ARRT Continuing Education (CE) Requirements

Although you will renew your certification with the ARRT each year, you will need to submit proof of continuing education activities every two years. There are three ways to satisfy the requirement of 24 hours of continuing education for that two-year period. The first is to attend 24 hours of continuing education courses that have met the criteria established by the ARRT. The second is to pass an entry-level exam in an area of radiologic technology in which you were not previously credentialed (e.g., radiation therapy, nuclear medicine, or sonography). Finally, you may pass one of the advanced-level exams offered by the ARRT. These advanced-level exams are described in Chapter 15.

You must begin to comply with the rules governing continuing education two years after you pass the radiography examination. In other words, passing the ARRT radiography exam satisfies the requirement for your first two years of certification. You need only renew your certification each year. After the first two years have elapsed, you will have two additional years (starting on the first day of the month in which you were born) to satisfy the requirement for 24 hours of continuing education. Thereafter, you will need to satisfy this requirement every two years.

Continuing education activities must be organized to expand the knowledge and skills needed by a radiologic technologist in clinical practice. In attempting to meet the requirement by attending 24 hours of continuing education, you should be aware that the ARRT organizes such activities within two categories.

Category A credits are awarded for classes or programs that have been approved by a recognized continuing education evaluation mechanism (RCEEM). Examples of RCEEMS are the American Society of Radiologic Technologists, the Society of Diagnostic Medical Sonographers, and the Society of Nuclear Medicine-Technologist Section. In addition, the ARRT will award Category A credits for programs approved by the American Medical Association as Category 1, and by the American Nurses Association if they pertain to the radiologic sciences. These are approval mechanisms that you will want to look for on program advertisements before you register for the program.

Category A credits are awarded, without RCEEM approval, for cardiopulmonary resuscitation (CPR) certification and approved postsecondary academic courses (e.g., biological, physical, radiological, medical, or social science courses; communications, math, computers, management, or education courses). For these two types of activities, the ARRT will accept a CPR card or college transcript as proof of attendance.

The ARRT will also accept CE credits that have been approved by the licensing agencies in certain states. Be sure to check with your state to determine if it is one of the approved CE providers.

Category B credits are continuing education activities that do not meet the Category A criteria and, consequently, must be individually approved.

The coordinator of a continuing education program will be happy to answer questions concerning the approval of the event. You, as a technologist, are not responsible for submitting a program for approval to obtain credit. The sponsor of the event seeks approval before the date of the presentation.

Of the 24 credits that you must earn every two years to meet ARRT requirements, at least 12 must be from Category A. The remaining 12 may be Category A or Category B credits. The 24 credit requirement remains the same, regardless of how many ARRT certificates you hold. If you are certified in more than one field, you are still required to earn a total of only 24 credits.

Credits are awarded on the basis of a contact hour. A contact hour is 50 to 60 minutes in length and is awarded 1 CE credit by the ARRT. Programs 30 to 49 minutes long are awarded one-half credit. Approved academic courses are awarded 16 CE credits for each semester credit (a grade of C or above must be earned). CPR is awarded 3 Category A credits for each area of certification, with no more than 6 credits allowed during each two-year cycle.

You may also receive credit for conducting a presentation. If the presentation has been approved as a Category A activity, you may be awarded 3 CE credits for the preparation and 1 CE credit per hour of the presentation. No more than 12 such credits may be accumulated during a two-year period.

The ARRT will place technologists who fail to meet the CE requirements on probationary status. Inquiries submitted to the ARRT by employers will receive a response that includes a notation of probationary status and may result in your rejection as a job applicant or loss of employment.

▲ Continuing Education Opportunities

There are multiple opportunities to obtain continuing education credits. The primary mission of your professional societies is continuing education. Be certain that you are an active member of the American Society of Radiologic Technologists (ASRT). Through its annual conference and numerous home study programs, as well as its directed readings in the journal *Radiologic Technology* you can obtain a considerable portion of your CE credits. The ASRT may be contacted at 15000 Central Avenue SE, Albuquerque, NM 87123-3917, (505) 298-4500.

The various state affiliate societies of the ASRT provide many continuing education opportunities every year. Ask your instructors or the radiologic technologists in clinical for membership information. As part of the state society, your local professional society probably has monthly or quarterly meeting that stress continuing education. Be certain to take advantage of these meetings.

If you choose a career in any of the radiologic specialties, in education, or in management, there are a number of other professional organizations to which you may belong. Each organization offers approved continuing education as part of its mission. Being an active member of a professional society will help to ensure that you are informed about the continuing education programs that will contribute most to your skill development.

As a registered technologist, it is your responsibility to know if the continuing education program you are attending has been approved and to obtain the necessary documentation proving your participation in the activity. At the end of each two-year period, you must submit proof that you have satisfied the requirement. Be sure to keep the original attendance documents for at least a year beyond the two-year period. The ARRT will conduct random audits to verify such documentation. The documentation will need to show the date of the program, the title and content, the number of contact hours, and the signature of an individual associated with the program, such as the speaker, instructor, or coordinator. The documentation should also include (if applicable) a CE reference number provided by the RCEEM.

Figure 14-1 shows the individual activity documentation form provided by the ARRT that you may use to track your credits. This form is kept in your personal file at home for your reference. Figure 14-2 shows the continuing education activity summary that will be submitted to the ARRT every two years. You may transfer the information from your individual activity forms to the summary form for submission. It would be wise to set up your own file for continuing education before you graduate so that it will be in place and ready for immediate use as soon as you are registered.

It is your responsibility to learn about modifications to the CE requirements. Be sure to read all of the information sent to you from the American Registry of Radiologic Technologists, particularly the annual report. Also, remain alert for changes to such requirements in your state.

Continuing education is a vital part of your medical radiography practice. View it as an opportunity to learn and enhance your skills rather than as an imposed obligation. Attend programs that you know will help you to become a better technologist. Take an active part in these events, both as an attendee and as a coordinator. Conduct your own presentation at such a meeting for a more complete learning experience. You will find that such activities enhance your

professional image and gain the respect and admiration of your colleagues.

Form 9403A

CONTINUING EDUCATION DOCUMENTATION FORM
INDIVIDUAL ACTIVITY

ARRT ID Number ☐☐☐☐☐☐ Birthdate ☐☐ ☐☐ ☐☐ ☐☐☐–☐☐–☐☐☐☐

MO   DA   YR   Social Security Number

Last Name ☐☐☐☐☐☐☐☐☐☐☐☐☐☐☐☐ First Name ☐☐☐☐☐☐☐☐☐☐☐☐☐ M.I. ☐

Date(s) of Attendance: _____ / _____ / _____

MO   DA   YR

Title of Activity: _____

Sponsor of the Activity: _____

Number of Actual Contact Hours: _____

_____

Signature of Authorized Representative of the Sponsor

Category (A) or (B)   (Circle appropriate category)

If Category A, indicate below the activity reference number provided by the sponsor of the activity and assigned by the evaluating agency (RCEEM).

CE Activity Reference Number: _____

Form 9403A

CONTINUING EDUCATION DOCUMENTATION FORM
INDIVIDUAL ACTIVITY

ARRT ID Number ☐☐☐☐☐☐ Birthdate ☐☐ ☐☐ ☐☐ ☐☐☐–☐☐–☐☐☐☐

MO   DA   YR   Social Security Number

Last Name ☐☐☐☐☐☐☐☐☐☐☐☐☐☐☐☐ First Name ☐☐☐☐☐☐☐☐☐☐☐☐☐ M.I. ☐

Date(s) of Attendance: _____ / _____ / _____

MO   DA   YR

Title of Activity: _____

Sponsor of the Activity: _____

Number of Actual Contact Hours: _____

_____

Signature of Authorized Representative of the Sponsor

Category (A) or (B)   (Circle appropriate category)

If Category A, indicate below the activity reference number provided by the sponsor of the activity and assigned by the evaluating agency (RCEEM).

CE Activity Reference Number: _____

Figure 14-1 Individual activity documentation form. From: The American Registry of Radiologic Technologists, Copyright © 1994.

THE AMERICAN REGISTRY OF RADIOLOGIC TECHNOLOGISTS
1255 Northland Drive, St. Paul, MN 55120-1155
Telephone: (612) 687-0048
BIENNIAL CONTINUING EDUCATION ACTIVITY SUMMARY
Form 9403B

ARRT ID Number ☐☐☐☐☐☐

Birthdate ☐☐ ☐☐ ☐☐ | ☐☐☐ – ☐☐ – ☐☐☐☐
MO   DA   YR   Social Security Number

Last Name ☐☐☐☐☐☐☐☐☐☐☐☐☐☐☐☐☐

First Name ☐☐☐☐☐☐☐☐☐☐☐☐☐

M.I. ☐

Biennium ☐☐ ☐☐   Through ☐☐ ☐☐
MO   YR   MO   YR

COMPLETE <u>EITHER SECTION</u> 1,2 or 3, <u>AND</u> SECTION 4 BELOW. Pencil in the circle within the section you have completed

SECTION 1

○ I have met the continuing education requirement by passing one of the approved examinations. I understand that the date the examination was administered must be during the biennium in which I am reporting compliance. The examination passed during this biennium and in which I have never previously passed is in the following area and through the following organization:

(Check one)
☐ Radiography/ARRT
☐ Nuclear Medicine Technology/ARRT
☐ Nuclear Medicine Technology/NMTCB
☐ Radiation Therapy Technology/ARRT
☐ Cardiovascular-Interventional Technology/ARRT
☐ Mammography/ARRT

☐ Computed Tomography/ARRT
☐ Magnetic Resonance Imaging/ARRT
☐ Diagnostic Medical Sonography/ARDMS
☐ Diagnostic Cardiac Sonography/ARDMS
☐ Vascular Technology/ARDMS

Date of exam administration ☐☐ ☐☐
MO   YR

SECTION 2

○ I have met the continuing education requirement by completing the following activities:
TWELVE (12) CREDITS OF CATEGORY A ACTIVITIES

DATE	TITLE OF ACTIVITY	CE REFERENCE #	# OF CE CREDITS

TWELVE (12) CREDITS OF CATEGORY B (or A) ACTIVITIES

DATE	TITLE OF ACTIVITY	CE REFERENCE #	# OF CE CREDITS

Total Category A credits_____
Total Category B credits_____
Total CE credits_____

ALL REGISTRANTS MUST COMPLETE SECTION 4 ON REVERSE SIDE

Figure 14-2 Continuing education activity summary. From: The American Registry of Radiologic Technologists, Copyright © 1994.

SECTION 3

◯ I have not met the continuing education requirements for this biennium. I am requesting probational status so that I may maintain my registration. I understand that I must now meet one of the requirements outlined in Section 1 or 2 within the 12 months which starts with the first day of my birthmonth. Further, I am not allowed to count any of the CE credits earned during this past biennium towards the probational requirements.

SECTION 4

By my signature below, I hereby certify that the information provided in this summary is true and correct. I further understand that the falsification or misrepresentation of any part of this documentation may lead to revocation of my registration with The American Registry of Radiologic Technologists.

_____   _____

Signature   Date

BIENNIAL CONTINUING EDUCATION ACTIVITY SUMMARY
(Form 9403B)

INSTRUCTIONS

1. The biennium dates during which your continuing education activities must be completed begin on the first day of your birthmonth in 1995 and extend through the last day of the month prior to your birthmonth in 1997. For example, with a birthdate of February 4, your biennium would extend from February 1, 1995 through January 31, 1997.

2. In order to comply with the ARRT continuing education requirements for renewal of registration, you must do one of the following during the biennium:

    *Complete twenty-four (24) continuing education credits over the 24 month period. Twelve (12) of these credits must be Category A activities. The remaining twelve (12) credits may be either Category A or Category B activities. Consult the document titled, "CE Requirements for Renewal of Registration" for details of these requirements.

    *Pass an entry-level examination in a discipline not previously passed and for which you are eligible [e.g., an ARRT examination in Radiography, Nuclear Medicine or Radiation Therapy; the Nuclear Medicine examination through the Nuclear Medicine Technology Certification Board (NMTCB); or a certification examination through the American Registry of Diagnostic Medical Sonographers (ARDMS)].

    *Pass an ARRT advanced-level examination not previously passed and for which you are eligible (e.g., an ARRT examination in Cardiovascular-Interventional Technology, Mammography, Computed Tomography or Magnetic Resonance Imaging).

3. The CE reference number is the number that has been assigned to the activity by the Recognized CE Evaluation Mechanism (RCEEM). The sponsor of the educational activity will provide this for you. If you do not have this number, put the name of the approving organization in the space for the reference number (e.g., SDMS for Society of Diagnostic Medical Sonographers; ASRT for American Society of Radiologic Technologists; or SNM-TS for Society of Nuclear Medicine-Technologist Section).

4. Your Individual Activity CE Documentation Forms verifying participation should **NOT** be returned with your renewal form. When the renewals have been received, a random sample of technologists will be requested to submit copies of their documentation in order to validate the Biennial Continuing Education Activity Summary form. The ARRT reserves the right to request the original documentation if there is any question as to the authenticity of a certificate. In such situations, the original will be returned to the registrant by the ARRT.

5. If you fail to include all requested information on your renewal form, your application for renewal will be considered incomplete. If you fail to meet the deadline for completion of your renewal, you will no longer be registered and you will be subject to a reinstatement fee. If a period of three or more years lapse without having satisfied the CE requirements, re-examination will be required.

Figure 14-2 Continuing education activity summary. From: The American Registry of Radiologic Technologists, Copyright © 1994.

Chapter 15

Radiologic Specialties

> *No one can predict to what height you can soar. Even you will not know until you spread your wings.*

▲ Preparing for Advanced-Level Examinations

As demand has increased for radiologic technologists with multispecialty capabilities, many radiography students, graduates, and practicing technologists are considering furthering their education. Currently, the radiologic specialties requiring advanced-level education are diagnostic medical sonography, nuclear medicine technology, and radiation therapy technology. This section addresses the educational opportunities available in those areas.

Other radiologic specialties such as computed tomography, angiography, magnetic resonance imaging, and mammography do not have specific additional educational requirements in order to become credentialed. Further, education programs offered in those areas do not undergo approval by the usual accrediting organizations. However, information concerning advanced-level examinations are available in these areas and such information is included in this chapter.

Information about each of the three major specialties presented in this chapter includes a brief summary of the educational program and the content specifications for the exam. The names and addresses of the professional organizations associated with that specialty are then provided. Finally, all accredited educational programs in each field are listed. This compilation is accurate as of the date of publication. Because certification requirements and educational programs are subject to change for a variety of reasons, the interested professional should use the resources found in this chapter to write for the most current program information.

Program Director
Radiation Therapy Program
Community Hospital
Your Town, New York

Date

Dear Program Director:

I am a second-year radiography student interested in pursuing additional education in radiation therapy technology. Please send a copy of your program's informational brochure/catalog along with an application form to me at the address below.

Thank you for your attention to my request.

Sincerely,

Student Radiographer
123 Main Street
My Town, Illinois 62650

Figure 15-1 Sample request for specialty program informational brochure.

When writing for information to one of the programs listed in this chapter, keep the letter brief. Program directors receive countless requests for informational brochures so being concise is extremely helpful. It is recommended that you write at the beginning of your second year of radiography studies if you are planning to enroll in a specialty program immediately after graduation. You may wish to use the sample letter shown in Fig. 15-1.

▲ Diagnostic Medical Sonography

Educational programs in sonography may be one, two, or four years in length, depending upon the inclusion of earned credit hours from an academic degree. The course of study will involve biology, sectional anatomy, patient care, physics and equipment of ultrasound, diagnostic procedures, imaging, and image evaluation. Clinical education will also constitute a major portion of the program.

The education program will prepare the student to take the certification exam which includes the following subject matter:

Content Specifications for the Examinations in Diagnostic Medical Sonography

RDMS EXAMS

Ultrasound Physics & Instrumentation

Elementary Principles 6% - 10%
A. Nature of ultrasound
  1. Definition of sound
    a. Propagation of vibration
      1) Compression
      2) Rarefaction
  2. Differentiation between audible sound and ultrasound
B. Frequency, wavelength, propagation speed
  1. Definition of terms
  2. Relationships
C. Properties of ultrasound waves
  1. Amplitude
  2. Pressure
  3. Power
  4. Intensity
D. Decibels
  1. Definition
    a. Related to intensity
    b. Related to amplitude
  2. Numerical examples
E. Physical units
  1. Scientific notation
  2. Engineering notation (e.g., micro, Mega)
  3. Common units

Propagation of Ultrasound through Tissues 14% - 18%
A. Speed of sound
  1. Average speed of sound in tissues
  2. Range of propagation speeds in the body
    a. Air
    b. Soft tissue (average)
    c. Soft tissue: specific tissues (e.g., muscle, fat, parenchyma)
    d. Bone
B. Reflection
  1. Characteristic of acoustic impedance—definition
  2. Reflection and transmission at specular interfaces
    a. Interface size, smoothness, and contour
    b. Dependence on angle
    c. Dependence on acoustic impedance mismatch

  3. Scattering
    a. Scatterer size dependence
    b. Frequency dependence (Rayleigh scattering)
C. Refraction
  1. Dependence of angle
    a. Scattering
    b. Absorption
  2. Dependence on velocity mismatch
  3. Numerical example
D. Attenuation
  1. Definition and sources of attenuation
  2. Typical values in soft tissue
  3. Variation with frequency—numerical example
  4. Effects on images
E. Useful diagnostic frequency range
  1. Numerical values
  2. Tradeoff: penetration vs. spatial resolution

Ultrasound Transducers 17% - 25%
A. The Piezoelectric Effect
  1. Definition and concept
  2. Curie point
B. Transducer construction and characteristics
  1. Thickness resonance of crystal
  2. Damping
  3. Matching layer—numerical example
C. Sound beam formation—near field and far field (Fresnel and Fraunhofer zones)
  1. Interference phenomena
    a. Huygen's principle
    b. Diffraction
  2. Length of near field
  3. Shape of near field and far field
  4. Dependence on frequency, transducer size, and bandwidth
D. Focusing
  1. Methods of focusing
    a. Lens
    b. Curved element
    c. Electronic
    d. Mirrors
  2. Focal zone characteristics
    a. Point of maximum intensity
    b. Depth of focus
    c. Focal area
E. Beam width and lateral resolution
  1. Frequency
  2. Transducer size and focal characteristics
  3. Range
  4. Attenuation
F. Pulse duration and axial resolution
  1. Numerical example
  2. Effect of damping
  3. Transducer frequency spectrum—relation to pulse length

4. Bandwidth
G. Transducer arrays
  1. Multiple elements
    a. Linear sequential arrays
    b. Linear phased arrays
    c. Annular arrays
  2. Beam steering
    a. Transit time delays
    b. Receive time delays
  3. Beam focusing
    a. Time delays
    b. Receive mode
    c. Multiple transmit foci

Pulse Echo Instruments 10% - 16%
A. Range equation—general concepts
B. Pulsing characteristics
  1. Pulse repetition frequency, pulse repetition period
  2. Duty factor
C. Output power control
  1. Effect of intensity on patient exposure
  2. Effects of pulser voltage
D. Receiver overall gain
E. Receiver swept gain (TGC)
  1. Attenuation with range
  2. Numerical example
  3. Effects on return signal and display
F. Reject
  1. Effect on displayed signal
G. Signal processing
  1. Steps in signal processing
  2. Dynamic range
    a. Definition
    b. Dynamic range of individual components
  3. Compression—numerical example
  4. Preprocessing

Principles of Pulse Echo Imaging 8% - 14%
A. Principal display modes (A-mode, B-mode, T-M-mode)
  1. Definition of each mode
  2. Information displayed on each mode
  3. Advantages and disadvantages of each mode
B. Principles of B-mode image formation
  1. Relationship between echo amplitude and B-mode display
  2. Positioning of echoes
C. Identification of major types of scanning equipment
  1. Manual (compound) static scanner
    a. Water path
    b. Articulated arm
  2. Real-time imagers
    a. Linear arrays (phased and mechanical)
    b. Sector (phased and mechanical)
    c. Annular
    d. Water path

D. Scanning speed limitations
  1. Applications of range equation and relationship to pulsing characteristics
  2. Real-time systems—relationships between
    a. Pulsing characteristics
    b. Frame rate and time required to generate one frame
    c. Number of lines per frame
    d. Field of view (e.g., sector angle)
    e. Depth to be imaged
  3. Temporal resolution, ability to evaluate rapid motion

Images, Storage, and Display 5% - 10%
A. General role and use of scan converters and digital memories
  1. Role in signal processing and display
  2. Associated terminology (e.g., pixels, analogue)
B. Basic concepts of digital systems
  1. Binary system
  2. Storage capacities
C. Image storage, resolution, and field of view
  1. Process of image storage
  2. Factors affecting image sharpness and spatial resolution
    a. Scan converter matrix
    b. Pixels
    c. TV lines
    d. Frequency
    e. Focal characteristics
D. Display devices and controls
  1. Devices
    a. CRTs and oscilloscopes
    b. TV monitors
  2. Controls affecting signal display
    a. Brightness
    b. Contrast
E. Post processing
  1. Effects on image
  2. Advantages and disadvantages
F. Recording techniques
  1. Hard copy film and paper
  2. Videotape player
  3. Adjustment of contrast/brightness controls

Doppler 3% - 8%
A. Physical principles
  1. Doppler effect
    a. Principle as related to sampling red blood cell movement
    b. Doppler equation
  2. Factors influencing the magnitude of the Doppler shift frequency
    a. Range of the Doppler shift frequency
    b. Effects of red blood cell concentration, angle of beam incidence, transmitted frequency, flow velocity

B. Instrumentation
1. Continuous wave and pulsed Doppler
   a. Differences
   b. Advantages and disadvantages of each
      1) Aliasing (Nyquist criteria)
      2) Range ambiguity
2. Duplex instruments and directional devices—definition and basic principles
3. Spectral analysis
   a. Purpose
   b. Fast fourier transform (FFT)
4. Correlation functions
5. Basic principles of color-flow imaging
   a. Sampling methods
   b. Display of Doppler information
   c. Advantages and limitations
   d. Artifacts

Image Features and Artifacts 5% - 10%
A. Definition of artifacts and role of artifact recognition in interpretation and performance of exams
B. Reverberation, refraction, and other artifacts (e.g., beam width, electronic noise)
1. Definitions
2. Mechanisms of production
3. Ultrasound appearance
C. Shadowing and enhancement
1. Definitions
2. Mechanism of production
3. Ultrasound appearance
D. Measurements of dimensions from images
1. Volumes
2. Circumferences
3. Areas
4. Diameters
5. Artifacts affecting measurement

Quality Assurance of Ultrasound Instruments 1% - 5%
A. General concepts regarding the need for and nature of a quality assurance program
B. Parameters to be evaluated and methods for evaluating each
1. Axial and lateral resolution
2. Depth calibration accuracy
3. System sensitivity
4. Gray scale display
5. Lesion detection
6. Doppler quality control
C. Preventive maintenance
D. Record keeping

Bioeffects and Safety 7% - 13%
A. Dosimetric quantities
1. Pressure
   a. Units (MPa, mmHg, atmospheres)

   b. Peak pressures (compressed, rarefied)
2. Relationships between pressure, intensity, power, area, etc., and units associated with each
3. Acoustic exposure
   a. Definition and concepts of prudent use
   b. Methods of reducing acoustic exposure
      1) Factors affecting acoustic exposure
      2) Equipment controls
4. Intensity
   a. Units (mW/cm2), W/cm2, etc.)
   b. Spatial and temporal considerations
   c. Average and peak intensities
   d. Methods of determining intensity
      1) Radiation forces
      2) Hydrophone probes
   e. Common intensities
      1) SPTA
      2) SATA
      3) SPTP
      4) SPPA
      5) Im
B. Typical values for diagnostic equipment
1. Intensity and power values for all modes of operation
C. Experimental biological effects studies
1. Animal studies
   a. Primary mechanisms of biological effect production
      1) Cavitation mechanisms and relevant acoustic parameters
      2) Thermal mechanism and relevant acoustic parameters
   b. Types of studies and effects reported
2. In vitro studies
   a. Primary mechanisms of biological effect production
      1) Cavitation: relevant acoustic parameters
   b. Types of studies and effects reported
3. Epidemiologic studies
   a. Limitations
   b. Types of studies and effects reported
D. AIUM statements
E. Electrical and mechanical hazards
1. Patient susceptibility to electrical hazard
2. Equipment components which could present a hazard

Obstetrics & Gynecology

Obstetrics (Total 50% - 60%)
A. First trimester 6% - 8%
1. Gestational sac
2. Yolk sac
3. Embryo (normal physiologic development/ sonographic appearance)
4. Ovaries (corpus luteum)
5. Cul-de-sac
6. Pregnancy failure

7. Ectopic pregnancy

B. Second/third trimester (normal anatomy) 8% - 12%
   1. Cranial
   2. Spine
   3. Heart
   4. Thorax
   5. Abdomen
      a. Gastrointestinal
      b. Genitourinary
      c. General
   6. Extremities
   7. Fetal position
   8. Other

C. Placenta 1% - 5%
   1. Development
   2. Position
   3. Anatomy
   4. Membranes
   5. Umbilical cord
   6. Abruption
   7. Previa
   8. Masses and lesions
   9. Maturity/grading
   10. Doppler
   11. Physiology

D. Assessment of gestational age 2% - 6%
   1. Gestational sac
   2. Embryonic size/crown-rump length
   3. Biparietal diameter
   4. Femur length
   5. Abdominal circumference
   6. Head circumference
   7. Transcerebellar measurements
   8. Binocular measurements
   9. Cephalic indices
   10. Fetal lung maturity
   11. Other

E. Complications 6% - 10%
   1. Intrauterine growth retardation
      a. Symmetrical
      b. Asymmetrical
      c. Nonstress test
      d. Biophysical profile
      e. Doppler flow studies
   2. Multiple gestations
      a. Diamniotic
      b. Monoamniotic
      c. Complications
   3. Maternal illness
      a. Gestational diabetes
      b. Diabetes mellitus
      c. Hypertension
      d. Other
   4. Antepartum
      a. Preterm labor

   b. Premature rupture of membranes
   c. RH isoimmunization
   d. Cervix related problems
   e. Other
   5. Fetal therapy
      a. Fetal blood sampling/transfusion
      b. Other
   6. Postpartum
      a. Hemorrhage
      b. Infection
      c. Cesarean section
      d. Other

F. Amniotic fluid 1% - 5%
   1. Assessment
   2. Polyhydramnios
   3. Oligohydramnios
   4. Fetal pulmonic maturity studies

G. Genetic studies 1% - 3%
   1. Maternal serum testing
   2. Amniotic fluid testing
   3. Chorionic villus sampling
   4. Dominant/recessive risk occurrence

H. Fetal demise 0% - 3%

I. Fetal abnormalities 10% - 15%
   1. Cranial
   2. Facial
   3. Neck
   4. Neural tube
   5. Abdominal wall
   6. Thoracic
   7. Genitourinary
   8. Gastrointestinal
   9. Skeletal
   10. Cardiac
   11. Syndromes
   12. Other

J. Coexisting disorders 0% - 3%
   1. Leiomyoma
   2. Cystic
   3. Trophoblastic disease
   4. Solid/mixed
   5. Myometrial contraction
   6. Other

Gynecology (Total 40% - 50%)
A. Normal pelvic anatomy 10% - 15%
   1. Uterus
      a. Corpus
      b. Endometrium
      c. Cervix
      d. Vagina
   2. Ovaries
   3. Fallopian tubes
   4. Supporting structures
   5. Cul-de-sac

6. Vasculature
7. Doppler flow
8. Gynecology related studies
   a. Gastrointestinal
   b. Genitourinary
B. Physiology 6% - 12%
  1. Menstrual cycle
  2. Pregnancy tests
  3. Human chorionic gonadotropin (hCg)
  4. Fertilization
C. Pediatric 1% - 5%
  1. Precocious puberty
  2. Hematometra/hematocolpos
  3. Sexual ambiguity
  4. Other
D. Infertility/Endocrinology 2% - 6%
  1. Contraception
  2. Causes
  3. Medications and treatment
  4. Ovulation induction (follicular monitoring)
  5. ART (Assisted Reproductive Technology), GIFT, IVF, ZIFT
E. Postmenopausal 6% - 10%
  1. Anatomy
  2. Physiology
  3. Therapy
    a. Hormonal replacement
  4. Pathology
    a. Hyperplasia
    b. Polyps
    c. Endometrial cancer
    d. Ovarian cancer
    e. Other
F. Pelvic pathology 6% - 10%
  1. Congenital uterine malformation
  2. Uterine masses
  3. Ovarian masses
  4. Endometriosis
  5. Polycystic ovarian disease
  6. Inflammatory disease
  7. Doppler flow studies
  8. Gynecology related studies
    a. Gastrointestinal
    b. Genitourinary
  9. Other
G. Extra-pelvic pathology associated with gyn 1% - 3%
  1. Ascites
  2. Liver metastasis
  3. Hydronephrosis
  4. Other

Patient Care Preparation/Technique (Total 1% - 5%)
A. Review charts
B. Explain examinations
C. Supine hypotensive syndrome

D. Bioeffects
E. Infectious disease control
F. Scanning techniques
G. Artifacts
H. Physical principles

Abdomen Content Outline

Liver 12% - 20%
A. Anatomy
B. Technique
C. Laboratory values
D. Indications
E. Parenchymal disease
F. Masses
G. Cysts
H. Abscesses
I. Hematomas

Biliary Tree 12% - 20%
A. Anatomy
B. Technique
C. Laboratory values
D. Indications
E. Dilatation
F. Masses
G. Cholelithiasis
H. Cholecystitis

Pancreas 12% - 20%
A. Anatomy
B. Technique
C. Laboratory values
D. Indications
E. Parenchymal disease (pancreatitis)
F. Masses
G. Cysts (pseudocysts)

Urinary Tract 16% - 24%
A. Anatomy
B. Technique
C. Laboratory values
D. Indications
E. Renal parenchymal disease
F. Masses
G. Cysts
H. Abscesses
I. Hematomas
J. Calculi
K. Obstructive disease
L. Infarctions
M. Anomalies
N. Transplants
O. Bladder
P. Prostate
Q. Scrotum

Spleen 1% - 3%
A. Anatomy
B. Technique
C. Laboratory values
D. Indications
E. Parenchymal disease
F. Masses
G. Cysts
H. Abscesses
I. Hematomas
J. Infarctions

Retroperitoneum 6% - 9%
A. Anatomy
B. Technique
C. Laboratory values
D. Indications
E. Masses, adenopathy
F. Hematomas
G. Adrenal

Abdominal Vasculature (including Doppler) 10% - 12%
A. Anatomy
B. Technique
C. Laboratory values
D. Indications
E. Aneurysms
F. Thrombus
G. Arteriovenous shunts
H. Doppler waveforms

GI Tract 3% - 6%
A. Anatomy
B. Technique
C. Laboratory values
D. Indications
E. Inflammatory disease
F. Masses
G. Obstruction
H. Hernia
I. Peritoneal fluid

Neck 2% - 5%
A. Anatomy
B. Technique
C. Laboratory values
D. Indications
E. Thyroid parenchymal disease
F. Thyroid masses
G. Thyroid cysts
H. Parathyroid masses
I. Abscesses
J. Lymph nodes
K. Carotid and jugular

Superficial Structures 1% - 3% (Breast, Musculoskeletal, Non-cardiac Chest)
A. Anatomy
B. Technique
C. Laboratory values
D. Indications
E. Masses
F. Cysts, fluid collection
G. Abscesses
H. Hematomas
I. Vessels
J. Breast
K. Non-cardiac chest

Instrumentation 1% - 3%
A. Technique
B. Transducers
C. Machine settings
D. Image recording
E. Artifacts
F. Quality assurance
G. Invasive procedures

Neurosonology

Physics & Instrumentation 1% - 5%
A. Effects of bone on ultrasonic energy
B. Effect of transducer frequency on image quality
C. Bone-induced artifacts
D. Effect of instrument controls on image quality
Technique in Neurosonography 10% - 20%
A. Rationale for selection of modality, instrument, and transducer for a specific examination
    1. Neonate
    2. Intraoperative
B. Scan-plane selection and identification
C. Adjustment of instrument controls
D. Recognition of normal anatomic structures and landmarks
    1. Cerebellum
    2. Cerebrum
    3. Brain stem
    4. Spinal cord
    5. Ventricular system
E. Examination protocol
F. Normal dimensions and measurement techniques
G. Sterile technique in intraoperative examination
H. Transcranial doppler techniques

Anatomy & Physiology 30% - 40%
A. Bones of the os cranium
B. Fontanelles and external landmarks

C. Gross topographical anatomy
    1. Cerebellum

2. Cerebrum
3. Brain stem
4. Spinal cord
D. Membranous partitioning of the intracranial space
E. Intra- and extracranial vascular structures
   1. Watershed areas
   2. Normal vascular structures
   3. ECMO effects
F. Gray/white matter organization of the brain and cord
G. The ventricular system
H. Origin, flow, and reabsorption of the cerebrospinal fluid
I. Principal functional tracts of the central nervous system

Recognition of Pathology and Differential
Diagnosis 40% - 50%
A. Midline displacements
B. Space-occupying lesions and mass effects in the brain
C. Inflammatory lesions
D. Ventricular enlargement
E. Intra- and extracranial hemorrhage
F. Atrophic lesions
G. Congenital lesions
H. Brain swelling (edema)
I. Lesions of the spine
J. Tethering of the spine
K. Vascular abnormalities
L. Trauma

Medical Care of the Neonate During Scanning 1% - 3%
A. Temperature maintenance
B. Asepsis and infection control
C. Scanning the neonate on a respirator
D. Care of the neonate with IVs
E. Seizure precautions

Ophthalmology

Physics 5% - 10%
A. Amplification
B. Transducer
C. Artifacts

Instrumentation 0% - 3%
A. Types of equipment
B. A-scan
C. B-scan

Exam Techniques 10% - 15%
A. A-scan
B. B-scan
C. M-scan
D. Doppler
E. Sterile
F. Contact scanning
G. Immersion scanning

H. Anesthesia
I. Pediatric
J. Kinetic
K. Ancillary diagnostic studies

Biometry 5% - 10%
A. Principles
   1. Normal ranges
   2. Formulas
   3. Velocities
   4. Transducer characteristics
B. Techniques
   1. Alignment
   2. Measuring modes
   3. Sources of error
C. Applications
   1. IOL power measurement
   2. Other ocular tissue measurement

Anatomy & Physiology 1% - 4%
A. Ocular
   1. Cornea
   2. Anterior chamber
   3. Lens
   4. Anterior uvea
   5. Vitreous
   6. Retina/choroid
   7. Sclera
B. Orbital
   1. Optic nerve
   2. Extraocular muscles
   3. Lacrimal gland
   4. Orbital wall
   5. Orbital FAT pad

Pathology 65% - 75%
A. Ocular
   1. Cornea
   2. Anterior chamber
   3. Iris
   4. Lens
   5. Ciliary body
   6. Vitreous
      a. Opacities
      b. Posterior hyaloid face
      c. Subhyaloid space
      d. Membranes
   7. Retina
      a. Detachment
      b. Degeneration
      c. Neovascularization
      d. Retinoblastoma
      e. Other retinal lesions
   8. Choroid
      a. Detachment

b. Degeneration
c. Tumors
   1) Malignant melanoma
   2) Metastatic carcinoma
   3) Hemangioma
   4) Nevus
   5) Other choroidal lesions
9. Sclera
  a. Contour abnormalities
  b. Scleritis
10. Phthisis bulbi
B. Orbital
  1. Optic nerve head
  2. Optic nerve
    a. Tumors
    b. Inflammation/edema
  3. Tumors/lesions
    a. Vascular
    b. Nonvascular
  4. Inflammatory processes
    a. Thyroid eye disease
    b. Myositis
    c. Pseudotumor
    d. Tenon's capsule
  5. Paranasal sinuses
  6. Lacrimal gland
  7. Lacrimal sac
C. Trauma ocular
  1. Penetrating trauma
  2. Blunt trauma
D. Trauma orbital
E. Glaucoma

RDCS EXAMS

Cardiovascular Principles & Instrumentation, Physics

Anatomy of the Heart (Review) 4% - 8%
A. Chambers and related septa
B. Valves and related apparatus
C. Arterial-venous system
D. Conduction system
E. Layers
F. Relational anatomy

Basic Embryology 1% - 3%
A. Primitive heart tube
  1. Formation from primitive vascular tube
  2. Sinus venosus
  3. Cardiac loop
  4. Aortic arches
  5. Septation
  6. Valve formation
B. Comparison of fetal and postnatal circulation

Congenital Defects 1% - 3%
A. Abnormalities of septation
B. Abnormal vasculature and resulting lesions
C. Persistence of normal fetal communication
D. Valvular anomalies

Cardiac Physiology 5% - 15%
A. Electrophysiology and the conduction system
  1. Propagation of electrical activity
  2. Excitation contraction coupling
B. Mechanical considerations and events
  1. Frank Starling law (length-tension relationship)
  2. Force-velocity relationship
  3. Interval-strength relationship
  4. Valve opening and closure
C. Phases of the cardiac cycle (electro-mechanical events)
  1. Passive filling phase (ventricular diastole)
  2. Atrial systole (p-wave on EKG; late diastole)
  3. Isovolumic contraction
  4. Ventricular ejection
  5. Isovolumic relaxation
D. Left ventricular function: indicators and normal values
  1. Stroke volume
  2. Ejection fraction
  3. Cardiac output
  4. Cardiac index
E. Pulmonary vs. systemic circulation: differences (e.g., pressure, oxygen content, etc.) and similarities (e.g., volumes)
F. Intracardiac pressures and principles of flow
  1. Normal values
  2. Changes during the cardiac cycle and relation to valve opening/closure
G. Maneuvers altering cardiac physiology (e.g., position)
H. Normal heart sound generation and timing
I. Cardiovascular circulation
  1. Normal metabolic needs and their variations
  2. Component parts of the circulation
  3. Control mechanisms
  4. Coronary circulation
  5. Properties of blood: composition

Cardiac Evaluation Methods 5% - 15%
A. Symptoms of cardiac diseases and common causes
B. Physical examination and signs
  1. General physical appearance and patient history
  2. Correlation of auscultatory findings
    a. Normal heart sounds
    b. Abnormal heart sounds and common causes
    c. Murmurs
      1) Timing, location, intensity
      2) Character, grading
      3) Murmurs associated with specific diseases
      4) Response to physiologic maneuvers (e.g., valsalva)

C. EKG
1. Basic principles and waveforms
2. Common abnormalities: basic pattern recognition
3. Exercise stress testing: basic principles
D. Phonocardiography
1. Basic principles and waveforms
2. Phonocardiographic configuration of common cardiac disease states/pattern recognition
E. Cardiac catheterization
1. Basic concepts of hemodynamic recordings
2. Determination of cardiac output
3. Determination of valve areas
4. Quantitation of shunt and regurgitant lesions
5. Oximetry
6. Coronary atriography
7. Evaluation and definition of gradients (e.g., peak-to-peak, mean, etc.)
8. Recognition of pressure wave forms in common disease states
9. Angiographic findings in common disease states
F. Other diagnostic modalities—correlation to echocardiography
1. Chest x ray
2. Nuclear cardiology
G. Relation of cardiac events as recorded on ECG, phonocardiogram, pressure tracings, etc.
H. Correlation and integration of information obtained with echocardiography and various methods of cardiac evaluation

Principles of Cardiac Hemodynamics 5% - 15%

A. Blood flow dynamics
1. Factors affecting blood flow (e.g., viscosity, cell number, etc.)
2. Laminar flow: definition, characteristics, and types
3. Disturbed flow: definition, characteristics (vortices, turbulence, etc.)
4. Relationships between pressure and velocity: Bernoulli principles and equations used
B. Effects of abnormal pressures and loading, volume concepts
1. Heart failure and shock
2. Valvular stenosis
3. Valvular regurgitation
4. Shunts
5. Pulmonary disease
6. Pericardial disease
7. Cardiomyopathies

Elementary Principles 4% - 8%

A. Nature of ultrasound: definitions, propagation, difference from audible sound
B. Frequency, wavelength, propagation speed: definitions and relationships
C. Properties of sound waves (e.g., amplitude, pressure, etc.)

D. Decibels: definition, relationships to amplitude, and intensity
E. Physical units
1. Scientific notation
2. Engineering notation (e.g., micro vs. Mega)
3. Common units

Propagation of Ultrasound Through Tissues 4% - 8%

A. Speed of sound
1. Average speed of sound in tissue
2. Range of propagation speeds in the body
3. Speeds in specific tissues (e.g., muscle, bone, fat)
B. Principles related to reflection
1. Characteristic acoustic impedance: definition
2. Reflection and transmission of specular interfaces
3. Scattering
C. Principles related to refraction
D. Principles related to attenuation
E. Useful diagnostic frequency range

Ultrasound Transducers 5% - 10%

A. The Piezoelectric effect
B. Transducer construction and characteristics
C. Sound beam formation: near and far fields (Fresnel and Frauhofer zones)
D. Focusing
1. Methods of focusing
2. Focal zone characteristics
E. Beam width and lateral resolution
F. Pulse duration and axial resolution
G. Transducer arrays
1. Multiple elements and their arrangements
2. Beam steering
3. Beam focusing

Pulse Echo Instruments 3% - 7%

A. Range equations: general concepts
B. Pulsing characteristics (e.g., pulse repetition frequency)
C. Output power control
D. Receiver overall gain
E. Receiver swept gain (TGC)
F. Reject
G. Signal processing
1. Steps in signal processing
2. Dynamic range
3. Compression
4. Preprocessing

Principles of Pulse Echo Imaging 5% - 10%

A. Principal display modes (A-mode, B-mode, T-M mode)
B. Principal of B-mode image formation
C. Identification of major types of imaging equipment
D. Scanning speed limitations
1. Applications of range equation and relationship to pulsing characteristics

2. Relationships between:
   a. Pulsing characteristics (e.g., PRF)
   b. Frame rate and time needed to generate one frame
   c. Number of lines per frame
   d. Field of view (e.g., sector angle)
   e. Depth to be imaged
3. Ability to evaluate rapid motion, temporal resolution

Images, Storage, and Display 1% - 5%
A. General role and use of scan converters and digital memories
B. Basic concepts of digital systems
C. Image storage, resolution, and field of view
D. Display devices and controls
E. Postprocessing
F. Recording techniques (e.g., videotape, stripchart, etc.)

Doppler 10% - 20%
A. Basic principles
   1. Doppler effect: principle as related to sampling red blood cell movement
   2. Scattering (from red blood cells)
      a. Frequency dependence
      b. Strength of emitted signal vs. returned signal
   3. Doppler equation
      a. Range of Doppler shift frequencies—audible
      b. Factors influencing magnitude of Doppler shift and special relationships
         1) Transducer frequency
         2) Angle of beam incidence
         3) Flow velocity
         4) Frequency conversion
B. Spectral analysis
   1. Purpose
   2. Fast fourier transform (FFT)
   3. Spectral display
      a. Axis identification (e.g., frequency and time)
      b. Assignment of gray shades represented on the spectrum
      c. Components of the spectrum
         1) Mean frequency (or velocity)
         2) Mode frequency (or velocity)
         3) Peak frequency (or velocity)
      d. Effect of wall filtering and gains
   4. Spectral broadening
      a. Influence of sample volume size
      b. Pulse width
      c. Flow disturbances
   5. Spectral artifacts
      a. Mirroring
      b. Aliasing
      c. Electrical interference
      d. Noise
   6. Methods of displaying Doppler information (e.g., visual and audio)

C. Instrumentation
   1. Continuous wave Doppler
      a. Transducer configurations
         1) Split crystals
         2) Arrays
      b. Lack of range resolution (range ambiguity)
      c. High velocity measurement capability
   2. Pulsed Doppler
      a. Transducers
         1) Single crystal
         2) Mechanical sector
         3) Arrays
      b. Range discrimination
         1) Sample volume
         2) Resolution compared to imaging resolution
      c. Aliasing (signal ambiguity): concept and factors influencing aliasing
         1) Pulse repetition frequency
         2) Nyquist frequency limit
         3) Maximum depth
         4) Baseline position
      d. High pulse repetition frequency
         1) Multiple sample volumes used
         2) Effect on maximum detectable Doppler shift
         3) Uses and limitations
   3. Color flow imaging
      a. Sampling methods
      b. Fundamental variables
         1) Packet size
         2) Line density
         3) Maximum depth
         4) Frame rate
         5) Echo vs. color threshold
      c. Evaluation of frequency content
         1) Methods of separating frequencies (e.g., auto-correlation algorithm)
         2) Estimation of frequencies represented
            a. Mean frequency
            b. Variance
      d. Color maps
      e. Artifacts
         1) Aliasing
         2) Ghosting
         3) Reverberation
         4) Drop angle due to beam angle
      f. Limitations
   4. Doppler output parameters (e.g., power, intensity)
      a. Continuous wave
      b. Pulsed
      c. Color flow
      d. Compared to imaging
   5. Roles and limitations of each Doppler modality

Image Features and Artifacts 1% - 5%
A. Artifacts: definition, role of recognition in performing and interpreting exams, understanding mechanism, and appearance
B. Reverberation, refraction and other artifacts (e.g., beam width, electronic noise)
C. Shadowing and enhancement
D. Measurements and dimensions from images (e.g., area)
E. Artifacts affecting measurement

Quality Assurance of Ultrasound Instruments 1% - 3%
A. General concepts regarding the need and nature of a quality assurance program
B. Quality assurance evaluation parameters and methods
C. Preventive maintenance
D. Record keeping

Bioeffects and Safety 2% - 6%
A. Dosimetric quantities (units and definitions)
   1. Pressure
   2. Intensities
   3. Power
   4. Relationship between pressure, intensity, power, and area
   5. Typical values for diagnostic equipment used in echocardiography in all modes of operation
B. Acoustic exposure
   1. Definition
   2. Factors affecting and methods of reducing acoustic exposure
C. Experimental biological effects studies
   1. Primary mechanisms of biological effect production
   2. Types of studies, their limitations and effects reported
      a. Animal studies
      b. In vitro studies
      c. Epidemiological
D. AIUM statements
E. Electrical and mechanical hazards

Pediatric Echocardiography

Instrumentation 5% - 10%
A. M-mode
B. Two-dimensional
C. Transducer/Doppler
D. Recording format
E. Ancillary recording modalities
   1. ECG
   2. Pulse
   3. Resp

Phases of the Cardiac Cycle 2% - 6%
A. Systolic events
B. Diastolic events

Normal Anatomy 10% - 20%
A. Semilunar valves/great vessels
B. Atrioventricular valves
C. Chambers/septa
D. Other related structures

Normal Hemodynamic 2% - 6%
A. Systemic—venous
B. Pulmonary venous
C. Systemic—arterial
D. Pulmonary—arterial
E. Atrioventricular events

Scanning Technique 5% - 10%
A. M-mode
B. Cross sectional
C. Contrast

Functional Assessment 5% - 10%
A. Volumes
B. Contractility
C. Time intervals

Congenital Pathology 50% - 60%
A. Left-volume overload
B. Right-volume overload
C. Left ventricular outflow obstruction
D. Left ventricular inflow obstruction
E. Right ventricular outflow obstruction
F. Right ventricular inflow obstruction
G. Aortic override
H. Tumors
I. Mitral valve prolapse (Idiopathic, Hunter's, Marfan's)
J. Malposition
K. Postop
L. Venous pathology

Acquired Pathology 3% - 10%
A. Pericardial effusion
B. Subacute bacterial endocarditis
C. Rheumatic heart disease
D. Miscellaneous
   1. Kawasaki
   2. Drugs
   3. Congestive cardiomyopathy

Adult Echocardiography

Anatomy and Physiology 5% - 10%
A. Ventricular wall segments (as recommended by American Society of Echocardiography)
B. Nomenclature
  1. Subdivisions of ventricles
    a. Inflow tract
    b. Outflow tract
  2. Valves
  3. Great vessels
C. Coronary sinus (vs. descending aorta)
D. Coronary arteries
E. Normal pressures (in all four cardiac chambers and great vessels)
  1. Phases of cardiac cycle
    a. Electrical/mechanical systole
    b. Filling phases of diastole
  2. Timing of events (relative to ECG)
F. Miscellaneous

Technique 10% - 20%
A. Use of equipment controls
B. Recognition of technical artifacts
C. Recognition of setup errors
D. Use of contrast agents
E. Provocative maneuvers
F. Best approach for Doppler studies
G. Miscellaneous
H. Two-dimensional study
I. M-mode patterns
J. CPR

Valvular Heart Disease 15% - 25%
A. Mitral valve
  1. Physiology/hemodynamics
  2. Mitral stenosis
    a. M-mode
    b. Two-dimensional study
    c. Doppler study
    d. Effects on:
      1) Atria
      2) Ventricles
      3) Cardiac vessels
  3. Mitral regurgitation
    a. M-mode
    b. Two-dimensional study
    c. Doppler study
    d. Effects on:
      1) Atria
      2) Ventricles
      3) Cardiac vessels
    e. Mitral prolapse
    f. Chordal rupture
    g. Flail leaflet
    h. Mitral annular calcification

    i. Mixed mitral valve disease (MA/MR)
B. Aortic valve
  1. Physiology/hemodynamics
  2. Aortic stenosis
    a. M-mode
    b. Two-dimensional study
    c. Doppler study
    d. Effects on:
      1) Atria
      2) Ventricles
      3) Cardiac vessels
    e. Etiologies
      1) Congenital
      2) Rheumatic
      3) Degenerative
    f. Mixed lesions (AS/AR)
    g. Distinctions between aortic stenosis and sclerosis
  3. Aortic regurgitation
    a. M-mode
    b. Two-dimensional study
    c. Doppler study
    d. Effects on:
      1) Atria
      2) Ventricles
      3) Cardiac vessels
    e. Etiologies
      1) Congenital
      2) Rheumatic
      3) Infectious
      4) Secondary (e.g., aortic root abnormality)
      5) Flail
    f. Mixed (AS/AR)
C. Tricuspid valve
  1. Physiology/hemodynamics
  2. Tricuspid stenosis
    a. M-mode
    b. Two-dimensional study
    c. Doppler study
    d. Effects on:
      1) Atria
      2) Ventricles
      3) Cardiac vessels
    e. Etiologies
      1) Rheumatic
    f. With mixed lesions
  3. Tricuspid regurgitation
    a. M-mode
    b. Two-dimensional Study
    c. Doppler study
    d. Effects on:
      1) Atria
      2) Ventricles
      3) Cardiac vessels
    e. Etiologies
      1) Rrheumatic

2) Carcinoid
3) Tricuspid prolapse
4) Chordal rupture
5) Flail leaflet
D. Pulmonary valve
1. Physiology/hemodynamics
2. Pulmonary stenosis
  a. M-mode
  b. Two-dimensional study
  c. Doppler study
  d. Effects on:
    1) Atria
    2) Ventricles
    3) Cardiac vessels
  e. Etiologies
    1) Congenital
    2) Carcinoid
3. Pulmonary regurgitation
  a. M-mode
  b. Two-dimensional study
  c. Doppler study
  d. Effects on:
    1) Atria
    2) Ventricles
    3) Cardiac vessels
  e. Etiologies
    1) Carcinoid
    2) Pulmonary hypertension
  f. Mixed PS/PI
E. Endocarditis
1. Physiology/hemodynamics
2. Involvement of adjacent cardiac structures
3. M-mode patterns
4. Two-dimensional study
F. Prosthetic valves
1. Mechanical
  a. Types
    1) Ball-and-cage
    2) Disc in cage
    3) Tilting-disc
  b. Dysfunction
    1) Stenosis
    2) Regurgitation
    3) Thrombosis
2. Tissue types (bioprostheses)
3. Means of evaluation
  a. M-mode
  b. Two-dimensional study
  c. Doppler study
  d. Other

Pericardial Disease 2% - 8%
A. Constrictive
1. Physiology/hemodynamics
2. Etiologies

3. Echocardiographic manifestations
B. Effusion
1. Physiology/hemodynamics
  a. Tamponade
2. Etiologies
3. Differentiation from pleural effusion
C. Tumor
1. Primary
2. Metastatic
D. Miscellaneous
1. Adhesions
2. Nonspecific thickening
3. False positives

Systemic & Pulmonary Hypertensive Heart Disease 1% - 3%
A. Systemic
1. Physiology/hemodynamics
2. Echocardiographic findings
B. Pulmonary
1. Physiology/hemodynamics
2. Doppler assessment
  a. From tricuspid regurgitant jet
  b. From pulmonary artery acceleration time
3. Image findings

Cardiomyopathies 5% - 15%
A. Hypertrophic
1. With/without obstruction
2. Associated abnormalities
  a. Mitral annular calcium
  b. Mitral regurgitant/left atrial enlargement
  c. Fibrous scarring of septum
  d. Thickening of anterior mitral valve leaflet
3. Methods of evaluation
  a. Provocative maneuvers
    1) Amyl nitrite
    2) Valsalva
  b. M-mode
  c. Two-dimensional study
  d. Doppler study (specifically for localizing site of obstruction and accessing LVOT gradients)
B. Dilated
1. Etiologies
  a. Idiopathic
  b. Ischemic
  c. Alcoholic
2. Associated findings
  a. Mitral regurgitation
  b. Other chamber enlargement
  c. Thrombus
C. Restrictive
1. Etiologies

Ischemic Heart Disease 10% - 20%
A. Wall motion abnormalities
B. Associated findings
  1. Thrombi
  2. Changes in appearance of involved myocardium
  3. Aneurysm
  4. Valve dysfunction
  5. Pericardial effusion
  6. Cardiomyopathy
  7. Ruptured myocardium
  8. Right ventricular involvement

Cardiac Tumors 2% - 5%
A. Benign (e.g., myxoma)
B. Malignant
  1. Primary vs. secondary (metastatic)
C. Pericardial involvement
D. Differentiation from other masses or artifacts

Miscellaneous 5% - 10%
A. Arrhythmias and conduction disturbances
  1. Effect on valve motion
  2. Production of wall motion abnormalities
  3. Effect on Doppler flow velocity waveforms
B. Parameters of left ventricular function
C. Other

Congenital Heart Disease in the Adult 2% - 8%
A. Categories
  1. Aortic valve
    a. Bicuspid
    b. Supravalvular/subvalvular stenosis
  2. Pulmonic stenosis
  3. Cleft mitral valve
  4. Atrial septal defect
    a. Types
    b. Means of assessing
      1) Contrast
      2) Doppler
    c. Physiology/hemodynamics
      1) Associated chamber enlargement
      2) Direction for shunt flow
  5. Ventricular septal defect
    a. Types
    b. Means of assessing
      1) Contrast
      2) Doppler
    c. Physiology/hemodynamics
      1) Associated chamber enlargement
      2) Directions for shunt flow
  6. Endocardial cushion defect
  7. Ebstein's anomaly
  8. Patent ductus arteriosus
  9. Tetralogy of Fallot
  10. Status, postoperative congenital heart disease
  11. Coarctation of the aorta

Diseases of the Aorta 3% - 8%
A. Marfan's syndrome
B. Miscellaneous aortic dilatation
C. Aortic aneurysm
D. Aortic dissection
E. Sinus of valsalva aneurysms
F. Coarctation of the aorta

Doppler 3% - 8%
A. General information
B. Formulas for measurement
  1. Modified Bernoulli equation
  2. Pressure half-time formula
  3. Doppler formula
C. Color flow mapping

RVT EXAMS

Vascular Physical Principles & Instrumentation

Ultrasound Physics 35% - 45%
A. Definition of sound (6% - 10%)
  1. Sound vs. ultrasound
  2. Propagation velocity
  3. Frequency
  4. Wavelength
  5. Frequency vs. depth
  6. Frequency ranges
B. Propagation of sound in tissue (6% - 10%)
  1. Speed of sound through tissue: air, bone, soft tissue
  2. Speed of sound through blood
  3. Acoustic impedance
  4. Reflection
  5. Refraction
  6. Absorption
  7. Attenuation
C. Transducers: ultrasound (6% - 10%)
  1. Piezoelectric effect
  2. Transducer characteristics
  3. Sound beam characteristics
    a. Effect of beam diameter on resolution
    b. Effect of transducer frequency on beam characteristics
    c. Beam focusing
    d. Near field
    e. Far field
  4. Lateral resolution
  5. Axial resolution
  6. Mechanical transducers
  7. Electronic transducers
D. Doppler signal processing (6% - 10%)
  1. Doppler effect

shift

itting frequency on Doppler fre-

ion angle on Doppler frequency shift
(velocity)

Doppler signal

er signal analysis

er waveform generation

ay characteristics

ne size

ments (6% - 10%)

wave instruments

ve instruments

nal Doppler

ional Doppler

w

anial

maging 15% - 25%

principles (10% - 14%)

de: definition

de: definition

time: definition

y scale display

namic range

ame rate

an converter

ain

Time gain compensation

Recording techniques
  a. Multi-imaging camera
  b. Video tape
  c. Thermal video printer
  d. Digital storage
1. Duplex instrumentation
2. Image resolution

Imaging artifacts (6% - 10%)
1. Artifact: definition
2. Origin of artifacts: technique
3. Origin of artifacts: instrumentation
4. Enhancement
5. Multiple reflections
6. Reverberation
7. Shadowing
8. Refraction

Physiology & Fluid Dynamic 10% - 20%
A. Arterial hemodynamics (7% - 11%)
  1. Energy gradient
  2. Effects of viscosity, friction, inertia
  3. Pressure/flow relationships
    a. Poiseuille's law
    b. Bernoulli's principle
  4. Velocity

5. Steady flow vs. pulsatile flow
6. Effects of stenosis on flow characteristics
  a. Direction, turbulence, disturbed flow
  b. Velocity acceleration
  c. Entrance/exit effects
  d. Diameter reduction
  e. Peripheral resistance
  f. Collateral effects
  g. Effects of exercise
  h. Occlusion
B. Venous hemodynamics (4% - 8%)
  1. Venous resistance
  2. Hydrostatic pressure
  3. Pressure/volume relationship
  4. Effects of edema
  5. Effects of muscle pump mechanism
    a. At rest
    b. Contraction
    c. Relaxation
C. Other (0% - 3%)
  1. Arteriovenous fistula (traumatic, congenital, access dialysis)
  2. Trauma (pseudoaneurysm)

Physical Principles 15% - 25%
A. General (3% - 7%)
  1. Energy
  2. Power
  3. Graphical recording
  4. Calibration
  5. AC/DC coupling
  6. Units of measure
B. Tissue mechanics/pressure transmission (1% - 5%)
  1. Venous occlusion by limb positioning
  2. Superficial venous occlusion by tourniquets
  3. Venous occlusion by cuffs
  4. Volume changes by blood inflow/outflow
  5. Arterial occlusion by cuffs
C. Plethysmography (1% - 5%)
  1. Displacement (pneumatic cuff)
  2. Photoplethysmography
  3. Oculoplethysmography - pressure
D. Pressure measurements (6% - 10%)
  1. Legs
  2. Arms
E. Other (0% - 3%)
  1. Skin temperature
  2. Transcutaneous oximetry

Ultrasound Safety & Quality Assurance 3% - 7%
A. Instrument performance (2% - 6%)
  1. Evaluation of image quality
  2. Evaluation of Doppler quality
  3. Preventive maintenance

B. Biological effects (0% - 3%)
1. Minimizing exposure time
2. Mechanisms of production
3. Scientific data
4. Preventing electrical hazards

Vascular Technology

Gross Anatomy (Vessel Routes, Variations, Collaterals)
5% - 15%
A. Central and peripheral arterial system (1% - 5%)
1. Aortic arch
2. Upper extremity
3. Thorax and abdomen
4. Lower extremity
B. Cerebral arterial system (1% - 5%)
1. Extracranial carotid and vertebral
2. Intracranial (circle of Willis)
C. Venous system (1% - 5%)
1. Upper extremity
   a. Deep veins
   b. Superficial veins
2. Lower extremity
   a. Deep veins
   b. Superficial veins
   c. Perforators
3. Central veins
   a. Vena cava
   b. Portal, mesenteric,, and renal veins
D. Microscopic anatomy (0% - 3%)
1. Arterial wall
2. Venous wall and valves

Test Validation 1% - 5%
A. Statistics (0% - 4%)
1. Sensitivity specificity
2. Positive predictive value, negative predictive value
3. Accuracy
B. Measurements (0% - 3%)
1. Diameter and area reduction

Therapeutic Intervention 1% - 3%
A. Arterial, cerebral, and venous disease
1. Medical therapy
2. Surgical therapy
3. Nonsurgical intervention (angioplasty, atherectomy)
4. Compression therapy for pseudoaneurysms

Arterial Disease Testing 20% - 30%
A. Patient history (2% - 6%)
1. Signs and symptoms
   a. Chronic occlusive disease (claudication, rest pain, tissue loss)
   b. Acute arterial occlusion
   c. Cold sensitivity

   d. Mesenteric ischemia
   e. Renovascular hypertension
2. Risk factors and contributing diseases
   a. Diabetes
   b. Hypertension
   c. Hyperlipidemia
   d. Smoking
3. Mechanisms of disease
   a. Atherosclerosis
   b. Embolism
   c. Aneurysm
   d. Nonatherosclerotic lesions (arteritis, vasopastic disorders, entrapment syndromes)
B. Physical examination (1% - 5%)
1. Skin changes
2. Palpation (pulses/aneurysms)
3. Auscultation (bruits)
C. Noninvasive tests (patient positioning, technique, interpretation, capabilities, limitations) (15% - 19%)
1. Doppler velocimetry (audible, analog, waveforms, spectral waveforms)
   a. Qualitative interpretation
   b. Quantitative measurements (pulsatility index, damping factor, transit time, acceleration time)
2. Pressures
   a. Upper extremity
   b. Lower extremity
   c. Penile (impotence, varicocele)
3. Plethysmography (venous occlusion technique, volume pulse measurements)
   a. Upper extremity
   b. Lower extremity
   c. Digits
4. Duplex imaging (B-mode image, Doppler, color)
   a. Upper extremity
   b. Lower extremity
   c. Abdomen (aortoiliac segment, renal arteries, visceral arteries)
   d. Bypass grafts
   e. Organ transplants (renal, liver)
   f. Penile
   g. Intraoperative monitoring
D. Invasive tests (0% - 3%)
1. Arteriography (methods, interpretation, limitations)

Cerebral Artery Disease Testing 27% - 33%
A. Patient history (3% - 7%)
1. Signs and symptoms
   a. Transient symptoms
   b. Stroke
2. Risk factors and contributing diseases
   a. Diabetes
   b. Hypertension
3. Mechanisms of disease
   a. Stenosis

b. Embolism

c. Thrombosis

d. Subclavian steal

B. Physical examination (1% - 5%)

1. Neurological

2. Pulses

3. Bruits

C. Noninvasive tests (patient positioning, technique, interpretation, capabilities, limitations) (17% - 23%)

1. Indirect tests

a. Periorbital Doppler

b. Pressure ocular plethysmography

2. Direct tests

a. Continuous wave Doppler (audible, analog waveforms, spectral waveforms)

b. Pulsed Doppler (audible, spectral waveforms)

c. Duplex imaging (B-mode image, Doppler, color)

d. Transcranial Doppler

e. Intraoperative monitoring

D. Invasive tests (0% - 4%)

1. Arteriography (methods, interpretation, limitations)

Venous disease testing 25% - 35%

A. Patient history (3% - 7%)

1. Signs and symptoms

a. Acute deep vein thrombosis

b. Chronic venous insufficiency

2. Risk factors and contributing diseases

a. Age

b. Cancer

c. Bedrest

d. Previous deep vein thrombosis

e. Trauma

f. Acute paraplegia

3. Mechanisms of disease

a. Thrombosis

b. Valvular incompetence

c. Ambulatory venous hypertension

B. Physical examination (1% - 5%)

1. Skin changes

2. Lymphedema

3. Varicose veins

4. Venous ulcers

C. Noninvasive tests (patient positioning, technique, interpretation, capabilities, limitations) (18% - 22%)

1. Continuous wave Doppler

2. Plethysmography (strain gauge, photo)

3. Duplex imaging (B-mode image, Doppler color)

a. Upper extremity

b. Lower extremity

c. Abdomen (vena cava, portal, hepatic, renal, mesenteric)

D. Invasive tests (0% - 4%)

1. Venography (methods, interpretation limitations)

Other Conditions 0% - 3%

A. Arteriovenous fistula (traumatic, congenital, vascular access)

B. Trauma

C. Compartment syndrome

D. Thoracic outlet syndrome

Content guidelines reprinted with permission from the American Registry of Diagnostic Medical Sonographers, 1995, Cincinnati, Ohio.

Professional Organizations

For information on a career as a diagnostic medical sonographer, contact:

Society of Diagnostic Medical Sonographers
12770 Coit Road, Suite 508
Dallas, Texas 75251
(214) 235-7367

For information on acquiring registration as a diagnostic medical sonographer, contact:

American Registry of Diagnostic Medical Sonographers
2368 Victory Parkway, Suite 510
Cincinnati, Ohio 45206
(513) 281-7111

Listing of Programs

ARIZONA

Gateway Community College
108 North 40th Street
Phoenix, AZ 85034

CALIFORNIA

Orange Coast College
2701 Fairview Road
Costa Mesa, CA 92628

Loma Linda University
School of Allied Health Professions
Loma Linda, CA 92350

University of California Medical Center-San Diego
UCSD, Ultrasound H-759
225 Dickinson Street
San Diego, CA 92103

COLORADO

Penrose Hospital
2215 North Cascade Avenue, P.O. 7021
Colorado Springs, CO 80933

DELAWARE

Delaware Technical and Community College-Wilmington
333 Shipley Street
Wilmington, DE 19801

FLORIDA

Broward Community College
3501 Southwest Davie Road
Davie, FL 33314

University of Miami-Jackson Memorial Medical Center
1611 Northwest 12th Avenue
Miami, FL 33136-1094

Valencia Community College
1414 S Kuhl Avenue
Orlando, FL 32806

Palm Beach Community College
3160 PGA Boulevard
Palm Beach Gardens, FL 33410

Hillsborough Community College
P.O. Box 30030
Tampa, FL 33630-3030

GEORGIA

Emory University
Department of Radiology
1364 Clifton Road
Atlanta, GA 30322

Grady Memorial Hospital
P.O. Box 26095, 80 Butler Street, SE
Atlanta, GA 30335

Medical College of Georgia
AE-1003
Augusta, GA 30912-0600

ILLINOIS

Wilbur Wright College
4300 North Narragansett Avenue
Chicago, IL 60634

Triton College
2000 Fifth Avenue
River Grove, IL 60171

IOWA

University of Iowa Hospitals and Clinics
Newton Road
Iowa City, IA 52242

KENTUCKY

West Kentucky State Vocational Technical
P.O. Box 7408, Blandville Road
Paducah, KY 42002-7408

LOUISIANA

Alton Ochsner Medical Foundation
880 Commerce Road West
New Orleans, LA 70123-3335

MARYLAND

Essex Community College
7201 Rossville Boulevard
Baltimore, MD 21237

University of Maryland Baltimore County
UMBC Office of Continuing Education
Baltimore, MD 21228

Montgomery College
7600 Takoma Avenue
Takoma Park, MD 21228

MASSACHUSETTS

Middlesex Community College
Springs Road
Bedford, MA 01730

MICHIGAN

Henry Ford Hospital
2799 West Grand Boulevard
Detroit, MI 48202

Jackson Community College
2111 Emmons Road
Jackson, MI 49201

Oakland Community College
22322 Rutland Drive
Southfield, MI 48075

MINNESOTA

Mayo Foundation
200 First Street, SW
Rochester, MN 55905

MISSOURI

St. Luke's Hospital of Kansas City
4400 Wornall Road
Kansas City, MO 64111

St. Louis Community College at Forest Park
5600 Oakland Avenue
St. Louis, MO 63110

NEBRASKA

University of Nebraska Medical Center
Radiology Department/Ultrasound
600 South 42nd Street
Omaha, NE 68198-1045

NEW JERSEY

Elizabeth General Medical Center
925 East Jersey Street
Elizabeth, NJ 07201

University of Medicine and Dentistry of New Jersey
School of Health-Related Professions
65 Bergen Street
Newark, NJ 07107-3006

Bergen County Community College
400 Paramus Road
Paramus, NJ 07652-1595

NEW MEXICO

University of New Mexico School of Medicine
Basic Medical Sciences - Box 528
Albuquerque, NM 87131

NEW YORK

SUNY Health Science Center-Brooklyn
College of Health-Related Professions
450 Clarkson Avenue
Brooklyn, NY 11203

New York University Medical Center
Basic Science Building
342 East 26th Street
New York, NY 10010

Rochester Institute of Technology
One Lomb Memorial Drive
P.O. Box 9887
Rochester, NY 14623-0887

NORTH CAROLINA

Pitt Community College
P.O. Drawer 7007
Greenville, NC 27835-7007

Caldwell Community College and Technical Institute
1000 Hickory Boulevard
Hudson, NC 28638

Forsyth Technical Community College
2100 Silas Creek Parkway
Winston-Salem, NC 27103

OHIO

Aultman Hospital
2600 Sixth Street, SW
Canton, OH 44710

MetroHealth Medical Center
2500 Metrohealth Drive
Cleveland, OH 44109

Kettering College of Medical Arts
3737 Southern Boulevard
Kettering, OH 45429

Central Ohio Technical College
1179 University Drive
Newark, OH 43055-1767

Michael J. Owens Technical College
P.O. 10000, Oregon Road
Toledo, OH 43699-1947

OKLAHOMA

University of Oklahoma at Oklahoma City
Box 26901
Oklahoma City, OK 73190

PENNSYLVANIA

Polyclinic Medical Center
2601 North Third Street
Harrisburg, PA 17110

Community College of Allegheny County-Boyce Campus
595 Beatty Road
Monroeville, PA 15146

Thomas Jefferson University
130 South Ninth Street, Room 1004
Philadelphia, PA 19107

TEXAS

Austin Community College
1020 Grove Boulevard
Austin, TX 78741-3300

Del Mar College
Corpus Christi, TX 78404

El Centro College
Main and Lamar
Dallas, TX 75202

El Paso Community College
P.O. Box 20500
El Paso, TX 79998

UTAH

Weber State University
Ogden, UT 84408-1602

VIRGINIA

Tidewater Community College
1700 College Crescent
Virginia Beach, VA 23456

WASHINGTON

Bellevue Community College
3000 Landerholm Circle, SE, Room 243
Bellevue, WA 98009-2037

Seattle University
Broadway and Madison
Seattle, WA 98122-4460

WEST VIRGINIA

West Virginia University Hospital
P.O. Box 6401
Morgantown, WV 26506

WISCONSIN

Chippewa Valley Technical College
620 West Clairemont Avenue
Eau Claire, WI 54701

University of Wisconsin Hospital and Clinics
Department of Radiology
600 Highland Avenue
Madison, MI 53792

St. Francis Hospital
3237 South 16th Street
Milwaukee, WI 53215

St. Luke's Medical Center
2900 West Oklahoma
Milwaukee, WI 53215

St. Mary's Hospital
2323 North Lake Drive
Milwaukee, WI 53201

▲ *Nuclear Medicine*

Educational programs in nuclear medicine technology may be one, two, or four years in length, depending upon whether credits from an academic degree are included. The course of study will involve biology, anatomy, patient care, nuclear physics and instrumentation, computer technology, biochemistry, radiopharmacology, radiation biology and health physics, immunology, radionuclide therapy and statistics. Diagnostic procedures, imaging, and image evaluation including extensive clinical education will also constitute a major portion of the program.

Test Specifications

The education program will prepare the student to take the certification exam which includes the following content categories, weighted as shown in Table 15-1.

Table 15-1 Content Specifications for the Examination in Nuclear Medicine Technology

Content Category	Percent of Test	Number of Questions
A. Radiation Protection	11%	22
B. Radiopharmaceutical	11%	22
C. Instrumentation Quality Control	14%	28
D. Diagnostic Procedures	57%	114
E. Patient Care	7%	14

Copyright ©1994, The American Registry of Radiologic Technologists.

Analysis of Category Components

An approximate number of questions for each of the major subject areas is shown in the detailed listing below.

Radiation Protection—22

A. Biological effects of radiation—1
1. Dose-effect relationships
2. Somatic effects

B. Personnel protection and monitoring—6
1. Basic concepts (or fundamental principles)
   a. Units of measurement
   b. Dose equivalent limits (formerly MPD)

c. ALARA
2. Personnel protection
   a. Principles of time, distance and shielding
   b. Shielding (e.g., gloves, lab coats)
3. Personnel monitoring devices
   a. Types
   b. Use, care, and placement
4. NRC regulations for personnel exposure
   a. Occupational
   b. Public
   c. Minors
   d. During pregnancy
   e. Nursing mothers
5. Review and maintenance of accumulative dose records

C. Area/facilities monitoring—4
1. Basic concepts
   a. Units of measurement (e.g., mR/hr, dps)
   b. Exposure rates
   c. Definition of contaminated area
2. Survey equipment and techniques
   a. Well counters
   b. Survey meters
   c. Wipe test technique
3. Federal regulations
   a. Frequency of surveys
   b. Classification of areas (e.g., restricted, controlled)
   c. Posting of signs (types, locations)
   d. Documentation of survey results

D. Packaging and storage of radioactive materials—3
1. Physical properties of radioactive materials
   a. Types of emissions
   b. Energies
   c. Decay rate and half-life
   d. Physical form (gas, solution, capsule)
2. Inspection of incoming and outgoing materials
   a. Shipping labels (e.g., Category I)
   b. Measurement of radiation dose rate
3. Storage of radiopharmaceuticals
   a. Temperature of storage environment
   b. Consequences of improper storage

E. Radioactive contamination—2
1. Contamination
   a. Definition
   b. Levels of radiation (e.g., background)
   c. Potential contaminants
2. Decontamination procedures
   a. Containing spills
   b. Isolating the area
   c. Materials (e.g., absorbers, ventilation)
   d. Personnel (e.g., showering)
   e. Reporting procedures

F. Disposal of radioactive waste—3
  1. Nomenclature (e.g., half-life, radiation level)
  2. Methods of disposal per regulations
    a. Release to environment (wastewater, atmosphere)
    b. Storage for decay (e.g., container labeling, duration)
    c. Incineration
    d. Transfer to authorized recipient
    e. Package or container label

G. Misadministrations and recordable events—3
  1. Definitions
  2. Regulations for reporting and notification

Radiopharmaceutical Preparation—22

A. Elution of Mo-99/Tc-99m generator—3
  1. Design and function of a Mo-99/Tc-99m generator
    a. Wet column
    b. Dry column
  2. Elution techniques
    a. Eluant
    b. Volume of eluate
    c. Materials needed
    d. Aseptic technique
  3. Calculation of concentration of eluant
  4. Intervals for elution
    a. Specific activity
    b. Time of equilibrium

B. Quality control of Tc-99m eluate—3
  1. Radionuclidic purity
    a. Mo-99 breakthrough (reasons, limits)
    b. Measurement and expiration time
  2. Chemical purity
    a. Alumina breakthrough (reasons, limits)
    b. Measurement (colorimetric technique)

C. Kit preparation—4
  1. Methodologies
    a. Volume maximum and minimum
    b. Activity maximum and minimum
    c. Shelf life
    d. Storage
  2. Tagging process
    a. Principles
      1) Oxidation/reduction
      2) pH
      3) Time for reaction
      4) Temperature
    b. Compounding techniques
      1) Venting
      2) Heating
      3) Mixing
    c. Interfering agents (e.g., bacteriostatic agents, oxidants)

3. Radiochemical purity (thin-layer chromatography)
  a. Principles
  b. Technique and materials
  c. Types of impurities
  d. Limits

D. Radiopharmaceutical identification—2
  1. Nomenclature
    a. Radiopharmaceutical name
    b. Abbreviations (e.g., MDP, DTPA, MAA)
  2. Labeling information
    a. Radiation symbols
    b. Date and time
    c. Lot number and expiration date
    d. Concentration
  3. Records management

E. Dosage determination—7
  1. Patient age
  2. Patient weight - calculations and conversions
  3. Volume determination
    a. Physical factors (e.g., formula, decay tables, concentration)
    b. Application factors (e.g., static, dynamic, kit preparation)
  4. Units - calculations and conversions
  5. Records management

F. Dosage preparation—3
  1. Preparation for administration
    a. Syringe and needle selection
    b. Uniform distribution (mixing, agitation)
  2. Technique
    a. Aseptic
    b. Venting
    c. Shielding
  3. Assay in dose calibrator
  4. Records management

Instrumentation Quality Control—28

A. Survey meter quality control—2
  1. Operating principles of survey meter
  2. Frequency and types of checks
    a. Daily for precision
    b. Annually and postservice for calibration
  3. Source selection
    a. Activity
    b. Energy
  4. Interpretation of results
B. Dose calibrator quality control—4
  1. Operating principles of dose calibrator
  2. Types of checks
    a. Zero setting
    b. Accuracy

c. Constancy (precision)

d. Linearity

e. Geometry

3. Frequency of checks

　a. Initial use

　b. Daily

　c. Quarterly

　d. Annually and postservice

4. Source selection

　a. Activity

　b. Energy

5. Interpretation of results

C. Scintillation detector system—5

1. Radionuclide source

　a. Energies

　b. Type of source

2. Principles and operation of NaI scintillation detectors (well counter and uptake probe)

3. Parameters

　a. Energy resolution

　b. Efficiency

　c. High voltage calibration

　d. Deadtime

　e. Sensitivity

　f. Energy linearity

　g. Scaler accuracy

D. Gamma camera quality control—13

1. Sources and phantoms

2. Performance characteristics

　a. Uniformity

　b. Linearity

　c. Spatial resolution

　d. Sensitivity

　e. Extrinsic versus intrinsic measurements

　f. Correction circuitry

3. Collimators

　a. Parallel hole

　b. Converging

　c. Diverging

　d. Pinhole

4. SPECT

　a. Axis of rotation

　b. Uniformity correction

　c. Phantom measurements

　d. Resolution

E. Gas and aerosol delivery systems—2

1. Design and function

2. Exhaust system (e.g., negative ventilation, gas traps)

3. NRC regulations

F. Documentation—2

1. NRC requirements

2. JCAHO standards

Diagnostic Procedures—114

A. Scintillation camera and collimator selection—3

1. Collimator selection

　a. Parameters (e.g., energy, sensitivity)

　b. Types (e.g., parallel hole, converging, diverging, pinhole)

2. Scintillation camera selection

　a. Planar (small, large, whole body)

　b. SPECT

　c. Mobile

B. Parameter selection—5

1. Detector system

　a. Information density

　b. Count or time mode

　c. Static or dynamic mode

　d. Detector orientation

　e. Photopeak energy setting and window width

2. Recording

　a. Media (e.g., film, computer disk, paper)

　b. Format (single, multiple)

　c. Intensity

3. Computer acquisition

　a. Demographic data

　b. Mode selection (byte, word, list)

　c. Framing (number and length)

　d. Gating

　e. SPECT

　f. Archiving

C. Radiopharmaceutical selection—7

1. Correspondence to ordered procedure

2. Method of localization

　a. Capillary blockade

　b. Active transport

　c. Phagocytosis

　d. Simple/exchange diffusion

　e. Compartmentalization

　f. Chemisorption

　g. Cell sequestration

3. Half-life

　a. Physical

　b. Biological

　c. Effective

4. Emission characteristics (type, energy)

5. Patient dosimetry

　a. Target organ

　b. Critical organ

　c. Units of absorbed dose

D. Administration of radiopharmaceuticals—3

1. Routes (oral, intravenous, other)

2. Intravenous injection techniques
3. Factors affecting biodistribution
4. Recording administrations

E. Patient-camera positioning and monitoring—3
  1. Orientation of patient and detector system
  2. Persistence oscilloscope
  3. Topographic anatomy
  4. Conditions requiring immobilization
    a. Patient's ability to cooperate
    b. Pediatric patients
    c. Involuntary patient movement
    d. Patient and employee protection
  5. Immobilization techniques
    a. Physical restraints
    b. Sedation
    c. Potential problems (e.g., restriction of circulation, attenuation, patient motion)

F. Image management—2
  1. Automatic film processing
  2. Image labeling
    a. Patient identification
    b. Procedural view (e.g., LAO)
  3. Evaluation for study completeness

G. Evaluation of image quality—6
  1. Instrumentation
    a. Camera
    b. Film development and processing
      1) Fog
      2) Chemical contamination
      3) Temperature
      4) Handling artifacts
    c. Electronic image production (e.g., CRT, computer)
  2. Patient considerations
    a. Contamination (e.g., injection site, catheter)
    b. Positioning (e.g., alignment, motion)
    c. Artifacts (e.g., pathology, extrinsic)
  3. Radiopharmaceutical factors
    a. Biodistribution (normal and abnormal)
    b. Pathology

H. Gated procedures —1
  1. Equipment
    a. Gating mechanism
    b. ECG
    c. Detector system
    d. Computer
  2. Attachment and placement of ECG leads
  3. Sources of error (patient arrhythmia; equipment malfunction, etc.)

I. Computerized data processing—3
  1. Analysis
    a. Region of interest selection
    b. Histograms
    c. Gated
    d. SPECT
  2. Computer artifacts

J. Specific diagnostic procedures—79 (Also refer to the following box.)
  1. Type of study
    a. Abscess/infection—4
    b. Bone—13
    c. Brain (e.g., static, blood flow)—3
    d. Cisternography—1
    e. Cardiac (e.g., first pass, gated, myocardial infarction, myocardial perfusion)—15
    f. Endocrine (e.g., thyroid function and morphology, parathyroid)—8
    g. Gastrointestinal (e.g., gastric emptying, GI bleed, Meckel's, shunt studies, salivary)—7
    h. Genitourinary (e.g., renal function and morphology, cystography, testicular)—9
    i. Liver, spleen, and biliary function—6
    j. Lung (e.g., ventilation, aerosol, perfusion)—7
    k. Tumor/antibody—3
    l. Venography—1
    m. Nonimaging procedures: thyroid uptake; Schilling's—2

Focus of Questions

Questions about a specific study or procedure may address any of the following factors:

1. Instrumentation
  • Detector system
  • Data acquisition
  • Image recording
  • Data analysis
  • Ancillary equipment

2. Radiopharmaceuticals
  • Selection
  • Dosage
  • Administration
  • Biodistribution

3. Patient preparation and monitoring

4. Imaging techniques
  • Views
  • Patient-detector alignment

5. Anatomy and pathophysiology

K. Selected therapeutic procedures—2
  1. Selection of radiopharmaceuticals
    a. I-131 (hyperthyroidism, thyroid cancer)
    b. Others (e.g., P-32, Sr-89)
  2. Parameters
    a. Preparation
    b. Administration
    c. Monitoring
    d. Regulations

Patient Care and Management—14

A. Patient scheduling—3
  1. Radiopharmaceuticals
    a. Time between administration and imaging
    b. Availability
  2. Ancillary supplies
  3. Length of time to complete imaging procedures
    a. Inpatient versus outpatient
    b. Additional or delayed images
  4. Contraindications
    a. Conflicting medications (e.g., anticoagulant therapy, contrast media)
    b. Pathology
    c. Medical history
    d. Concerns for pregnant or nursing patients
  5. Sequencing of procedures

B. Patient identification and requisition forms—2
  1. Methods of patient identification
  2. Procedures requiring consent form
    a. Investigational drugs
    b. Patient age
  3. Compatibility of ordered procedure with technical capability
  4. Medical abbreviations

C. Patient considerations —2
  1. Route of radiopharmaceutical administration
  2. Preparation
    a. NPO, hydration, cleansing enemas, etc.
    b. Apparel
    c. Exercise
    d. Medications (e.g., sedation, timing)
  3. Specimen collection

D. Patient transport—1
  1. Hospital transport equipment (e.g., wheelchairs, carts, mobile lifting units)
  2. Body mechanics and patient transfer
  3. Special patient care needs (e.g., physical limitations, patient isolation, attached medical equipment)

E. Support systems—1
  1. Types (e.g., IVs, oxygen tanks, suction, indwelling catheters, chest tubes, ECG)
  2. Monitoring (e.g., subcutaneous infiltration, gauges on oxygen tanks)

F. Monitoring vital signs—1
  1. Normal ranges of vital signs
  2. Use of equipment (e.g., sphygmomanometer, stethoscope)

G. Emergency situations and adverse reactions—2
  1. Signs and symptoms of distress (e.g., shock, cardiac or respiratory arrest, seizure)
  2. Management (e.g., CPR, first aid)

H. Infection control —2
  1. Mechanism of transmission
  2. Aseptic and sterile technique
  3. Disinfection and cleaning
  4. Types of isolation
    a. Wound
    b. Enteric
    c. Reverse
    d. Respiratory
  5. Disposal of biohazardous materials

Professional Organizations

For information on a career as a nuclear medicine technologist, contact:

Society of Nuclear Medicine-Technologist Section
136 Madison Avenue
New York, New York 10016

For information on acquiring registration as a nuclear medicine technologist, contact:

American Registry of Radiologic Technologists
1255 Northland Drive
St. Paul, Minnesota 55120-1155
(612) 687-0048
or
Nuclear Medicine Technology Certification Board
2970 Clairmont Road, NE, Suite 610
Atlanta, Georgia 30329-1634
(404) 315-1739

Listing of Programs

ALABAMA

University of Alabama at Birmingham
School of Health Related Professions
UAB Station SHRP 214
Birmingham, AL 35294-1270

ARIZONA

Gateway Community College
108 North 40th Street
Phoenix, AZ 85034

ARKANSAS

Baptist Medical System
11900 Colonel Glenn Road, Suite 1000
Little Rock, AR 72210-2820

St. Vincent Infirmary Medical Center
Two St. Vincent Circle
Little Rock, AR 72205-5499

University of Arkansas for Medical Sciences
4301 West Markam, Slot 714
Little Rock, AR 72205

CALIFORNIA

California State University-Dominguez Hills
1000 East Victoria Street
Carson, CA 90747

Loma Linda University
Office of the Dean
Loma Linda, CA 92350

Charles R. Drew University of Medicine and Science
College of Allied Health Medical Imaging Technology
1621 East 120th Street
Los Angeles, CA 90059

Los Angeles County-USC Medical Center
1200 North State Street, P.O. Box 2082
Los Angeles, CA 90033

VA Medical Center of West Los Angeles-Wadsworth Division
Wilshire and Sawtelle Boulevards
Los Angeles, CA 90073

Sutter Community Hospitals
2801 L Street
Sacramento, CA 95816

University of California Medical Center-San Diego
200 West Arbor Drive
San Diego, CA 92103-8758

University of California-San Francisco
505 Parnassus Avenue
San Francisco, CA 94143

Cancer Foundation of Santa Barbara
300 West Pueblo Street, P.O. Box 837
Santa Barbara, CA 93105

COLORADO

Community College of Denver-Auraria Campus
P.O. Box 173363, Campus Box 950
Denver, CO 80217-3363

St. Anthony Hospitals
4231 West 16th Avenue
Denver, CO 80204

CONNECTICUT

St. Vincent's Medical Center
2800 Main Street
Bridgeport, CT 06606

Middlesex Community College
100 Training Hill Road
Middletown, CT 06457

Gateway Community-Technical College
60 Sargent Drive
New Haven, CT 06511

DELAWARE

Delaware Technical and Community College
Stanton-Wilmington Campus
333 Shipley Street
Wilmington, DE 19801

DISTRICT OF COLUMBIA

George Washington University Medical Center
2300 I Street, NW, Room 617
Washington, DC 20037

FLORIDA

Santa Fe Community College
3000 Northwest 83rd Street
Gainesville, FL 32606-6200

University of Miami-Jackson Memorial Medical Center
1611 Northwest 12th Avenue
Miami, FL 33136

Mt. Sinai Medical Center of Greater Miami
4300 Alton Road
Miami Beach, FL 33140

Valencia Community College
1800 South Kirkman Road
Orlando, FL 32811

Hillsborough Community College
P.O. Box 30030
Tampa, FL 33630

GEORGIA

Medical College of Georgia
Augusta, GA 30912

ILLINOIS

College of Du Page
Lambert Road and 22nd Street
Glen Ellyn, IL 60137-6599

Edward Hines Jr. VA Hospital
Fifth Avenue and Roosevelt Road
Hines, IL 60141

Triton College
2000 Fifth Avenue
River Grove, IL 60171

INDIANA

Ball State University
c/o Methodist Hospital of Indiana
1701 North Senate Boulevard
Indianapolis, IN 46202

Indiana University School of Medicine
541 Clinical Drive, CL 120
Indianapolis, IN 46202

IOWA

University of Iowa
Department of Radiology
Iowa City, IA 52242-1009

KENTUCKY

Lexington Community College
Cooper Drive-Oswald Bldg
Lexington, KY 40506-0235

University of Louisville
Health Sciences Center
Louisville, KY 40292

LOUISIANA

Alton Ochsner Medical Foundation
1516 Jefferson Highway
New Orleans, LA 70121

Delgado Community College
501 City Park Avenue
New Orleans, LA 70119

Overton Brooks VA Medical Center
510 E Stoner Avenue
Shreveport, LA 71101-4295

MARYLAND

Essex Community College
7201 Rossville Boulevard
Baltimore, MD 21237

Naval School of Health Sciences-MD
Bethesda, MD 20889-5611

Prince George's Community College
301 Largo Road
Largo, MD 20772

MASSACHUSETTS

Bunker Hill Community College
New Rutherford Avenue
Boston, MA 02129

Massachusetts College of Pharmacy and Allied Health
179 Longwood Avenue
Boston, MA 02215

Salem State College
352 Lafayette Street
Salem, MA 01970

Springfield Technical and Community College
One Armory Square
Springfield, MA 01105

University of Massachusetts Medical Center/
Worcester State College
University of Massachusetts Medical Center
55 Lake Ave North
Worcester, MA 06655

MICHIGAN

Ferris State University
200 Ferris Drive, VFS 411
Big Rapids, MI 49307

St. John Hospital and Medical Center
22101 Moross Road
Detroit, MI 48236

William Beaumont Hospital
3601 West 13 Mile Road
Royal Oak, MI 48073-6769

MINNESOTA

Mayo Foundation
School of Health-Related Sciences
200 First Street, SW
Rochester, MN 55905

St. Mary's College
700 Terrace Heights, #10
Winona, MN 55987-1399

MISSISSIPPI

University of Mississippi Medical Center
2500 North State Street
Jackson, MS 39216

MISSOURI

University of Missouri-Columbia
One Hospital Drive
Columbia, MO 65211

Research Medical Center
2316 East Meyer Boulevard
Kansas City, MO 64132

St Luke's Hospital of Kansas City
4400 Wornall Road
Kansas City, MO 64111

St Louis University
1504 South Grand Boulevard
St Louis, MO 63104

NEBRASKA

University of Nebraska Medical Center
600 South 42nd Street
Omaha, NE 68198-1045

NEVADA

University of Nevada
4505 Maryland Parkway
Las Vegas, NV 89154

NEW JERSEY

University of Medicine and Dentistry of New Jersey
School of Health-Related Professions
150 Bergen Street, Room H41
Newark, NJ 07103

Riverview Medical Center
One Riverview Plaza
Red Bank, NJ 07701

Gloucester County College
Deptford Township
Sewell, NJ 08080

Overlook Hospital
99 Beauvoir Avenue
Summit, NJ 07902-0220

NEW MEXICO

University of New Mexico School of Medicine
Health Science and Service Building, Room 214
Albuquerque, NM 87131

NEW YORK

CUNY Bronx Community College
University Ave and West 181st Street
Bronx, NY 10453

SUNY Health Science Center-Brooklyn
450 Clarkson Avenue
Brooklyn, NY 11203

SUNY at Buffalo
105 Parker Hall
Buffalo, NY 14226

Institute of Allied Medical Professions
23D 106 Central Park South
New York, NY 10019

New York University Medical Center
550 First Avenue
New York, NY 10016

St. Vincent's Hospital and Medical Center of New York
153 West 11th Street
New York, NY 10011

Northport VA Medical Center #632C
Middleville Road
Northport, NY 11768

Manhattan College
Manhattan College Parkway
Riverdale, NY 10471

Rochester Institute of Technology
One Lomb Memorial Drive, Box 9887
Rochester, NY 14623

Molloy College
1000 Hempstead Avenue
Rockville Centre, NY 11570

SUNY Health Science Center at Syracuse
750 East Adams Street
Syracuse, NY 13210

NORTH CAROLINA

University of North Carolina Hospitals
101 Manning Drive
Chapel Hill, NC 27514

Pitt Community College
P.O. Drawer 7007
Greenville, NC 27835-7007

Forsyth Technical Community College
2100 Silas Creek Parkway
Winston-Salem, NC 27103

OHIO

Aultman Hospital
2600 Sixth Street, SW
Canton, OH 44710

University of Cincinnati Medical Center
234 Goodman Street
Cincinnati, OH 45267

Ohio State University Hospitals
410 West 10th Avenue
Columbus, OH 43210

The University of Findlay
1000 North Main Street
Findlay, OH 45840

St. Elizabeth Hospital Medical Center
1044 Belmont Avenue
Youngstown, OH 44501

OKLAHOMA

University of Oklahoma at Oklahoma City
P.O. Box 26901
Oklahoma City, OK 73190

OREGON

Veterans Administration Medical Center
P.O. Box 1034 (115)
Portland, OR 97207

PENNSYLVANIA

Cedar Crest College
100 College Drive
Allentown, PA 18104-6196

Harrisburg Hospital
South Front Street
Harrisburg, PA 17101

Hospital of the University of Pennsylvania
3400 Spruce Street
Philadelphia, PA 19104

Temple University Hospital
3401 North Broad Street
Philadelphia, PA 19140

Community College of Allegheny County
Allegheny Campus
808 Ridge Avenue
Pittsburgh, PA 15212

Western Pennsylvania Hospital
4800 Friendship Avenue
Pittsburgh, PA 15224

Wilkes-Barre General Hospital
North River and Auburn Streets
Wilkes-Barre, PA 18764

PUERTO RICO

University of Puerto Rico
G.P.O. Box 5067
San Juan, PR 00936

RHODE ISLAND

Rhode Island Hospital
593 Eddy Street
Providence, RI 02902

SOUTH CAROLINA

Midlands Technical College
P.O. Box 2408
Columbia, SC 29202

SOUTH DAKOTA

Southeast Technical Institute
2301 Career Place
Sioux Falls, SD 57107

TENNESSEE

University of Tennessee Medical Center at Knoxville
1924 Alcoa Highway
Knoxville, TN 37920

Baptist Memorial Hospital
899 Madison Avenue
Memphis, TN 38146

Methodist Hospital of Memphis
1265 Union Avenue
Memphis, TN 38104

Vanderbilt University Medical Center
Radiology Department-Room R1317 MCN
21st and Garland, CCC-1124 MCN
Nashville, TN 37232-2675

TEXAS

Galveston College-University of Texas
4015 Avenue Q
Galveston, TX 77550

Baylor College of Medicine
1200 Moursund Street
Houston, TX 77030

Houston Community College System
3100 Shenandoah Street
Houston, TX 77021-1042

Incarnate Word College
4301 Broadway Street
San Antonia, TX 78209

UTAH

Weber State University
Odgen, UT 84408-1602

University of Utah Health Sciences Center
50 North Medical Drive
Salt Lake City, UT 84132

VERMONT

University of Vermont
004 Rowell Building
Burlington, VT 05405

VIRGINIA

University of Virginia Health Sciences Center
Jefferson Park Avenue, Box 486
Charlottesville, VA 22908

Old Dominion University
Norfolk, VA 23529-0287

Medical College of Virginia/
Virginia Commonwealth University
Department of Radiation Sciences
Box 495, MVC Station
Richmond, VA 23298-0495

Carilion Health Systems
Roanoke Memorial Hospitals
Belleview at Jefferson
Roanoke, VA 24033

WASHINGTON

Bellevue Community College
3000 Landerholm Circle, SE
Box 92700
Bellevue, WA 98009-2037

WEST VIRGINIA

West Virginia State College
P.O. Box 183
Institute, WV 25112

West Virginia University Hospital
Medical Center Drive, Box 6401
Morgantown, WV 26506

Wheeling Jesuit College
316 Washington Avenue
Wheeling, WV 26003

WISCONSIN

St. Joseph's Hospital
611 St. Joseph Avenue
Marshfield, WI 54449

Milwaukee County Medical Complex
8700 West Wisconsin Avenue
Milwaukee, WI 53226

St Luke's Medical Center
2900 West Oklahoma Avenue
Milwaukee, WI 53215

St Mary's Hospital
2323 North Lake Drive
Milwaukee, WI 53211

▲ *Radiation Therapy Technologist*

Educational programs in radiation therapy technology may be one, two, or four years in length, depending upon the inclusion of earned credit hours from an academic degree. The course of study will involve biology, radiation oncology, pathology, radiation biology, physics and equipment of radiation therapy, dosimetry, computer technology, hyperthermia, and quality assurance.

Test Specifications

The educational program will prepare the student for the certification exam in radiation therapy technology. The subject areas covered in the education program and the exam are shown in Table 15-2.

Table 15-2 Content Specifications for the Examination in Radiation Therapy Technology

Content Category	Percent of Test	Number of Questions
A. Radiation Protection and Quality Assurance	20%	40
B. Treatment Planning and Delivery	65%	130
C. Patient Care, Management, and Education	15%	30
	100%	200

Copyright ©1994, The American Registry of Radiologic Technologists.

Analysis of Category Components

An approximate number of questions for each of the major subject areas is shown in the detailed listing below.

Radiation Protection and Quality Assurance—40

A. Radiation protection—10
  1. Biological effects of radiation
    a. Somatic
    b. Genetic
  2. Monitoring of patients and radiation workers
    a. ALARA
    b. Dose equivalent limits
      1) Occupational
      2) Nonoccupational
    c. Personnel monitoring devices
    d. Documentation of accumulative occupational exposure
  3. Monitoring of area
    a. Controlled
    b. Uncontrolled
    c. Area monitoring devices
    d. Documentation of area monitoring
  4. Units of radiation
  5. Federal protection standards (e.g., NRC, NCRP, FDA)
  6. Basic methods of radiation protection
    a. Time
    b. Distance
    c. Shielding

B. Theory and principles of equipment operation—12
  1. Treatment units

a. Linear accelerators (photons, electrons)
b. Cobalt-60
c. Superficial/orthovoltage
d. Brachytherapy
2. Imaging units
a. Simulators
b. Linear accelerators
3. Production of radiation
a. Characteristics of radiation
b. Interactions with matter

C. Quality assurance procedures and assessment—12
1. Warm-up and troubleshooting of treatment units, automatic processors, and simulator
a. Interlock systems (e.g., door, filter)
b. Safety lights
c. Emergency switches (e.g., table, door, main circuit breaker)
d. Critical machine parameters (e.g., pressure, temperature)
e. Potential radiation and nonradiation hazards (e.g., electrical, mechanical)
2. Radiation output verification
a. Absorbed dose versus exposure dose
b. Methods for verifying radiation output
c. Frequency of output verification
d. Effect of barometric pressure, temperature, and humidity on ionization chambers
3. Light field, radiation field, and collimator indicator agreement
4. Rotation check
a. Safety procedures
b. Operation of gantry/console
5. Sidelight/laser check
a. Verification of isocenter
b. Techniques for verifying accuracy
6. Evaluation of quality assurance results
a. Significance of quality assurance results
b. Documentation and notification
c. Action plan

D. Environmental protection—6
1. Handling and disposal of toxic and hazardous materials (e.g., metals, chemicals)
a. Procedures
b. Regulations
2. Handling and disposal of radioactive materials
a. Procedures
b. Regulations

Treatment Planning and Delivery—130

A. Factors affecting simulation and treatment—28
1. Clinical concepts in radiation oncology
a. Radiosensitivity
b. Tissue tolerance and radiation pathology
c. Time, dose, and volume relationships
2. Principles of oncology (*The following may be covered: breast, head and neck, respiratory, reproductive, digestive, hematopoietic, urinary, nervous, bone, connective tissue, skin, endocrine, and pediatric.*)
a. Symptoms and signs
b. Histopathology
c. Staging principles (*Staging is covered only for true vocal cord, cervix, and Hodgkin's Disease.*)
d. Patterns of metastases
e. Multimodal treatment methods
7. Treatment results
3. Utilization of diagnostic information
a. Results of physical examination
b. Imaging studies (e.g., CT, MRI)
c. Surgical reports
d. Histologic reports

B. Treatment volume localization—29
1. Treatment techniques and anatomic relationships (*The following may be covered: breast, head and neck, respiratory, reproductive, digestive, hematopoietic, urinary, nervous, bone, connective tissue, skin, endocrine, and pediatric.*)
a. Radiation therapy techniques
b. Anatomy and physiology
c. Topographic and three-dimensional anatomy
d. Critical organs
e. Patient positioning and immobilization
1) Anatomical position
2) Positioning aids
3) Immobilization devices
4) Protective devices and techniques
2. General radiographic procedures
a. Film types
b. Cassettes/screens
c. Film placement
d. Exposure factors
e. Film processing
f. Film labeling
g. Magnification factors
h. Contrast media
1) Types and techniques
2) Contraindications
3) Risks and emergency procedures
3. Contours
a. Purpose
b. Devices and materials
c. Technique
1) Obtain contour
2) Mark and label contour
3) Transfer information from contour device
4. Documentation of simulation procedure
a. Anatomic position

b. Equipment orientation

c. Accessory equipment

d. Field parameters

e. Setup diagrams or photographs

C. Elements of treatment planning—25

1. Treatment prescription
   a. Total tumor dose
   b. Fractionation schedules
   c. Radiation energy
   d. Types of radiation
   e. Treatment volume
   f. Number of fields
   g. Fixed versus rotational fields
   h. Field weighting
   i. Field orientation
   j. Treatment unit capabilities and limitations
   k. Modifications

2. Geometric parameters and patient measurements
   a. Field size and shape
   b. Tumor depth
   c. Patient thickness
   d. SSD, SAD
   e. Collimator setting

3. Factors involved in dose calculation
   a. Equivalent square
   b. Backscatter factor
   c. Percentage depth dose
   d. TAR, TMR
   e. SSD, SAD
   f. Mayneord's F factor
   g. Roentgen to cGy (rad) conversion factor
   h. Wedges (e.g., wedge angle or factor)
   i. Off-axis calculation (e.g., scatter functions, scatter/air ratios)
   j. Field shape correction factors
   k. Isodose curves and their characteristics (e.g., penumbra)
   l. Factors for beam modifiers (e.g., tray factor, bolus, compensator)
   m. Tissue transmission factors
   n. Rotational factors

4. Calculation of doses
   a. Selection of energy/radiation tables
   b. Equivalent square tables
   c. Depth dose, TAR or TMR data
   d. Machine output data (e.g., cGy/min)
   e. Units of dose measurement
   f. Calculation procedure

5. Calculation verification
   a. Documentation of calculations
   b. Accuracy
   c. Legal aspects

D. Dose to critical structures—15

1. Radiation tolerance of tissues and organs
   a. Radiobiological factors (e.g., dose, time, volume, energy, OER, RBE)
   b. Biological factors (e.g., age, physical status, concurrent medications)
   c. Contribution of dose from brachytherapy
   d. Contribution of effect from chemotherapy or radiation effect modifiers
   e. Contribution of dose from other fields (e.g., prior fields, gap calculations)

2. Effect of anatomical or physiological variation on dose distribution

3. Adverse effects of dose

E. Treatment accessories —5

1. Types of devices (e.g., immobilization devices, compensating filters, bolus, blocks)

2. Fabrication methods

3. Fabrication materials

4. Parameters necessary for fabrication
   a. SSD, SAD
   b. Source-film distance (SFD)
   c. Collimator settings
   d. Source-to-block tray distance (STD)
   e. Patient thickness
   f. Block thickness, half-value layer (HVL), half-value thickness (HVT)

F. Setup of treatment machine—9

1. Machine operation
   a. SSD, SAD
   b. Collimator or cone settings
   c. Optical or mechanical distance indicator
   d. Gantry angle
   e. Collimator angle
   f. Field light
   g. Treatment couch
   h. Console controls

2. Use of auxiliary setup devices and beam modifiers (e.g., alignment lasers, wedges, compensators, positioning aids, blocks)

G. Monitoring patient and treatment room—3

1. Patient monitoring systems
   a. Direct visual
   b. Indirect visual (mirror, TV monitor)
   c. Two-way voice communication system
   d. Backup systems

2. Monitoring regulations

H. Monitoring treatment machine—4

1. Identification and management of machine malfunctions
   a. Radiation

   b. Electrical
   c. Mechanical
   2. Documentation and reporting of malfunctions

I. Verification imaging—3
   1. Purpose
   2. Labeling
   3. Enacting change

J. Radiation treatment record keeping—9
   1. Treatment documentation
      a. Prescription verification
      b. Dmax dose (daily and accumulated)
      c. Monitor units or time
      d. Tumor dose (daily and accumulated)
      e. Energy and type of radiation
      f. Date
      g. Time of day for b.i.d. treatment
      h. Fraction
      i. Elapsed days
      j. Field number and description
      k. Doses to other points of interest
      l. Setup instructions
   2. Elements of record keeping
      a. Accuracy and legibility
      b. Documentation of variance from original prescription (errors, prescription changes)
      c. Notification requirements, including misadministrations, reportable events, equipment malfunctions
   3. Legal issues
      a. Accountability (e.g., signatures)
      b. Informed consent
      c. Reconstruction of treatment
      d. Patient identification

Patient Care, Management, and Education—30

A. Ethics —2
   1. Patients' bill of rights
   2. Professional code of ethics

B. Professional interactions —4
   1. Communication
      a. Patient
      b. Patient's family and friends
      c. Other health care professionals
   2. Identification of patient concerns and special needs
   3. Patient education regarding simulation and treatment
      a. Positioning and immobilization (including skin marks)
      b. Duration of treatment
      c. Patient comfort
      d. Auditory and visual communication
      e.

   Machine characteristics (e.g., type, movement, noises, patient contact)
      f. Auxiliary equipment
   4. Referral to available resources

C. Assessment, care, and management—12
   1. Treatment side effects
      a. Physiological
      b. Emotional
      c. Radiation-induced
   2. Skin care
      a. Maintenance of marks
      b. Bathing techniques
      c. Potential skin irritants
   3. Blood studies
      a. Normal hematological values
         1) WBC
         2) RBC, hematocrit, and hemoglobin
         3) Platelet
      b. Factors affecting blood values during treatment
         1) Radiation
         2) Chemotherapy
         3) Overall medical status
   4. Nutrition and dietary counseling
      a. Causes of abnormal nutritional status
      b. Routes of nutrition (e.g., oral, IV, feeding tubes, total parenteral nutrition)
      c. Nutritional groups (e.g., carbohydrates, fats, proteins)
      d. Significance of weight change
      e. Identification of needs
      f. Dietary management (e.g., supplements, low-residue diets)
      g. Referral

D. Physical assistance of patients —3
   1. Effect of patient condition
      a. Age of patient
      b. Extent of disease
      c. Physical and mental limitations
   2. Body mechanics
   3. Patient transfer
   4. Positioning and monitoring of accessory medical equipment
      a. Infusion catheters and pumps
      b. Chest tubes
      c. Oxygen delivery systems
      d. Nasogastric and gastrostomy tubes
      e. Urinary catheters
      f. Tracheostomy tubes
      g. Pacemakers
      h. Other

E. Universal precautions and infection control—5
   1. Sterile technique

2. Isolation procedures
3. Reverse isolation procedures
4. Handling and disposal of contaminated material (e.g., body fluids)
    a. Protective technique and devices
    b. Regulations

F. Medical emergencies—4
    1. Allergic reactions
    2. Cardiac or respiratory arrest
        a. CPR
        b. Code status (DNR)
    3. Physical injury
    4. Other medical disorders (e.g., seizures, diabetic reactions)

Copyright ©1994, The American Registry of Radiologic Technologists.

Professional Organizations

For information on a career as a radiation therapist, contact:

American Society of Radiologic Technologists
15000 Central Avenue, SE
Albuquerque, New Mexico 87123
(505) 298-4500

For information on acquiring registration as a radiation therapist, contact:

American Registry of Radiologic Technologists
1255 Northland Drive
St. Paul, Minnesota 55120-1155
(612) 687-0048

Listing of Programs

ALABAMA

University of Alabama at Birmingham
School of Health-Related Professions
UAB Station
Birmingham, AL 35294-1270

Mobile Infirmary Medical Center
P.O. Box 2144
Mobile, AL 36652

ARIZONA

University Medical Center
1501 North Campbell Avenue
Tucson, AZ 85724

ARKANSAS

Northwest Arkansas Community College
P.O. Box 1408
Bentonville, AR 72712

CARTI School of Radiation Therapy Technology
Markham and U, Box 5210
Little Rock, AR 72215

CALIFORNIA

City of Hope National Medical Center
1500 East Duarte Road
Duarte, CA 91010

Loma Linda University
Office of the Dean
Loma Linda, CA 92350

California State University-Long Beach
1250 Bellflower Boulevard
Long Beach, CA 90840-4902

Foothill Community College
12345 El Monte Road
Los Altos Hills, CA 94022

Los Angeles County-USC Medical Center
1200 North State Street
Los Angeles, CA 90033

Radiology Association of Sacramento Medical Group
1800 I Street
Sacramento, CA 95814

U of California Medical Center-San Diego
225 Dickinson Street
San Diego, CA 92103-8757

City College of San Francisco
50 Phelan Avenue
San Francisco, CA 94112

Cancer Foundation of Santa Barbara
300 East Pueblo Street
Santa Barbara, CA 93105

COLORADO

Community College of Denver-Auraria Campus
P.O. Box 173363, Campus Box 950
Denver, CO 80217-3363

CONNECTICUT

Hartford Hospital
80 Seymour Street
Hartford, CT 06115

Gateway Community-Technical College
60 Sargent Drive
New Haven, CT 06511

DISTRICT of COLUMBIA

George Washington University Medical Center
901 23rd Street, NW
Washington, DC 20037

Howard University Hospital
2041 Georgia Avenue, NW
Washington, DC 20059

FLORIDA

Broward Community College
1000 Coconut Creek Boulevard, Building 41
Coconut Creek, FL 33066

Halifax Medical Center
303 North Clyde Morris Boulevard
P.O. Box 2830
Daytona Beach, FL 32115-2830

Radiation Therapy Regional Centers
7341 Gladiolus Drive
Fort Meyers, FL 33908

Santa Fe Community College
P.O. Box 1530
Gainesville, FL 32606-6206

St. Vincent's Medical Center
1800 Barrs Street, P.O. Box 2982
Jacksonville, FL 32203

Miami-Dade Community College
950 Northwest 20th Street
Miami, FL 33127

Florida Hospital Medical Center
College of Health Sciences
601 East Rollins
Orlando, FL 32803

Valencia Community College
P.O. Box 3028
Orlando, FL 32802

Hillsborough Community College
P.O. Box 30030
Tampa, FL 33630

GEORGIA

Grady Memorial Hospital
80 Butler Street, SE
P.O. Box 26095
Atlanta, GA 30335-3801

Medical College of Georgia
Building HK-MCG
Augusta, GA 30912-3965

Armstrong State College
11935 Abercorn Street
Savannah, GA 31419

IDAHO

St. Luke's Regional Medical Center
Mountain State Tumor Institute
151 East Bannock Street
Boise, ID 83712

ILLINOIS

Parkland College
2400 West Bradley Avenue
Champaign, IL 61821-1899

Chicago State University
9501 South King Drive
Chicago, IL 60628

University of Chicago Hospital
Roosevelt University
5841 South Maryland Avenue, Box 442
Chicago, IL 60637

St. Joseph Hospital
77 North Airlite Street
Elgin, IL 60123

National-Louis University
2840 North Sheridan Road
Evanston, IL 60201

Edward Hines Jr. VA Hospital
Fifth Avenue and Roosevelt Road
Hines, IL 60141

Swedish American Hospital
1400 Charles Street
Rockford, IL 61104

INDIANA

Welborn Baptist Hospital
700 North Burkhardt Road
Evansville, IN 47715

Indiana University School of Medicine
535 Barnhill Drive, Route 071
Indianapolis, IN 46223

Methodist Hospital of Indiana, Inc.
I-65 at 21st Street
Indianapolis, IN 46206

Memorial Hospital of South Bend
615 North Michigan Avenue
South Bend, IN 46601

IOWA

University of Iowa Hospitals and Clinic
200 Hawkins Drive, W1892 GH
Iowa City, IA 52242

KANSAS

University of Kansas Medical Center
3901 Rainbow Boulevard
Kansas City, KS 66160

Washburn University
1700 College Avenue
Topeka, KS 66621

KENTUCKY

University of Kentucky Chandler Medical Center
800 Rose Street, Room N-13
Lexington, KY 40536-0084

James Graham Brown Cancer Center
529 South Jackson Street
Louisville, KY 40202

St. Anthony Medical Center
1313 St. Anthony Place
Louisville, KY 40204

LOUISIANA

Alton Ochsner Medical Foundation
880 Commerce Road West
New Orleans, LA 70123-3335

MAINE

Southern Maine Technical College
2 Fort Road
South Portland, ME 04106

MARYLAND

Essex Community College
7201 Rossville Boulevard
Baltimore, MD 21237

MASSACHUSETTS

Laboure College
2120 Dorchester Avenue
Boston, MA 02124

Massachusetts College of Pharmacy and Allied Health
179 Longwood Avenue
Boston, MA 02115

Springfield Technical and Community College
One Armory Square
Springfield, MA 01105

University of Massachusetts Med Center/
Worcester State College
55 Lake Avenue North
Worcester, MA 01605

MICHIGAN

University of Michigan Medical Center
Box 0010, Room B2C490
Ann Arbor, MI 48109

Wayne State University
Shapero Annex, Room 121
Detroit, MI 48202

Henry Ford Hospital
2799 West Grand Boulevard
Detroit, MI 48202

Lansing Community College
Department of Health Careers - 34
P.O. Box 40010
Lansing, MI 48901

MINNESOTA

University of Minnesota Health Science Center
Harvard Street at East River Rodd
Box 494, Unit J
Minneapolis, MN 55455

Mayo Foundation
School of Health-Related Sciences
200 First Street, SW
Rochester, MN 55905

MISSISSIPPI

University of Mississippi Medical Center
2500 North State Street
Jackson, MS 39216

MISSOURI

St. Luke's Hospital of Kansas City
4400 Wornall Road
Kansas City, MO 64111

Barnes Hospital
One Barnes Hospital Plaza
St Louis, MO 63110

NEBRASKA

University of Nebraska Medical Center
600 South 42nd Street
Omaha, NE 68198-1045

NEW JERSEY

Cooper Hospital/University Medical Center
One Cooper Plaza
Camden, NJ 08103

St. Barnabas Medical Center
Old Short Hills Road
Livingston, NJ 07039

St. Peter's Medical Center
254 Easton Avenue
New Brunswick, NJ 08901

NEW MEXICO

University of New Mexico School of Medicine
Health Sciences and Services Building
Albuquerque, NM 87131

NEW YORK

Montefiore Medical Center
111 East 210th Street
Bronx, NY 10467

Methodist Hospital of Brooklyn
506 Sixth Street
Brooklyn, NY 11215

Erie Community College
121 Ellicott Street-City Campus
Buffalo, NY 14203

Nassau Community College
Stewart Avenue
Garden City, NY 11530

Memorial Sloan-Kettering Cancer Center
1275 York Avenue
New York, NY 10021

University of Rochester
601 Elmwood Avenue, P.O. Box 647
Rochester, NY 14642

Staten Island University Hospital-North
475 Seaview Avenue
Staten Island, NY 10305

SUNY Health Science Center at Syracuse
750 East Adams Street
Syracuse, NY 13210

NORTH CAROLINA

University of North Carolina hospitals
101 Manning Drive
Chapel Hill, NC 27514

Pitt Community College
P.O. Drawer 7007
Greenville, NC 27835-7007

Forsyth Technical Community College
2100 Silas Creek Parkway
Winston-Salem, NC 27103

OHIO

Aultman Hospital
2600 Sixth Street, SW
Canton, OH 44710

University of Cincinnati
234 Goodman Street
Cincinnati, OH 45267

Cleveland Clinic Foundation
One Clinic Center
9500 Euclid Avenue
Cleveland, OH 44195-5130

University Hospitals of Cleveland
School of Radiation Therapy Technology
2074 Abington Road
Cleveland, OH 44106

Ohio State University Hospitals
Arthur G. James Cancer Hospital and Research Institute
300 West 10th Avenue
Columbus, OH 43210-1228

Michael J. Owens Technical College
P.O. 10000, Oregon Road
Toledo, OH 43699-1947

OKLAHOMA

University of Oklahoma at Oklahoma City
Box 26901
Oklahoma City, OK 73190

OREGON

Oregon Health Sciences University
3181 Southwest Sam Jackson Park Road
Portland, OR 97201

PENNSYLVANIA

Mercy Regional Health System
2500 Seventh Avenue
Altoona, PA 16603-2099

Geisinger Medical Center
North Academy Avenue
Danville, PA 17822-2007

Gwynedd-Mercy College
Sumneytown Pike
Gwynedd Valley, PA 19437

Community College of Allegheny County
Allegheny Campus
808 Ridge Avenue
Pittsburgh, PA 15212

Western Pennsylvania Hospital
4800 Friendship Avenue
Pittsburgh, PA 15224

RHODE ISLAND

Rhode Island Hospital
593 Eddy Street
Providence, RI 02902

SOUTH CAROLINA

Medical University of South Carolina
College of Health-Related Professions
171 Ashley Avenue
Charleston, SC 29425

TENNESSEE

Chattanooga State Technical Community College
4501 Amnicola Highway
Chattanooga, TN 37406-1097

Baptist Memorial Hospital
809 Madison Avenue, #285A
Memphis, TN 38146

Methodist Hospital of Memphis
1265 Union Avenue
Memphis, TN 38104

Vanderbilt University Medical Center
Radiation Oncology
The Vanderbilt Clinic-B902
Nashville, TN 37232-5671

TEXAS

Amarillo College
2200 South Washington, P.O. Box 447
Amarillo, TX 79178-0001

Shiver Cancer Center
2600 East Martin Luther King Boulevard
Austin, TX 78702

Baylor University Medical Center
3500 Gaston Avenue
Dallas, TX 75246

El Paso Community College
P.O. Box 20500
El Paso, TX 79998

Moncrief Radiation Center
1450 Eighth Avenue
Fort Worth, TX 76104

Galveston College-University of Texas
4015 Avenue Q
Galveston, TX 77550

University of Texas M. D. Anderson Cancer Center
1515 Holcombe Boulevard, Box 701
Houston, TX 77030

Methodist Hospital
3615 19th Street
Lubbock, TX 79410

Cancer Therapy and Research Center
4450 Medical Drive
San Antonio, TX 78229

UTAH

Weber State University
Ogden, UT 84408-1602

LDS Hospital
8th Avenue and C Street
Salt Lake City, UT 84143

University of Utah Health Sciences Center
50 North Medical Drive
Salt Lake City, UT 84132

VERMONT

University of Vermont
004 Rowell Building
Burlington, VT 05405

VIRGINIA

University of Virginia Health Science Center
Jefferson Park Avenue, Box 383
Charlottesville, VA 22908

Sentara Norfolk General Hospital
600 Gresham Drive
Norfolk, VA 23507

Medical College of Virginia/
Virginia Commonwealth University
Department of Radiation Sciences
Box 495, MCV Station
Richmond, VA 23298-0495

Carilion Health Systems
Roanoke Memorial Hospitals
Belleview at Jefferson Street
Roanoke, VA 24033

WASHINGTON

Bellevue Community College
3000 Landerholm Circle, SE
Bellevue, WA 98007-6484

WEST VIRGINIA

West Virginia University Hospital
1244 University Hospital
Morgantown, WV 26506-8150

WISCONSIN

University of Wisconsin Hospital and Clinics
600 Highland Avenue (K4/B100)
Madison, WI 53792

Medical College of Wisconsin
8701 Watertown Plank Road
Milwaukee, WI 53226

St. Joseph's Hospital
5000 West Chambers Street
Milwaukee, WI 53210

St. Luke's Medical Center
2900 West Oklahoma Avenue, P.O. Box 2901
Milwaukee, WI 53201-2901

▲ *Advanced-Level Examinations*

The American Registry of Radiologic Technologists offers examinations leading to certificates of advanced qualifications in the radiologic specialties of computed tomography, magnetic resonance imaging, cardiovascular-interventional technology, and mammography. These examinations do not lead to certification because there are, as yet, no formal educational requirements to enter these specialties.

In the following sections, the general requirements for taking each exam are listed along with the content specifications for each exam. For full details concerning advanced-level examinations the reader should contact:

The American Registry of Radiologic Technologists
1255 Northland Drive
St. Paul, MN 55120-1155
(612) 687-0048

Computed Tomography

Candidates must be in compliance with the "Rules of Ethics" which are part of the *Standards of Ethics* of the ARRT and must meet all requirements as stated in the *Examinee Handbook*. In addition, candidates must be registered in radiography or radiation therapy technology with at least one year having elapsed since passing the certification exam. Content specifications for the computed tomography exam are provided in Table 15-3.

Table 15-3 Content Specifications for the Examination in Computed Tomography

Content Category	Number of Questions
A. Patient Care	30
B. Imaging Procedures	75
C. Physics and Instrumentation	45
	150

Copyright ©1994, The American Registry of Radiologic Technologists.

Analysis of Category Components

An approximate number of questions for each of the major subject areas is shown in the detailed listing below.

Patient Care—30

A. Patient preparation—4
  1. Screening/consent
  2. Patient education

B. Assessment and monitoring—6
  1. History
  2. Physical status
    a. Level of consciousness
    b. Respiration
    c. Conscious sedation
  3. Life-threatening situations
  4. Lab values
    a. BUN
    b. Creatinine
    c. PT
    d. PTT
    e. Platelet

C. IV procedures—8
  1. Aseptic and sterile technique
    a. Butterfly
    b. Angiocatheter
  2. Site selection
  3. Injection rate
    a. Manual
      1) Bolus
      2) Drip
    b. Automatic
      1) Volume
      2) Rate

D. Contrast agents—9
  1. Types
    a. Ionic
    b. Nonionic
    c. Barium sulfate
    d. Water soluble
  2. Administration route
    a. IV
    b. Oral
    c. Rectal
    d. Catheter
  3. Dose calculations
    a. IV
    b. Oral
  4. Special considerations
    a. Allergy preparation
    b. Pathologic processes
    c. Contraindications

d. Indications
5. Adverse reactions
   a. Symptoms
   b. Treatment

E. Radiation safety—3
   1. Technical factors affecting patient dose
   2. Gonadal shielding
   3. Fetal-embryonic effects

Focus of Questions

Questions about each of the studies listed may focus on any of the following relevant factors:

1. Anatomy and physiology
   • Sagittal plane
   • Transverse plane
   • Coronal plane
   • Off-axis (oblique)
   • Landmarks

2. Contrast Media
   • Types of agents
   • Indications
   • Contraindications
   • Dose calculation
   • Administration route
   • Effects on image

3. Scanning procedures
   • Scout
   • Acquisition methods (e.g., spiral, dynamic, high resolution, conventional)
   • Parameter selection (e.g., slice thickness, mA, time, algorithm)
   • Recognition of pathology or trauma

4. Special procedures
   • Three-dimensional studies
   • Biopsies
   • Radiation therapy planning
   • Stereotaxis
   • Drainage and aspiration

Imaging Procedures—75 (Also refer to the above box).

A. Type of study
   1. Head —15
      a. Cranial nerves
      b. Internal auditory canal
      c. Petrous pyramid
      d. Pituitary
      e. Orbit
      f. Sinuses
      g. Maxillofacial
      h. Temporomandibular joint
      i. Posterior fossa
      j. Supratentorium
   2. Neck—3
      a. Larynx
      b. Soft tissue neck
   3. Spine—11
      a. Cervical
      b. Thoracic
      c. Lumbosacral
      d. Post myelography
   4. Chest—15
      a. Vascular
      b. Mediastinum
      c. Lung
      d. Heart
   5. Abdomen —15
      a. Liver
      b. Spleen
      c. Pancreas
      d. Adrenals
      e. Kidneys
      f. Peritoneum
      g. Retroperitonem
      h. GI tract
      i. Vascular
      j. Gall bladder
   6. Pelvis —12
      a. Bladder
      b. Rectum
      c. Ovary
      d. Uterus
      e. Prostate
      f. Testes
   7. Musculoskeletal —4
      a. Upper extremity
      b. Lower extremity
      c. Sternum
      d. Pelvic girdle; hips

Physics and Instrumentation—45

A. System operation and components—9
   1. Tube
   2. Detector
   3. Collimation
   4. Computer and array processor

B. Image processing and display—16
   1. Image reconstruction
      a. Filtered back projection reconstruction
      b. Reconstruction filter
      c. Raw data versus image data
      d. Retrospective reconstruction

2. Image display
   a. Pixel, voxel
   b. Matrix
   c. Image magnification
   d. Field of view (scan, reconstruction and display)
   e. Attenuation coefficient
   f. CT number
   g. Partial volume averaging
   h. Window level, window width
   i. Plane specification (x, y, z coordinates)
3. Post-processing
   a. Multiplanar reformation
   b. Three-dimensional surface rendering
4. Data management
   a. Hard copy (film)
   b. Storage/archival copy

C. Image quality —11
   1. Spatial resolution
   2. Contrast resolution
   3. Noise
   4. Quality assurance

D. Artifacts—9
   1. Beam hardening
   2. Partial volume artifact
   3. Motion
   4. Metallic
   5. Edge gradient
   6. Equipment-induced
      a. Rings
      b. Streaks
      c. Tube arcing
   7. Artifact reduction

Magnetic Resonance Imaging

Candidates must be in compliance with the "Rules of Ethics" which are part of the *Standards of Ethics* of the ARRT and must meet all requirements as stated in the *Examinee Handbook*. In addition, candidates must be registered in radiography, radiation therapy technology, or nuclear medicine technology with at least one year having elapsed since passing the certification exam. Content specifications for the magnetic resonance imaging examination are provided in Table 15-4.

Table 15-4 Content Specifications for the Examination in Magnetic Resonance Imaging

Content Category	Number of Questions
A. Patient Care and MRI Safety	17
B. Imaging Procedures	53
C. Data Acquisition and Processing	62
D. Physical Principles of Image Formation	43
	175

Analysis of Category Components

An approximate number of questions for each of the major subject areas is shown in the detailed listing below.

Patient Care and MRI Safety—17

A. Screening—3
   1. Patients
   2. Ancillary equipment
   3. Personnel

B. Assessment and monitoring—3
   1. Sedated patients
   2. Adverse reactions to contrast
   3. Life-threatening situations

C. Safety precautions—6
   1. Placement of electrical conductors (e.g., ECG leads, coils, cables)
   2. Environmental considerations
      a. Temperature
      b. Humidity
      c. Gauss lines (5G, 10G)
      d. Magnetic shielding
      e. RF shielding
   3. Emergency procedures
      a. Quench
      b. Evacuation

D. Biological considerations—5
   1. Radio frequency
      a. FDA guidelines
      b. Specific absorption rate

c. Potential biological effects
2. Static field strength
   a. FDA guidelines
   b. Tesla
   c. Potential biological effects
3. Gradient field
   a. FDA guidelines
   b. Time-varying magnetic fields
   c. Potential biological effects

Focus of Questions

Questions about each of the studies listed may focus on any of the following factors:

1. Anatomy and physiology
   - Sagittal plane
   - Transverse plane
   - Coronal plane
   - Off-axis (oblique)

2. Patient positioning
   - Coil selection and position
   - Patient orientation
   - Landmarking
   - Physiologic gating and triggering

3. Indications for contrast
   - Type of agent (FDA approved)
   - Contraindications
   - Dose calculation
   - Administration route
   - Mechanism of action
   - Effects on image

Imaging Procedures—53 (Also refer to the box above.)

A. Type of Study
   1. Head and neck—14
      a. Brain
      b. Internal auditory canal
      c. Pituitary
      d. Orbit
      e. Cranial nerves
      f. Soft tissue neck
   2. Spine—10
      a. Cervical
      b. Thoracic
      c. Lumbosacral
   3. Thorax—3
      a. Brachial plexus
      b. Cardiovascular
      c. Breast
   4. Abdomen—7
      a. Liver, spleen, pancreas
      b. Kidneys, adrenals
      c. Retroperitoneum
   5. Pelvis—5
      a. Female
      b. Male
   6. Musculoskeletal—10
      a. Temporomandibular joint
      b. Upper extremities
      c. Lower extremities
   7. Vascular—4
      a. Head and neck
      b. Body
      c. Extremities

Data Acquisition and Processing—62

A. Pulse sequences - 12
   1. Spin echo
      a. Conventional spin echo
      b. Fast spin echo
   2. Inversion recovery
   3. Gradient recall echo
      a. Conventional gradient echo
      b. Fast gradient echo

B. Data manipulation—6
   1. K-space mapping and filling
   2. Fourier transformation
   3. Maximum intensity projection
   4. Multiplanar reconstruction

C. Special procedures - 6
   1. MR angiography
      a. Flow dynamics
      b. Time-of-flight principles
      c. Phase contrast principles
   2. Cine
      a. Cardiac
      b. Musculoskeletal

Focus of Questions

Questions will address the interdependence of the imaging parameters and options listed, and how those parameters and options affect image quality and contrast.

1. Image quality
   - Contrast-to-noise
   - Signal-to-noise
   - Spatial resolution
   - Acquisition time

2. Contrast
   - T_1 weighted
   - T_2 weighted
   - Spin (proton) density

D. Sequence parameters and options—38 (Also refer to the box above.)

1. Imaging parameters
   a. TR
   b. TE
   c. T_1
   d. Number of signal averages
   e. Flip angle
   f. FOV
   g. Matrix
   h. Number of slices
   i. Slice thickness and gap
   j. Phase and frequency
   k. Echo train length
   l. Effective TE (target TE)

2. Imaging options
   a. Dimensionality (two-dimensional versus three-dimensional)
   b. Bandwidth
   c. Slice order
   d. Saturation pulse
   e. Gradient moment nulling
   f. Fat suppression
   g. Physiologic gating and triggering

Physical Principles of Image Formation—43

A. Instrumentation—15
   1. Electromagnetism
      a. Faraday's law
      b. Types of magnets (superconductive, permanent, resistive)
   2. Radiofrequency system
      a. Coil configuration
      b. Transmit and receive coils
      c. Transmit and receive bandwidth
      d. Coil tuning
      e. Pulse profile
   3. Gradient system
      a. Coil configuration
      b. Amplitude (+, -)
      c. Rise time

B. Fundamentals —20
   1. Nuclear magnetism
      a. Equilibrium
      b. Vectors
      c. X, Y, Z coordinate system
   2. Larmor frequency
      a. Precession
      b. Gyromagnetic ratio
      c. Resonance
      d. RF pulse
   3. Tissue characteristics
      a. T_1 relaxation
      b. T_2 relaxation
      c. Spin density
      d. Flow and motion
   4. Spatial localization
      a. Physical and logical gradient
      b. Slice select gradient
      c. Phase-encoding gradient
      d. Frequency (readout) gradient
      e. K-space (raw data)

C. Artifacts—6
   1. Cause and appearance of artifacts
      a. Aliasing
      b. Gibbs, truncation
      c. Chemical shift
      d. Magnetic susceptibility
      e. Radiofrequency
      f. Motion and flow
      g. Partial volume averaging
   2. Compensation for artifacts

D. Quality control—2
   1. Slice thickness
   2. Spatial resolution
   3. Contrast resolution
   4. Signal-to-noise
   5. RF shielding
   6. Field homogeneity and shimming

Cardiovascular-Interventional Technology

Candidates must be in compliance with the "Rules of Ethics" which are part of the *Standards of Ethics* of the ARRT and must meet all requirements as stated in the *Examinee Handbook*. In addition, candidates must be registered in radiography with at least one year having elapsed since passing the certification exam. The content specifications for the cardiovascular-interventional technology exam are shown in Table 15-5.

Table 15-5 Content Specifications for the Examination in Cardiovascular-Interventional Technology

Content Category	Number of Questions
A. Patient Care and MRI Safety	17
B. Imaging Procedures	53
C. Data Acquisition and Processing	62
D. Physical Principles of Image Formation	43
	175

Copyright ©1994, The American Registry of Radiologic Technologists.

Analysis of Category Components

An approximate number of questions for each of the major subject areas is shown in the detailed listing below.

Maintenance of Equipment and Supplies

A. Specialized equipment instrumentation—25
  1. Cine camera
    a. Basic operation
    b. Film transport

  2. Automatic film changers/spot film devices
    a. Types (e.g., cut film, cassette, programmer, single plane, biplane)
    b. Function
  * c. Operation
    d. Cleaning, preventive maintenance

  3. Intensifying screens
    a. Selection
  * b. Cleaning, preventive maintenance

  4. Basic principles of digital

  5. Automatic pressure injectors
    a. Parts
    b. Function
    c. Operation
  * d. Cleaning, preventive maintenance

  6. Catheters, guidewires, needles
    a. Identification
    b. Construction
    c. Use

* In specifications, but not tested

Patient Preparation, Medication, Monitoring and Follow-Up Care

A. Patient care and management—4
  1. Gaining patient cooperation
    a. Explanation of exam
    b. Discussion of needed patient cooperation
  2. Consent form
    a. Verbal explanation
    b. Patient reaction
    c. Legal implications
  3. Taking and recording procedural data

B. Pharmacology—7
  1. Contrast media
    a. Types
      1) Low osmolarity
      2) Ionics
      3) Lipid based
    b. Dose limits
    c. Adverse reactions
      1) Allergic-type
      2) Hemodynamic
      3) Nephrotoxicity
      4) CNS toxicity
  2. Medications
    a. Preparation and administration
    b. Uses
      1) Preprocedural
      2) Intraprocedural
      3) Desired and adverse effects

C. Physiologic monitoring—11
  1. Parts, function and operation of transducers
  2. ECG electrodes
  3. Specialized techniques
    a. Cardiac output measurements
    b. Ventricular volume analysis
  4. Cardiac monitoring
    a. Normal rhythm

b. Basic cardiac arrhythmias
   1) Atrial
   2) Ventricular
5. Maintaining accessory medical equipment (e.g., oxygen, IVs, chest tubes, Foley catheters, drainage bags)

D. Emergency care—10
1. Adverse reactions to contrast media
   a. Symptoms
      1) Allergic-type
      2) Hemodynamic responses
   b. Medications
      1) Types (e.g., steroids, histamines)
      2) Indications
      3) Serious contraindications
2. Symptoms of life-threatening complications
   a. TIA
   b. Embolism
   c. Thrombosis
   d. Myocardial infarction
   e. Congestive heart failure
   f. Cardiac arrhythmias
   g. Vasovagal response
   h. Anaphylaxis
   i. Hypotensive episodes
   j. Hypertensive episodes
3. Single-rescuer cardiopulmonary resuscitation

General Procedural Considerations

A. Intravenous therapy
   1. IV solution preparation
   2. IV control
   3. Complications
      a. Symptoms
      b. Corrective action

B. Sterile technique
   1. Sterilization
      a. Types (e.g., autoclave, gas)
      b. Utilization
   2. Sterile fields
      a. Patient preparation
      b. Procedural tray
      c. Maintenance of sterile fields
   3. Gowning and gloving

C. Isolation procedures—1
   1. Infection control
      a. Knowledge of transmittable diseases
      b. Levels of isolation
      c. Precautions
   2. Reverse isolation

D. Image enhancement—4
   1. Subtraction (first order only)
      a. Mask

b. Film
c. Equipment
d. Technique
2. Principles of compensation filtration
3. Magnification
   a. Application
   b. Procedure

Specific Procedural Studies

A. Circulatory System
(*Note: In addition to the anatomy linked to the specific studies, the circulatory system in general may be covered as outlined here. The questions are classified into the chart on the following pages [Fig. 15-2].*)

1. Structure of blood vessels
   a. Arteries
   b. Veins
   c. Capillaries
   d. Lymphatic system
2. Anatomical parts of the heart
3. Hemodynamics and blood pressure
   a. Systolic, diastolic phases
   b. Total body blood volume values
4. Conduction (electrical path)
5. Pulse rate and rhythm
   a. Normal
   b. Abnormal
6. Basic vascular anatomy and physiology
   a. Cardiac circulation
   b. Pulmonary circulation
   c. Visceral circulation
   d. Peripheral circulation
   e. Coronary circulation
   f. Cerebral circulation
7. Basic vascular pathology
   a. AVM
   b. Aneurysms
   c. Arteriosclerosis
   d. Fibromuscular dysplasia
   e. Spasm
   f. Traumatic
   g. Congenital
   h. Neoplasm

B. Basic anatomy and physiology of the central nervous system
(*Note: In addition to the anatomy linked to the specific studies, the basic anatomy and physiology of the CNS may be covered as outlined here. The questions are classified into the chart on the following pages [Fig. 15-2].*)

1. Brain
2. Spinal cord

	# of Questions	1. Normal Anatomy	2. Variant Anatomy	3. Surgical Anatomy (e.g., transplants, grafts)	4. Indications	5. Contraindications	6. Access Method (e.g., catheterization, needle placement, Seldinger Technique, assisting, guidewires)	7. Patient Management During Procedure	8. Contrast Media	9. Equipment (e.g., filming media, automatic injectors, film changers)	10. Patient Positioning	11. Exposure Technique	12. Image Enhancement	13. Complications
A. Neurologic														
1. Angiography														
a. intracranial	6													
b. extracranial	4													
2. Other														
a. myelography	1													
B. Lymphatic														
1. Lymphangiography	1			X										
C. Pulmonary														
1. Angiography														
a. pulmonary arteriograms	3													
2. Other														
a. pulmonary pressure measurement	2			X					X			X	X	

NOTE: All studies may be covered in terms of cut film, digital, and/or cinee.
X = Not Applicable

Figure 15-2 Classification of specific procedural studies questions on the cardiovascular-interventional exam. From: The American Registry of Radiologic Technologists, Copyright © 1994.

	# of Questions	1. Normal Anatomy	2. Variant Anatomy	3. Surgical Anatomy (e.g., transplants, grafts)	4. Indications	5. Contraindications	6. Access Method (e.g., catheterization, needle placement, Seldinger Technique, assisting, guidewires)	7. Patient Management During Procedure	8. Contrast Media	9. Equipment (e.g., filming media, automatic injectors, film changers)	10. Patient Positioning	11. Exposure Technique	12. Image Enhancement	13. Complications
D. GU														
1. Angiography														
a. renal	6													
b. adrenal	2													
2. Interventional														
a. nephrostomy	3													
b. urethral stents	1													
c. precutaneous stone extraction	1													
d. embolizations	2													
e. renal-arterial angioplasty	2													
3. Other														
a. venous sampling	1													

Figure 15-2 (cont'd) Classification of specific procedural studies questions on the cardio-vascular-interventional exam. From: The American Registry of Radiologic Technologists, Copyright © 1994.

	# of Questions	1. Normal Anatomy	2. Variant Anatomy	3. Surgical Anatomy (e.g., transplants, grafts)	4. Indications	5. Contraindications	6. Access Method (e.g., catheterization, needle placement, Seldinger Technique, assisting, guidewires)	7. Patient Management During Procedure	8. Contrast Media	9. Equipment (e.g., filming media, automatic injectors, film changers)	10. Patient Positioning	11. Exposure Technique	12. Image Enhancement	13. Complications
E. GI														
1. Angiography														
a. selective visceral	10													
2. Interventional														
a. pharmacoangiography (e.g., pitressin injection)	1								✕					
b. embolization	2													
c. angioplasty	2													
d. stone extraction	2													
e. percutaneous transhepatic cholangiogram	2													
f. biliary drainages	2													
3. Other														
a. hepatic wedge	1													

Figure 15-2 (cont'd) Classification of specific procedural studies questions on the cardio-vascular-interventional exam. From: The American Registry of Radiologic Technologists, Copyright © 1994.

	# of Questions	1. Normal Anatomy	2. Variant Anatomy	3. Surgical Anatomy (e.g., transplants, grafts)	4. Indications	5. Contraindications	6. Access Method (e.g., catheterization, needle placement, Seldinger Technique, assisting, guidewires)	7. Patient Management During Procedure	8. Contrast Media	9. Equipment (e.g., filming media, automatic injectors, film changers)	10. Patient Positioning	11. Exposure Technique	12. Image Enhancement	13. Complications
F. Peripheral														
1. Angiography														
a. abdominal aortography	3													
b. thoracic aortography	3													
c. upper extremity	2													
d. lower extremity	4													
e. inferior vena cava	2													
f. superior vena cava	2													
2. Interventional														
a. revascularization: PTA, lasers, atherectomy	5													
b. revascularization: thrombolytic therapy (e.g., streptokinase, urokinase, TPA)	2													
c. caval filter placement	1													
d. foreign body retrieval	1													
3. Other														
a. pressure measurements	2									✗				

Figure 15-2 (cont'd) Classification of specific procedural studies questions on the cardio-vascular-interventional exam. From: The American Registry of Radiologic Technologists, Copyright © 1994.

	# of Questions	1. Normal Anatomy	2. Variant Anatomy	3. Surgical Anatomy (e.g., transplants, grafts)	4. Indications	5. Contraindications	6. Access Method (e.g., catheterization, needle placement, Seldinger Technique, assisting, guidewires)	7. Patient Management During Procedure	8. Contrast Media	9. Equipment (e.g., filming media, automatic injectors, film changers)	10. Patient Positioning	11. Exposure Technique	12. Image Enhancement	13. Complications
G. Cardiac														
1. Angiography														
a. coronary	4													
b. ventriculography	2													
c. root injections	1													
2. Interventional														
a. revascularization: angioplasty	2													
3. Other														
a. temporary pacemakers	1								X				X	
b. pressure measurements	1													
c. cardiac output	2								X			X	X	
H. Miscellaneous Studies														
1. Biopsies	2								X					
2. Abscess drainages	2								X					

Figure 15-2 (cont'd) Classification of specific procedural studies questions on the cardio-vascular-interventional exam. From: The American Registry of Radiologic Technologists, Copyright © 1994.

Mammography

Candidates must be in compliance with the "Rules of Ethics" which are part of the *Standards of Ethics* of the ARRT and must meet all requirements as stated in the *Examinee Handbook*. In addition, candidates must be registered in radiography with at least one year having elapsed since passing the certification exam. The content specifications for the mammography examination may be found in Table 15-6.

Table 15-6 Content Specifications for the Examination in Mammography

Content Category	% Weight	Number of Questions
A. Patient Education	14%	14
B. Clinical Breast Examination	9%	9
C. Instrumentation	21%	21
D. Anatomy, Physiology, Pathology	18%	18
E. Positioning	19%	19
F. Mammography Techniques	19%	19
	100%	100

Copyright ©1994, The American Registry of Radiologic Technologists.

Analysis of Category Components

An approximate number of questions for each of the major subject areas is shown in the detailed listing below.

Patient Education

A. Risk factors for breast cancer—2
  1. Major
    a. Aging
    b. Personal or family history of breast cancer
    c. Nulliparity
    d. First birth after age 30
  2. Minor
    a. Obesity
    b. Early menstruation
    c. Late menopause

B. American Cancer Society (ACS) guidelines for mammograms (for asymptomatic female without personal or family history of breast cancer)
  1. Baseline between ages 35 to 40
  2. Every 1 to 2 years between 40 and 49
  3. Annual after 50

C. Breast disease—3
  1. Signs and symptoms
    a. Breast lump
    b. Thickening of breast tissue or skin
    c. Swelling of breast
    d. Dimpling
    e. Skin irritation/inflammation
    f. Nipple discharge
    g. Pain or tenderness
    h. Acute onset nipple inversion/retraction
    i. Lymph node enlargement
  2. Benign and malignant conditions
    a. Breast cancer
    b. Cysts
    c. Fibroadenomas
    d. Other benign conditions
  3. Treatment options (basic information on surgery, chemotherapy, radiation therapy)

D. Risk versus benefit of mammography—2
  1. Natural incidence of breast cancer
  2. Induced cancers from high doses of radiation
  3. Comparative risks
  4. Benefits of early detection
  5. Typical dose levels

E. Breast self-examination—3
  1. Frequency of BSE
  2. Methods and patterns of search (spiral, grid)
  3. General technique (e.g., flats of fingers)
  4. Rationale for BSE

F. Other breast diagnostic procedures (basic information necessary to respond to patient questions)—3
  1. Ultrasound
  2. Cyst aspirations
  3. Galactograms
  4. Fine needle aspirations
  5. Pneumocystogram
  6. Xeromammography

Clinical Breast Examination

A. Localization conventions—2
  1. Quadrant system
  2. Clock-face system

B. Visual inspection—2
 1. Positions
 2. Characteristics of interest (e.g., moles, scars)
 3. Verification of patient preparation (e.g., removal of deodorant)

C. Palpation—2
 1. Positions
 2. Areas of interest (perimeter, nipples, lymph nodes)
 3. Methods of examination
 4. Patterns of search

D. Medical history—3
 1. Soliciting information
 2. Factors relevant to performing/interpreting the exam
   a. Symptoms (e.g., mass, discharge, dimpling)
   b. Personal or family history of breast cancer
   c. Age at onset and cessation of menses
   d. Menstrual status (pre-, peri-, post-)
   e. Hormone ingestion (e.g., birth control, fertility, length of time)
   f. Radiation treatment to breasts
   g. Prior mammograms, breast surgeries, recent aspirations, breast sonography
   h. Parity
 3. Informed procedural consent

Instrumentation
(*Note: Because everyone taking this test will understand the basic operation of an x-ray unit by virtue of their certification in radiography, differences from standard radiographic units will be emphasized here.*)

A. Characteristic of dedicated film screen mammography unit—10
 1. kVp
   a. Range (20 to 35 kVp)
   b. Rationale for low kVp
   c. Why standard radiographic units are not used
 2. Mammography tube
   a. Target
     1) Material (molybdenum versus tungsten)
     2) Angle
   b. Focal spot size (measured)
     1) Standard mammography (0.3-0.6 mm)
     2) Magnification (0.1-0.2 mm)
   c. Window/inherent filtration
 3. Compression
   a. Characteristics
   b. Devices
   c. Pressure settings
   d. Hand versus foot pedal
 4. Phototiming
 5. Grid versus no grid
   a. Rationale for use

   b. Characteristics
   c. Effect on dose
 6. Filters
 7. Collimation devices
 8. Machine positioning features
 9. Source-to-image distance (SID)

B. Image receptor—3
 1. Single-emulsion versus double-emulsion
 2. Cassettes
 3. Screens

C. Quality control tests—8
 1. Automatic Processor
   a. Dedicated versus nondedicated
   b. Regular development cycle versus extended development cycle
 2. Accessory equipment (cassettes, view boxes, screens)
 3. Radiographic unit (kVp, mA, timers, leakage, image quality)
 4. Darkroom integrity
 5. Retake/reject analysis
 6. Artifact identification

Anatomy, Physiology, Pathology

A. Surface anatomy—3
 1. Nipple
 2. Areola
 3. Inframammory crease
 4. Axillary prolongation (tail)
 5. Base

B. Deep anatomy—4
 1. Tissues
   a. Adipose (fatty)
   b. Glandular
   c. Fibrous or connective
 2. Blood vessels
 3. Lymph nodes
 4. Retromammary space
 5. Pectoralis major muscle

C. Tissue composition classification—3
 1. Fibro-glandular breast
 2. Fibro-fatty breast
 3. Fatty breast
 4. Impact on radiographic quality

D. Physiology—3
 1. Normal involution
 2. Fatty infiltration
 3. Factors affecting tissue composition (e.g., age, pregnancy, lactation)

E. Pathology—5
1. Mammographic appearances of benign and malignant processes
1. Areas of occurrence

Positioning
(*Note: Questions on the structure best demonstrated, the patient position, part position, central ray orientation, patient instructions and criteria for evaluating the mammogram may be covered for each of the projections listed below.*)

A. Routine projections—8
1. Craniocaudal
2. Mediolateral oblique

B. Special projections - 7
1. Exaggerated craniocaudal (medially or laterally)
2. 90-degree mediolateral
3. Caudocranial
4. 90-degree lateromedial
5. Axillary (AP)
6. Axillary (Cleopatra)
7. Cleavage (valley)
8. Rolled view
9. Tangential view (including localization of skin calcifications)
10. Lateromedial oblique

C. Special situations—4
1. Patients with breast implants (Eklund projection)
2. Postmastectomy patients
3. Postradiation therapy patients

Mammography Techniques

A. Breast compression—3
1. Provides more uniform optical density
2. Spreads out breast tissue
3. Reduces breast radiation dose
4. Reduces scatter, improves subject contrast
5. Reduces motion and geometric blur

B. Spot compression—2

C. Magnification—3

D. Selection of technical factors—3
1. Factors affecting selection
2. Automatic exposure control

E. Radiopaque markers—1
1. Conventions for placing (toward axilla)
2. Skin lesion markers

F. Use of grids—2

G. Setup for localization procedure—2
H. Specimen radiography methods—1
I. Localization of skin lesions and calcifications—2

Copyright ©1994, The American Registry of Radiologic Technologists.

Additional advanced-level examinations are being explored. As can be seen from this chapter, there are many opportunities to specialize and obtain advanced-level credentials in the field of radiologic technology. Take advantage of all that is offered and there will be little that you cannot achieve!

Chapter 16

Advanced Academic Degrees

> *Y*ou cannot discover new
> oceans unless you have the
> courage to lose sight
> of the shore.

▼

▲ Factors Influencing Degree Program Selection

An increasing number of radiography students and technologists are interested in pursuing higher level academic degrees. This is particularly true for those individuals seeking a career in radiology management or education. Some wish to pursue degrees because they enjoy learning or will find the achievement fulfilling. Others hope to expand their earning potential or to raise the level of their professional status. The baccalaureate degree is now considered the professional level for radiologic technologists.

The United States Departments of Education and Labor have ample data to support the contention that earnings and employment opportunities are greater for those with increased levels of education. Regardless of the motivation, such career planning and goal setting must be based on accurate information.

This section provides a listing of postsecondary institutions offering degrees or completion degrees in radiologic technology at the baccalaureate, master's, and doctoral levels. *The listing is current as of the date of publication; however, college and university enrollment statistics and governing board decisions exert a constant influence on degree availability.* Those interested in pursuing such degrees should request the latest edition of the college or university catalog to determine that the curriculum is offered.

As with other health professions, an advanced degree within the discipline of radiologic technology is not required for career advancement. However, baccalaureate and master's degrees in business, management, and education have become increasingly important in recent years. This is particularly significant in view of the fact that there are relatively few advanced degree programs available in radiologic technology itself. Therefore, one should carefully define career goals and pursue advanced education that is specific enough to provide skills in certain areas but broad enough to allow for flexibility.

If your career goals include teaching in radiologic technology, then you should plan to pursue, successively, a baccalaureate and a master's degree in education. If you plan to become a director of radiology, begin working on a baccalaureate degree in health care administration or business, with a master's degree in health care administration or business administration to follow. In most cases, rising to these levels of responsibility no longer depends upon moving up through the ranks. A solid college education is required.

If an advanced degree is among your career goals, begin planning now. Keep in mind that requests for information take time to process and to be mailed. The sooner you acquire the needed information, the sooner you will be able to establish your plans for further education. Figure 16-1 shows a sample letter that may be used to request a college or university catalog from the department of admissions and registration of any of the institutions listed in this chapter.

The program listing that follows may, as indicated earlier, change at any time. Be sure to enlist the help of your reference librarian or career guidance office at a local community college or university for updates to the listing. This listing does not include the many off-campus degree completion programs available to health care professionals. Such programs are frequently advertised in monthly, bimonthly, or quarterly journals in radiologic technology.

Be sure to interview radiologic technologists at your clinical sites who are currently enrolled in degree completion programs. They can provide you with helpful information about the college or university in which they are enrolled.

Today's Date

Office of Registration and Admissions
State University
College Town, IL   65432

Please forward one copy of the latest undergradu-
ate (graduate) catalog. I am particularly interested
in pursuing a major in (subject area) and would appreciate any additional degree information or program brochures that may be available in that area.

Thank you in advance for this information.

Sincerely,

Interested Technologist
123 Main St
My Town, IL   12345

Figure 16-1 Sample catalog request letter.

▲ *Advanced Degree Programs*

Baccalaureate Degree Programs in Radiologic Technology

University of Alabama-Birmingham
University Station-University Center
Birmingham, AL 35294

University of the Ozarks
415 College Avenue
Clarksville, AR 72830

University of Central Arkansas
Conway, AR 72032

University of Arkansas for Medical Sciences
College of Pharmacy
4301 West Markham
Little Rock, AR 72205

California State University-Northridge
18111 Nordhoff Street
Northridge, CA 91330

California State University at Long Beach
1250 Bellflower Boulevard
Long Beach, CA 90840

Quinnipiac College
Mt. Carmel Avenue
Hamden, CT 06518

University of Hartford
200 Bloomfield Avenue
West Hartford, CT 06117

The George Washington University
2121 I Street, NW, Suite 089
Washington, DC 20052

University of Central Florida
P.O. Box 25000
Orlando, FL 32816

Medical College of Georgia
1120 Fifteenth Street
Augusta, GA 30912

Boise State University
1910 University Drive
Boise, ID 83725

Idaho State University
P.O. Box 8054
Pocatello, ID 83209

Chicago State University
95th Street at King Drive
Chicago, IL 60628

National-Louis University
2840 Sheridan Road
Evanston, IL 60201

Roosevelt University
430 South Michigan Avenue
Chicago, IL 60605

Indiana University-Purdue University at Indianapolis
Cavanaugh Hall, Room 129
425 University Boulevard
Indianapolis, IN 46202-5143

Marian College
3200 Cold Spring Road
Indianapolis, IN 46222

Briar Cliff College
3303 Rebecca Street
Sioux City, IA 51104-2100

Southwestern College
100 College Street
Winfield, KS 67156

University of Kansas
126 Strong Hall
Lawrence, KS 66045

McNeese State University
Lake Charles, LA 70609

Northeast Louisiana University
700 University Avenue
Monroe, LA 71209

Northwestern State University of Louisiana
College Avenue
Natchitoches, LA 71497

St. Joseph's College
Windham, ME 04062-1198

Andrews University
Berrien Springs, MI 49104

Madonna University
36600 Schoolcraft Road
Livonia, MI 48150

St. Mary's College
Commerce and Orchard Lake Roads
Orchard Lake, MI 48324

Wayne State University
100 Antoinette-Room 165
Detroit, MI 48202

William Carey College
Tuscan Avenue
Hattiesburg, MS 39401

Avila College
11901 Wornall Road
Kansas City, MO 64145

Southwest Missouri State University
901 South National
Springfield, MO 65804

University of Missouri-Columbia
130 Jesse Hall
Columbia, MO 65211

University of Nevada-Las Vegas
4505 Maryland Parkway
Las Vegas, NV 89154

Fairleigh Dickinson University-Madison
285 Madison Avenue
Madison, NJ 07940

Thomas Edison State College
101 West State Street
Trenton, NJ 08608-1176

Long Island University-C.W. Post Campus
Northern Boulevard-College Hall
Greenvale, NY 11548

SUNY Health Science Center-Syracuse
155 Elizabeth Blackwell Street
Syracuse, NY 13210

Queens College
1900 Selwyn Avenue
Charlotte, NC 28274

University of North Carolina-Chapel Hill
Campus Box 2200
Chapel Hill, NC 27599-2200

University of Mary
7500 University Drive
Bismark, ND 58504

Minot State University
Minot, ND 58707

Ohio State University-Columbus
1800 Cannon Drive-1210 Lincoln Tower
Columbus, OH 43210

University of Oklahoma-Health Science Center
P.O. Box 26901
Oklahoma City, OK 73190

Oregon Institute of Technology
Klamath Falls, OR 97601

College Misericordia
301 Lake Street
Dallas, PA 18612

LaRoche College
9000 Babcock Boulevard
Pittsburgh, PA 15237

Rhode Island College
Providence, RI 02908

Medical University of South Carolina
171 Ashley Avenue
Charleston, SC 29425

Midwestern State University
3400 Taft Boulevard
Wichita Falls, TX 76308

University of Texas Medical Branch-Galveston
1212 Asbel Smith Building-Suite 1
Galveston, TX 77555-1305

University of Vermont
194 South Prospect Street
Burlington, VT 05401-3596

Alderson-Broaddus College
Philippi, WV 26416

Marian College of Fond Du Lac
45 South National Avenue
Fond Du Lac, WI 54935

Master's Degree Programs in Radiologic Technology

University of California-Irvine
UCI College of Medicine
Medical Sciences I-E112
Irvine, CA 92717

University of Washington
Seattle, WA 98195

Doctoral Programs in Radiologic Technology

University of California-Irvine
UCI College of Medicine
Medical Sciences I-E112
Irvine, CA 92717

As you begin planning for an advanced degree, be sure to inquire about advanced standing or credit for prior learning from your radiologic technology education. Many institutions will award two full years of college credit, while others are more selective. Your program director may have advice about writing a portfolio of educational and work experiences to help you receive additional college credit for what you already know and have accomplished.

The work environment of the twenty-first century will require you to have as much knowledge and as many credentials as possible in order to advance in your career. Now is a good time to begin planning and setting goals for a lifetime of learning!

Answers to Review Questions

Chapter 2

1. C
2. D
3. E
4. D
5. C
6. B
7. B
8. E
9. D
10. B
11. E
12. D
13. A
14. B
15. C
16. E
17. A
18. C
19. D
20. A
21. B
22. A
23. D
24. C
25. B
26. A
27. C
28. A
29. D
30. D
31. E
32. B
33. A
34. B
35. C
36. D
37. B
38. E
39. D
40. E
41. A
42. B
43. C
44. C
45. B
46. A
47. E
48. A
49. C
50. D
51. E
52. C
53. B
54. D
55. A
56. A
57. E
58. A
59. C
60. A
61. D
62. A
63. C
64. A
65. D
66. A
67. B
68. A
69. C
70. A
71. D
72. E
73. E
74. B
75. A
76. C
77. D
78. B
79. B
80. C
81. E
82. A
83. C
84. A
85. B
86. C
87. A
88. E
89. E
90. B
91. A
92. C
93. E
94. B
95. A
96. E
97. C
98. B
99. D
100. D

Chapter 3

1. C
2. A
3. C
4. D
5. A
6. B
7. A
8. D
9. C
10. D
11. B
12. A
13. C
14. A
15. D
16. D
17. C
18. C
19. B
20. A
21. C
22. D
23. B
24. A
25. C
26. D
27. B
28. C
29. D
30. B
31. A
32. C
33. D
34. B
35. A
36. E
37. D
38. E
39. C
40. E
41. A
42. D
43. B
44. C
45. B

46. D
47. B
48. B
49. A
50. D
51. A
52. E
53. C
54. D
55. A
56. C
57. B
58. D
59. C
60. A
61. D
62. B
63. C
64. D
65. C
66. A
67. B
68. D
69. C
70. A
71. B
72. E
73. E
74. D
75. A
76. A
77. B
78. C
79. A
80. E
81. A
82. B
83. D
84. B
85. C
86. E
87. C
88. A
89. D
90. B
91. E
92. C
93. D
94. A
95. D
96. C
97. D
98. B
99. C
100. A

Chapter 4

1. E
2. D
3. B
4. D
5. C
6. D
7. E
8. D
9. E
10. B
11. E
12. A
13. E
14. C
15. D
16. A
17. C
18. A
19. C
20. B
21. D
22. C
23. E
24. C
25. B
26. D
27. A
28. D
29. B
30. A
31. B
32. E
33. C
34. D
35. D
36. C
37. E
38. D
39. A
40. C
41. E
42. A
43. B
44. D
45. E
46. A
47. E
48. E
49. B
50. C
51. A
52. E
53. D
54. A

55. D
56. A
57. D
58. A
59. A
60. D
61. D
62. A
63. D
64. E
65. C
66. B
67. C
68. D
69. A
70. B
71. E
72. C
73. B
74. A
75. E
76. E
77. D
78. D
79. C
80. A
81. B
82. E
83. C
84. D
85. A
86. B
87. C
88. E
89. D
90. B
91. A
92. C
93. D
94. E
95. A
96. E
97. A
98. D
99. A
100. D

Chapter 5

1. D
2. A
3. D
4. C
5. B
6. A

7. D
8. A
9. B
10. C
11. D
12. E
13. C
14. A
15. B
16. D
17. E
18. A
19. C
20. D
21. B
22. B
23. B
24. A
25. D
26. C
27. B
28. E
29. C
30. B
31. A
32. C
33. B
34. D
35. A
36. D
37. A
38. E
39. B
40. C
41. E
42. A
43. B
44. D
45. C
46. A
47. D
48. D
49. E
50. B
51. D
52. C
53. A
54. B
55. C
56. D
57. C
58. A
59. D
60. A
61. E

62. D
63. B
64. C
65. A
66. C
67. B
68. D
69. B
70. C
71. A
72. E
73. E
74. B
75. D
76. C
77. A
78. D
79. E
80. C
81. D
82. B
83. E
84. A
85. E
86. D
87. A
88. C
89. B
90. B
91. D
92. C
93. A
94. C
95. D
96. C
97. A
98. E
99. B
100. C

Chapter 6

1. D
2. C
3. D
4. D
5. B
6. B
7. E
8. E
9. A
10. B
11. A
12. B
13. D

14. C
15. E
16. D
17. A
18. B
19. E
20. C
21. A
22. B
23. D
24. C
25. B
26. A
27. A
28. D
29. C
30. A
31. B
32. C
33. A
34. B
35. C
36. A
37. B
38. D
39. E
40. B
41. B
42. D
43. B
44. E
45. A
46. C
47. B
48. C
49. B
50. E
51. E
52. D
53. A
54. B
55. C
56. D
57. E
58. C
59. A
60. C
61. E
62. A
63. D
64. B
65. A
66. E
67. B
68. C

69. D
70. E
71. A
72. B
73. C
74. E
75. A
76. E
77. E
78. E
79. E
80. B
81. E
82. A
83. B
84. E
85. C
86. A
87. D
88. C
89. E
90. A
91. B
92. C
93. B
94. A
95. B
96. B
97. A
98. B
99. B
100. B

Chapter 7

1. D
2. C
3. E
4. B
5. E
6. A
7. C
8. C
9. E
10. B
11. A
12. C
13. B
14. D
15. C
16. D
17. E
18. E
19. A
20. B

21. C
22. B
23. D
24. A
25. B
26. C
27. B
28. E
29. E
30. C
31. A
32. D
33. C
34. A
35. B
36. E
37. D
38. E
39. C
40. D
41. B
42. A
43. D
44. E
45. A
46. B
47. C
48. D
49. B
50. D
51. A
52. C
53. D
54. E
55. A
56. A
57. B
58. C
59. D
60. E
61. D
62. A
63. C
64. E
65. D
66. B
67. D
68. E
69. B
70. D
71. B
72. E
73. A
74. C
75. A

76. B
77. B
78. B
79. A
80. A
81. B
82. A
83. A
84. B
85. B
86. B
87. D
88. A
89. A
90. A
91. D
92. D
93. A
94. C
95. B
96. A
97. B
98. B
99. A
100. A
101. A
102. C
103. B
104. B
105. C
106. B
107. B
108. A
109. C
110. C
111. A
112. D
113. D
114. C
115. B
116. A
117. E
118. D
119. E
120. A
121. E
122. C
123. C
124. B
125. A
126. D
127. B
128. A
129. E
130. A

131. B
132. B
133. E
134. C
135. B
136. D
137. C
138. E
139. B
140. A
141. C
142. A
143. D
144. D
145. E
146. B
147. C
148. A
149. B
150. D
151. B
152. E
153. C
154. C
155. B
156. D
157. C
158. E
159. B
160. A
161. E
162. B
163. B
164. C
165. A
166. B
167. E
168. C
169. C
170. A
171. E
172. C
173. E
174. B
175. A
176. B
177. C
178. D
179. E
180. A
181. B
182. C
183. D
184. A
185. E

186. B
187. E
188. C
189. D
190. D
191. B
192. E
193. C
194. E
195. A
196. B
197. C
198. B
199. D
200. E

Bibliography

Allied health education directory 1994-1995, Chicago, 1994, American Medical Association.

Annual report to registered technologists, The American Registry of Radiologic Technologists, 1994.

Ballinger, P.: Merrill's atlas of radiographic positions and radiologic procedures, ed 8, St. Louis, 1995, Mosby–Year Book, Inc.

Ballinger, P: Pocket guide to radiography, ed 3, St. Louis, 1995, Mosby–Year Book, Inc.

Bontrager, K.: Textbook of radiographic anatomy and positioning, ed 3, St. Louis, 1992, Mosby-Year Book, Inc.

Bushong, S.: Radiologic science for technologists, ed 5, St. Louis, 1993, Mosby-Year Book, Inc.

Callaway, WJ: Graduate technologists and customer service: a 1991 survey, Radiology Management, 14:2, 50-55, 1992.

Callaway, WJ: Clinical education checklist, Associate Degree Radiography Clinical Handbook: 3-4, 1994.

Chronicle four-year college datebook for 1993-1994 school year, 1993, New York, Chronicle Guidance Publishers, Inc.

Cullinan, A & Cullinan, J: Producing quality radiographs, ed 2, Philadelphia, 1994, J.B. Lippincott Company.

Darby, M & Bushee, E: Mosby's comprehensive review of dental hygiene, ed 2, St. Louis, 1991, Mosby-Year Book, Inc.

Dowd, S: Practical radiation protection and applied radiobiology, Philadelphia, 1994, W. B. Saunders Company.

Educator's handbook, St. Paul, 1990, American Registry of Radiologic Technologists.

Eisenberg, R & Dennis, C: Comprehensive radiographic pathology, ed 2, St. Louis, 1995, Mosby-Year Book, Inc.

Ehrlich, R & McCloskey, E: Patient care in radiography, ed 4, St. Louis, 1993, Mosby-Year Book, Inc.

Examinee handbook for examinations in radiography, radiation therapy, and nuclear medicine, 1995, St. Paul, American Registry of Radiologic Technologists.

Examinee handbook for examinations in mammography, cardiovascular-interventional technology, computed tomography, magnetic resonance imaging, 1995, St. Paul, American Registry of Radiologic Technologists.

Gurley, L & Callaway, W: Introduction to radiologic technology, ed 3, St. Louis, 1992, Mosby-Year Book, Inc.

Hiss, S: Understanding radiography, ed 3, Springfield, 1993, Charles C. Thomas Publisher.

Laudicina, P: Applied pathology for radiographers, Philadelphia, 1989, W.B. Saunders Co.

Limitation of exposure to ionizing radiation, NCRP Report No. 116, Bethesda, 1993, National Council on Radiation Protection and Measurements.

Mace, J & Kowalczyk, N: Radiographic pathology for technologists, St. Louis, 1994, Mosby-Year Book, Inc.

Malott, J & Fodor, J: The art and science of medical radiography, ed 7, St. Louis, 1993, Mosby-Year Book, Inc.

Medical x-ray, electron beam and gamma-ray protection for energies up to MeV (equipment design, performance and use), NCRP Report No. 102, Bethesda, 1989, National Council on Radiation Protection and Measurements.

Mosby's medical nursing and allied health dictionary, ed 4, St. Louis, 1994, Mosby-Year Book, Inc.

Quality assurance for diagnostic imaging, NCRP Report No. 99, Bethedsa, 1988, National Council on Radiation Protection and Measurements.

Radiation protection for medical and allied health personnel, NCRP Report No. 105, Bethesda, 1989, National Council on Radiation Protection and Measurements.

Saxton, D: Mosby's comprehensive review of nursing, ed 14, St. Louis, 1993, Mosby-Year Book, Inc.

Selman, J: The fundamentals of x-ray and radium physics, ed 8, Springfield, 1994, Charles C. Thomas Publisher.

Thompson, M: Principles of imaging science and protection, Philadelphia, 1994, W.B. Saunders Company.

Torres, L: Basic medical techniques and patient care for radiologic technologists, ed 4, Philadelphia, 1993, J.B. Lippincott Company.